This book is due for return on or before the last date shown below.

Perioperative
medicine

Tel: 020

D0682200

Perioperative medicine

Managing surgical patients with medical problems

edited by
Anthony Nicholls
Consultant Physician/Nephrologist,
Royal Devon and Exeter Hospital

and

Iain Wilson
Consultant in Anaesthetics and Intensive Care,
Royal Devon and Exeter Hospital

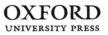

OXFORD
UNIVERSITY PRESS

*This book has been printed digitally and produced in a standard specification
in order to ensure its continuing availability*

OXFORD
UNIVERSITY PRESS

Great Clarendon Street, Oxford OX2 6DP

Oxford University Press is a department of the University of Oxford.
It furthers the University's objective of excellence in research, scholarship,
and education by publishing worldwide in

Oxford New York

Auckland Cape Town Dar es Salaam Hong Kong Karachi
Kuala Lumpur Madrid Melbourne Mexico City Nairobi
New Delhi Shanghai Taipei Toronto
With offices in
Argentina Austria Brazil Chile Czech Republic France Greece
Guatemala Hungary Italy Japan South Korea Poland Portugal
Singapore Switzerland Thailand Turkey Ukraine Vietnam

Oxford is a registered trade mark of Oxford University Press
in the UK and in certain other countries

Published in the United States
by Oxford University Press Inc., New York

© A. J. Nicholls and I. H. Wilson, 2000

ISBN 0-19-921173-6

Printed and bound by CPI Antony Rowe, Eastbourne

Preface

Anthony Nicholls and Iain Wilson

This book is written for trainees in surgery (and its sub-disciplines) who deal with the day-to-day medical problems arising in surgical patients. Anaesthetists, more senior surgeons, medical students and nursing staff may also find this book helpful, as it complements many of the larger texts dealing with the influence of medical disorders on surgical and anaesthetic practice. The specialized areas of paediatric, cardiac and neurosurgery, obstetrics and organ transplantation are not specifically covered.

Surgical wards contain many patients with complex medical disorders treated by an array of potent medications. The implications for surgery and anaesthesia are important and wide-ranging. Morbidity and mortality may be increased; therapy may need modification in the perioperative period; and medical complications may arise postoperatively. Medical management often needs modification from that described in standard medical texts due to surgical and anaesthetic factors. We have invited physician and anaesthetic colleagues to develop sound pragmatic guidelines about perioperative medical care based on the best evidence available and their wide clinical experience.

We believe this book will prove invaluable to those many trainee surgeons who often improvise medical strategies for their patients. The advice here is clear, practical and logically arranged. We hope it leads to simpler and safer care for patients whose medical conditions make surgery particularly hazardous.

January 2000   AJN, IHW
                                                                    Exeter

Acknowledgements

This book has evolved with help, encouragement and ideas from many of our colleagues, all of whom have been willing to assist with reading early drafts of various chapters. Omisions and errors were frequently spotted; we are responsible for those that remain.

We would like to record our thanks to the following people (mostly colleagues at the Royal Devon and Exeter Hospital) who agreed either to write sections of the book or to read chapters and comment on them (or both!): Alison Authers, Reuben Ayres, Pat Backwell, Paul Ballard, Colin Berry, Bruce Campbell, David Conn, Tawfique Daneshmend, Chris Day, John Dean, Alasdair Dow, Julia Gamlen, Jim Gilbert, Richard Hardie, Andrew Hattersley, Tom Irvin, Andrew Knox, Richard Lee, Ken MacLeod, Marina Morgan, Julia Munn, Richard Pocock, John Purday, John Saddler, Simon Satchell, Peter Schranz, John Searle, Chris Sheldon, Mark Stott, Rachel Sturley, Richard Telford, Paul Thomas, Will Woodward.

Our wives, Catriona and Carol, deserve our gratitude for forbearance and total support.

Note

Drug doses indicated in the text have been scrupulously checked, but we cannot guarantee that an error has slipped through unnoticed. *All doses, interactions, and precautions for unfamiliar drugs should be checked in the current BNF before prescription.*

Contents

List of contributors

Alison Authers Cancer Nurse Specialist, former Ward Manager, Royal Devon and Exeter Hospital

Colin Berry Consultant Anaesthetist, Royal Devon and Exeter Hospital

Bruce Campbell Consultant Surgeon, Royal Devon and Exeter Hospital

David Conn Consultant Anaesthetist, Royal Devon and Exeter Hospital

Tawfique Daneshmend Consultant Gastroenterologist, Royal Devon and Exeter Hospital

Chris Day Consultant Anaesthetist, Royal Devon and Exeter Hospital

John Dean Consultant Cardiologist, Royal Devon and Exeter Hospital

Alasdair Dow Consultant Anaesthetist, Royal Devon and Exeter Hospital

Julia Gamlen Physiotherapist, Royal Devon and Exeter Hospital

Jim Gilbert Consultant in Palliative Medicine, Royal Devon and Exeter Hospital

Richard Hardie Consultant Neurologist, Atkinson Morley Hospital, Epsom

Andrew Hattersley Professor of Molecular Medicine, University of Exeter and Consultant Endocrinologist, Royal Devon and Exeter Hospital

Richard Lee Consultant Haematologist, Royal Devon and Exeter Hospital

Paul Marshall Consultant Anaesthetist, Royal Devon and Exeter Hospital

Marina Morgan Consultant Microbiologist, Royal Devon and Exeter Hospital

Julia Munn Consultant Anaesthetist, Royal Devon and Exeter Hospital

Julie Murdoch Pain Control Nurse Specialist, Royal Devon and Exeter Hospital

Anthony Nicholls Consultant Renal Physician, Royal Devon and Exeter Hospital

John Purday Consultant Anaesthetist, Royal Devon and Exeter Hospital

John Saddler Consultant Anaesthetist, Royal Devon and Exeter Hospital

John Searle Consultant Anaesthetist, Royal Devon and Exeter Hospital

Chris Sheldon Consultant Chest Physician, Royal Devon and Exeter Hospital

Richard Telford Consultant Anaesthetist, Royal Devon and Exeter Hospital

Paul Thomas Specialist Registrar in Anaesthesia, Royal Devon and Exeter Hospital

Iain Wilson Consultant Anaesthetist, Royal Devon and Exeter Hospital

Will Woodward Consultant Anaesthetist, Royal Cornwall Hospital, Truro

List of abbreviations

+ve	positive
–ve	negative
ACE	angiotensin converting enzyme
ACh-R	acetylcholine receptor
ACTH	adrenocorticotrophic hormone
ADH	antidiuretic hormone
AED	anti-epileptic drug
AF	atrial fibrillation
AICD	automatic implantable cardioverter defibrillator
AIDS	acquired immmune deficiency syndrome
AMI	acute myocardial infarction
AP	abdomino-perineal
APT(T)R	activated partial thromboplastin time ratio
ARDS	acute respiratory distress syndrome
ASA	American Society of Anaesthesiologists
ATN	acute tubular necrosis
ATP	adenosine triphosphate
AV	atrioventricular
BAPEN	British Association of Parenteral and Enteral Nutrition
BBV	blood-borne virus
bd	*bis die* (twice daily)
BMI	body mass index
BNF	British National Formulary
BP	blood pressure
Ca	calcium
Ca^{2+}	ionized calcium
CAPD	continuous ambulatory peritoneal dialysis
CBW	current body water
CCF	congestive cardiac failure
CCU	coronary care unit
CF	cystic fibrosis
CK	creatine (phospho) kinase
CMV	cytomegalovirus

CNS	central nervous system
CO_2	carbon dioxide
COHb	carboxyhaemoglobin
COPD	chronic obstructive pulmonary disease
CPAP	continuous positive airways pressure
CPR	cardiopulmonary resuscitation
CRP	C-reactive protein
CSF	cerebrospinal fluid
CSU	catheter specimen of urine
CT	computed tomography
CTZ	chemoreceptor trigger zone
CVE	cerebrovascular event
CVP	central venous pressure
CXR	chest radiograph
DC	direct current
DDAVP	desmopressin
DIC	disseminated intravascular coagulation
DNR	do not resuscitate
2,3-DPG	diphosphoglycerate
DRVVT	direct Russell viper venom time
DTs	delirium tremens
DVT	deep venous thrombosis
EBM	evidence-based medicine
ECF	extracellular fluid
ECG	electrocardiogram
EDTA	ethylene diamine tetra-acetic acid
EEG	electroencephalogram
EMG	electromyogram
EMRSA	epidemic MRSA
ENT	ear, nose, and throat
ERCP	endoscopic retrograde cholangio-pancreatography
ESR	erythrocyte sedimentation rate
FBC	full blood count
FDP	fibrin degradation product
FEV_1	forced expiratory volume in 1 s
FFP	fresh frozen plasma
FiO_2	inspired oxygen tension (partial pressure of oxygen in inspired air)
FVC	forced vital capacity
γ-GT	gamma-glutamyl transpeptidase
G&S	group and save (blood)
G6PD	glucose-6-phosphate dehydrogenase
GA	general anaesthetic
GCS	Glasgow coma scale
GFR	glomerular filtration rate
GI	gastrointestinal
GKI	glucose, potassium, and insulin

GTN	glyceryl trinitrate
HAS	human albumin solution
Hb	haemoglobin
HbS/β-thal	β-thalassaemia
HBV	hepatitis B virus
HCO_3^-	bicarbonate
Hct	haematocrit
HCV	hepatitis C virus
HDU	high dependency unit
HDV	hepatitis D virus (delta agent)
HIB	*Haemophilus influenzae* type B
HIV	human immunodeficiency virus
HLA	human leucocyte antigen
HOCM	hypertrophic obstructive cardiomyopathy
HRT	hormone replacement therapy
ht	height
5HT	5-hydroxytryptamine
IBD	inflammatory bowel disease
ICU	intensive care unit
IDDM	insulin-dependent diabetes mellitus
IHD	ischaemic heart disease
i/m	intramuscular
INR	international normalized ratio
IPC	intermittent pneumatic compression
IPPB	intermittent positive pressure breathing
IPPV	intermittent positive pressure ventilation
ISC	intermittent self-catheterization
ITP	immune (idiopathic) thrombocytopenic purpura
i/v	intravenous(ly)
JVP	jugular venous pressure
K^+	potassium
KCl	potassium chloride
L	left
LDH	lactate dehydrogenase
LFTs	liver function tests
LMWH	low molecular weight heparin
LV	left ventricular, left ventricle
LVF	left ventricular failure
M,C&S	microscopy, culture and sensitivity
MCV	mean cell volume
MDMA	3,4-methylenedioxymethamphetamine ('ecstasy')
MG	myasthenia gravis
Mg^{2+}	ionized magnesium
MI	myocardial infarction
MLSO	medical laboratory scientific officer
MRSA	methicillin-resistant *Staphylococcus aureus*
MSU	mid-stream urine

n/g	nasogastric
Na^+	ionized sodium
NADH	nicotinamide adenine dehydrogenase
NBM	nil-by-mouth
NBW	normal body water
NCEPOD	National Confidential Enquiry into Perioperative Deaths
NIDDM	non insulin-dependent diabetes mellitus
NIPPV	non-invasive positive pressure ventilation
NSAID	non-steroidal anti-inflammatory drug
NTS	nucleus of the tractus solitarius
od	once daily
OSA	obstructive sleep apnoea
PA	postero-anterior
$PaCO_2$	partial pressure of carbon dioxide in arterial blood
PaO_2	partial pressure of oxygen in arterial blood
PCA	patient controlled analgesia
PCP	*Pneumocystis carinii* pneumonia
PD	peritoneal dialysis
PD	Parkinson's disease
PE	pulmonary embolism
PEA	pulseless electrical activity
PEFR	peak expiratory flow rate
PEG	percutaneous endoscopic gastrostomy
PEP	positive expiratory pressure
po	*per os* (by mouth)
PO_4	phosphate
PONV	postoperative nausea and vomiting
pr	*per rectum*
prn	*pro re nata* (as required)
PSS	progressive systemic sclerosis
qds	*quater die sumendum* (4 times daily)
R	right
RA	rheumatoid arthritis
RTA	road traffic accident
SaO_2	oxygen saturation (arterial blood)
s/c	subcutaneous(ly)
SBE	subacute bacterial endocarditis
SCD	sickle cell disease
SHO	senior house officer
SLE	systemic lupus erythematosus
SOB	shortness of breath
SOL	space occupying lesion
SpO_2	oxygen saturation (pulse oximetry)
SVT	supraventricular tachycardia
T_3	tri-iodothyronine
T_4	thyroxine

TB	tuberculosis
TBW	total body water
TCRE	transcervical resection of the endometrium
tds	*ter die sumendum* (3 times daily)
TENS	transcutaneous electrical nerve stimulation
TIA	transient ischaemic attack
TIPSS	transporto-systemic shunt
TPN	total parenteral nutrition
TPR	temperature, pulse, respiratory rate
TSH	thyroid stimulating hormone
TT	thrombin time
TTP	thrombotic thrombocytopenic purpura
TURP	transurethral resection of prostate
U&E	urea and electrolytes (commonly includes creatinine)
V/Q	ventilation/perfusion
VAS	visual analogue scale
VF	ventricular fibrillation
VPB	ventricular premature beat
VRE	vancomycin-resistant enterococci
VRS	verbal rating scale
VRSA	vancomycin-resistant *Staphylococcus aureus*
VT	ventricular tachycardia
vWD	von Willebrand's disease
WBC	white blood cell
WCC	white cell count
WPW	Wolff–Parkinson–White
wt	weight

Introduction

Anthony Nicholls and Iain Wilson

Who is this book for?

This book is primarily for junior surgeons and anaesthetists who are often faced with the perioperative medical management of patients undergoing surgery. It is not a guide to surgical management, but deals specifically with medical care of the surgical patient.

Most medical care for surgical patients is routine, but increasing numbers of medically compromised patients are presenting for both elective and emergency surgery. Medical practice is also becoming more specialized and it is common for more than one doctor to be involved with the care of a complicated surgical patient. In this book we have attempted to draw together relevant advice from specialist physicians, anaesthetists, and surgeons to improve the medical care of the surgical patient. Often referral to other specialists is involved in perioperative care and we have made specific suggestions as to when we feel this would be appropriate.

Much of the acute medical care in surgical patients revolves around assessment, first line management, reassessment, and seeking advice and help from relevant personnel in devising appropriate action plans. Early expert advice is often basic but produces a good outcome, preventing further deterioration. Other patients need immediate intervention and expert assessment, which may be life-saving. We have tried to indicate in the acute medical sections where we feel this is appropriate.

We have not attempted to cover all areas of medical and surgical practice, but hope that we have covered most of the common difficulties. The book is designed to be manageable in size and practical in nature, and we have tried not to repeat what is available in other handbooks. We hope that we have succeeded. Like all other handbooks of clinical practice it will gradually become out of date, so space is available for notes to be added by the user.

Section 1: General medical issues on surgical wards

The first part of this book addresses a range of medical issues common to all patients undergoing surgery such as consent, risk management, resuscitation decisions, cross-infection, blood-borne viruses, and venous thrombosis. Although hospitals may have local policies in place, in the absence of such guidance this book provides simple, safe advice.

- How to prepare a patient for day surgery.
- Who needs HDU/ICU?
- How to control pain and nausea postoperatively.
- When to ask for physiotherapy.
- How to prescribe antibiotics.
- How to prevent malnutrition.

These are subjects that are seldom taught effectively at medical school. The junior doctor may learn by mistakes and experience, but we hope this book will prove to be a practical guide.

Section 2: Perioperative care of chronic medical disorders

Underlying medical problems affect fitness for surgery and anaesthesia. This is particularly true with major surgery in the elderly population. Careful optimization of their underlying problems gives these patients the best chance of survival.

Medical practice is continually evolving and becoming more specialized. Patients with more complex illnesses often see a variety of specialists within the hospital before presenting for surgery. It is difficult to keep up to date, and the number of journals published makes this even more difficult. Although we use the available literature, we also rely on our colleagues to help us out, often in the corridor:

'got a patient with factor IX deficiency coming in next week – anything special I should organize for him?'

'... woman with a prosthetic aortic valve on warfarin, what regime of anticoagulation should we use?'

- Who is at special risk?
- What sort of risk?
- What tests should be done?

- What is their significance?
- What drugs can be stopped while the patient is nil-by-mouth?
- And which are vital to continue?

These issues are addressed in section 2. This book does not refer to anaesthetic techniques used for specific problems: these are well covered elsewhere in standard textbooks of anaesthetics.

Section 3: Postoperative complications

All junior doctors will have experienced a feeling of dismay when late at night they are faced with a desperately sick patient recovering from major surgery who develops a potentially life-threatening complication. How much was this event predictable? Should warning signs have been identified sooner? And how can the patient's life be saved or complication treated?

Studies have shown that even after routine surgical procedures such as transurethral resection of the prostate, knee replacement, hip replacement, and colectomy the mortality is 3% with a major complication rate of 17%. Cardiac arrest in surgical patients is often preceded by physiological abnormalities such as tachypnoea, hypotension, tachycardia, or a sudden fall in consciousness. Airway problems remain common and are potentially life-threatening.

This is the rationale for the third section of the book. It looks at the range of medical emergencies that may arise postoperatively:

- Why is my patient oliguric?
- Why has the blood pressure fallen abruptly?
- How do I recognize a pulmonary embolism?
- What is the source of fever?

These difficult problems face all junior doctors, and this book offers guidance.

Section 4: Sensible prescribing

The last section of the book is a table of perioperative prescribing for virtually any drug that is likely to be encountered in general surgical practice. The BNF should always be referred to for doses, interactions, side-effects, and special precautions, but this book supplements the it with simple guidance for safe prescribing around the time of surgery.

Why use guidelines?

Antony Nicholls and Iain Wilson

Doctors are busy, and need easy sources of quick information. Guidelines provide rapid assistance to clinical care, and have become a fact of modern medical life. They are not intended to supplant major textbooks or original research, but when properly written and used, they may improve the quality of care and the efficiency of health care provision. They may also decrease costs, reduce liability and risk, provide medical education, and help in determining legal standards of care. This book contains guidelines intended to improve the care of the surgical patient.

Legal considerations

The legal status of guidelines has been made unnecessarily controversial. Guidelines such as those in this book legally constitute hearsay. That is, they cannot be quoted in court as being explicit instructions to act in a certain fashion. For example, if a patient were to allege that care was negligent because it did not follow a certain set of guidelines, the courts would still rely on expert evidence to determine what was acceptable practice. Guidelines have never been used in the courts as a substitute for expert opinion. However, we believe that the guidelines contained in this book offer safe, pragmatic, and acceptable practice and would be consistent with expert opinion in the areas covered.

Any practitioner who does not adhere to guidelines should be able to justify his or her actions to a court, including supporting these actions by citing a reasonable body of opinion that would have adopted the same strategy.

Methodological issues

National societies have taken the lead in producing simple guidelines for common conditions such as asthma, hypertension, osteoporosis, and breast cancer, but there are still many gaps in clinical practice. the assembly of relevant, valid evidence to inform medical decision-making is said to be central to the production of guidelines. This is the most difficult step in many clinical areas, as the necessary research evidence base may be inadequate. In these circumstances expert advice and experience has to substitute for evidence. In clinical situations where the evidence base from research is lacking, the production of guidelines is even more important to develop a consensus on how to deal with particular situations. Junior doctors should not have to make up clinical practice for themselves as they go along. This book, we hope, will provide practical advice on managing many of the medical aspects of surgical care.

Further reading

Berger JT, Rosner F (1996). The ethics of practice guidelines. *Archives of Internal Medicine* 1996, **156**:2051–6.

Collins J (1998). Guidelines in clinical practice. *Journal of the Medical Defence Union* 14(2):4.

Jackson R, Feder G (1998). Guidelines for clinical guidelines. *British Medical Journal* 317:427–8.

What about evidence-based protocols?

Anthony Nicholls and Iain Wilson

This book is largely based on the tried and tested principles of experience, reasoning, and common sense, together with evidence-based medicine where that evidence exists. We support the principles underlying evidence-based medicine, but realize their limitations in many situations.

Grades of evidence

The main methodology of evidence-based medicine is to base clinical decision-making upon the results of randomized clinical trials or meta-analyses of several trials. For example, the United States Preventive Services Taskforce rates the value of evidence from randomized controlled trials as grade 1 and evidence from non-randomized trials as grade 2, but evidence from the opinions of respected authorities is only grade 3. On this basis, we would claim that most of the clinical practice described in this book might be grade 2 or 3. We believe, however, that the guidelines described here are just as relevant to safe clinical practice as those of grade 1 status.

Limitations of randomized controlled trials

Much of the surgical and medical practice covered in this book is well established (e.g. that oxygen and β_2 agonists are useful in acute asthma), although many have not been formally assessed in a double-blind placebo-controlled setting (nor should they be). Although randomized controlled trials have the potential to prevent worthless treatments and confirm the value of effective treatments, they can only be expected to cover a limited range of clinical issues.

Patients can only realistically give consent to entry to a randomized trial if the treatment options offer the potential for equal benefits – that is, where there is genuine doubt about the value of different interventions. However, it would be unethical to randomize patients to interventions that (from simple clinical observation) might offer either very great benefits or major risks. Much of clinical practice, and in particular, surgical practice, faces this dilemma. Grade 1 evidence may be unobtainable because of these ethical requirements, and clinical recommendations for many scenarios will have to be based on the principles of clinical experience, clinical observation, lessons from past mistakes, clinical judgment, extrapolation from basic science, the views of patients, and simple common sense – all of which predate evidence-based medicine.

Further problems arise even when there is a clinical trial related to the patient's problem. Most patients entering trials represent a selected group of those with the disorder. Exclusions from clinical trials are legion, usually by virtue of multiple pathology or previous medication. Real-life decision-making includes complex patients who would never have been entered into a clinical trial, so even when an evidence-based recommendation may seem clear-cut (the use of anticoagulants, for example), medical decision-making will draw heavily on clinical judgement, experience, and extrapolation from basic science.

Further reading

Charlton BG, Miles A (1998). The rise and fall of EBM. *Quarterly Journal of Medicine* 91:371–4.

Kerridge I, Lowe M, Henry D (1998). Ethics and evidence based medicine. *British Medical Journal* 316:1151–3.

Part 1

Medical issues in perioperative care

This first section of the book addresses a range of issues in perioperative care which are common to many surgical procedures, and reflect the impact of medical factors on surgical and anaesthetic care. The principles of risk management and the lessons of the National Confidential Enquiry into Peroperative Deaths (NCEPOD) influence the preparation of patients for surgery: informed consent can only be given if the enhanced risk conferred by medical disorders is explained to the patient.

Some patients will need preoperative optimization in HDU/ICU, and others need intensive care postoperatively. Pain control, anti-emesis, nutrition, fluid balance, DVT prophylaxis, infection control, and physiotherapy are all discussed, and the basic principles outlined.

In essence, this section covers the range of issues facing junior surgical staff in the provision of safe perioperative management.

Risk management

Bruce Campbell

Definitions

Risk is defined as 'the possibility of incurring misfortune or loss' and affects any health service in a variety of ways, including risks to patients, staff, visitors, buildings, and property. Risk management concerns the harnessing of information about possible risks, and taking steps to minimize them. The steps include:

- *risk identification*: what could go wrong? how could it happen?
- *risk analysis*: how likely is an adverse event? how serious would it be?
- *risk control*: how can a risk be eliminated, or its effect reduced?
- *risk funding*: optimal insurance against inevitable risks
- *clinical incident reporting*: when untoward events happen.

Doctors are concerned primarily with the risks to patients (clinical risk management). They need to recognize the risks a procedure poses to each individual patient, and balance these risks against the likely benefits. The patient must be properly informed and accept these risks. The practice of clinical risk management has become increasingly important in recent years, driven by the demands of patients for safe treatment, and by the threat of legal action if outcomes do not meet their expectations.

Clinical decisions: balancing risks and benefits

Making decisions about surgical procedures involves identification, analysis, and control of risks. In practical terms this means considering the following questions.

- *How necessary is the procedure* in this case? If all goes well, is the patient likely to gain real benefit?
- *What will be the impact of surgery* on the patient's quality of life in the short and longer term?
- *What are the usual risks of the procedure* in terms of morbidity and mortality (from published series, or preferably from the audit of the individual surgeon for major and high-risk operations)?
- *Does the medical condition of that particular patient increase their degree of risk?* This judgement demands a thorough and relevant history, supplemented by examination and often by other investigations. It is not adequate simply to know, for example, that a patient has angina: how often do they get chest pain? What precipitates it? How active can they be? What treatments do they take? What else limits them? Is their medical treatment optimal?
- *Would it be helpful to involve other specialists* in the assessment of the patient, to decide on the balance of risks and benefit?
- *Does the patient want the procedure*, having had a simple explanation of the benefits and risks?
- If there is doubt about the wisdom of intervention, *could the decision about intervention be delayed?* Would conservative management with observation be reasonable, keeping the possibility of surgery in reserve?

Informed consent

Informed consent is a fundamental part of clinical risk management, and is dealt with in more detail in Chapter 9. Patients who have been counselled thoroughly about the need for intervention, possible alternatives, and risks are much less likely to take action against their medical attendants if problems ensue. It is equally important to involve close relatives in discussions about risk – they are often responsible for complaint or litigation if things 'go wrong' which they did not anticipate. All counselling must be done in a way that individual patients and their families can grasp. 'Counselling' implies that the patient asks questions and shares their concerns: it is not simply one-way transmission of information.

Documentation

The main elements of these discussions must be recorded in the patient's notes, particularly when decisions have been difficult or when the risks are high. This is a vital part of the record of informed consent. The notes must make mention that the following have been explained to the patient (and specify family members or others who were present):

- what the procedure involves, including type of anaesthesia
- specified risks (with percentages for important risks)
- alternative treatments.

Most hospitals insist on the signing of consent forms, but these generally contain little specific information apart from the name of the procedure, and records of counselling are therefore a very important part of clinical risk management. This is often most easily done in a clinic letter.

Written information for patients

Whenever possible, patients should be given written information about procedures and their risks. Provision of an information booklet should be recorded in the notes. Copies of information booklets should be kept on file when they are updated, so that there is clear evidence of the precise written information given to a patient who takes action some time after they were treated.

Seniority of surgeon

A surgeon who is able to do the operation, and who can answer questions with authority, should counsel patients. Trainees need to consider carefully when they should involve a more senior member of the team, especially when making decisions about emergency operations. They have to be able to justify why they decided to proceed unsupervised, if problems occur.

Damage limitation when adverse events occur

Obtain senior advice at the earliest opportunity. It is often helpful to inform relatives in detail immediately after any procedure from which a patient may not make a straightforward recovery: this is appreciated as courtesy if all goes well, and helps to avoid complaint if problems do occur. When adverse events happen, early and thorough counselling of the patient and their family is important: this guards against later feelings of a 'cover up', which is often the stimulus for complaint or litigation.

Clinical incident reporting

All hospitals should have systems for the rapid reporting of clinical incidents. Part of the process of risk management is to recognize situations when reporting a clinical incident may help to minimize its impact, by involving senior clinicians and managers formally at an early stage. It is sometimes beneficial to submit a clinical incident report (or an informal warning) when patients or their relatives are antagonistic or unreasonably dissatisfied about treatment. Early reporting of potential medicolegal problems or complaints enables:

- proper and early counselling of patients and their relatives
- action to minimize clinical damage and optimize further treatment
- checking the completeness of clinical records

- written accounts by the staff involved, while events are fresh in their minds
- those dealing with the media to be properly informed
- early guidance from legal advisors.

Throughout all dealings with patients, preservation of confidentiality is fundamental.

Further reading

NHS Executive (1994). *Risk management in the NHS*. Department of Health.

The National Confidential Enquiry into Perioperative Deaths (NCEPOD)

Bruce Campbell

Background

The National Confidential Enquiry into Perioperative Deaths (NCEPOD) is a collaborative review of surgery, anaesthesia and gynaecology, which began data collection in 1985. The reports (listed in Table 5.1) are based on anonymous and confidential questionnaires completed by surgeons and anaesthetists about patients who have died under their care. Panels of peer reviewers assess questionnaires and the data are recorded on computer. The data are protected against use in medicolegal actions, but destruction of questionnaires is an essential part of this protection and no copies should be kept.

Each year NCEPOD gathers information about different groups of patients, which is then presented in a detailed report, with a summary of findings and recommendations. The publication of each report is accompanied by substantial publicity. The benefits of NCEPOD include:

- public demonstration that surgeons and anaesthetists engage in audit
- recommendations which discourage substandard or unsafe practices
- recommendations which add impetus to the development of services.

NCEPOD has been criticized because:

- the data are anecdotal
- the recommendations are based on the prejudices of the authors
- vignettes have been published which are potentially identifiable.

Despite these reservations, NCEPOD has become an influential force in surgical practice, and there is an expectation for all surgeons and anaesthetists to participate. The main recommendations of the NCEPOD reports are summarized below, in sections on preoperative, operative, and postoperative management, with a section on administrative and other matters. Many of the reports highlight the hazards of inadequate assessment or preparation of patients with complex underlying medical disorders, and this underscores the importance of the chapters in section 2 of this book. The year(s) of the relevant NCEPOD reports are shown in parentheses.

Preoperative management

- thorough preoperative assessment and resuscitation are important (1987)
- decisions about operating on very sick and elderly patients should be taken at a senior level; often by consultation between consultant surgeons and anaesthetists (1987)

Table 5.1 The main themes of NCEPOD reports

1987	All patients who died within 30 days of operation
1989	Children aged 10 years or under
1990	A 20% sample of all deaths, plus 'index' survivors
1991/2	Specified conditions
1992/3	Deaths of patients aged 6–70 years
1993/4	Deaths on the day of operation, or within 3 days
1994/5	Operations performed over seven 24 h periods
1995/6	Who operates when?
1996/7	Deaths following gynaecological, head and neck, minimally invasive, oesophageal, spinal, and urological surgery

- appropriate decisions should be made not to operate on moribund patients (1987)
- no trainee should operate on a child without talking to their consultant (1989)
- appropriately trained staff should accompany seriously ill patients during transfer (1992/3)
- there is a need to develop and enforce standards of practice for many common acute conditions (e.g. head injuries, aortic aneurysm, colorectal cancer, gastrointestinal bleeding) (1992/3)
- certain patients need individual attention by consultant anaesthetists and surgeons – those over 90 years old; with aortic stenosis; needing radical pelvic surgery; needing transfer to neurosurgical units; and needing emergency vascular operations (1994/5)
- both surgeons and patients' relatives should recognize the limits of surgery for advanced malignant disease (1996/7).

The authors of the 1995/6 report were concerned about the lack of preoperative preparation of many of the patients who died, in particular:

- low use of intravenous fluids
- infrequent use of objective cardiac assessment
- patchy use of thromboembolic prophylaxis.

They recommended that the condition of all patients should be optimized prior to anaesthesia and surgery, and that development of local protocols be considered, addressing issues such as:

- required duration of preoperative starvation
- use of emergency admission units/wards
- preoperative use of critical care services
- management of co-morbidities by other specialists
- fluid management
- analgesia
- special facilities for the elderly.

Operative management

Operations should be classified (1987) as:

- Emergency: immediate operation, resuscitation simultaneous with surgical treatment (e.g. ruptured aneurysm, chest, head, and abdominal injuries). Operation usually within 1 h.
- Urgent: delayed operation as soon as possible after resuscitation (e.g. intestinal obstruction, embolism, perforation, major fractures). Operation usually within 24 h.
- Scheduled: an early operation but not immediately lifesaving (e.g. cancer, cardiovascular surgery). Operation usually within 1– 3 weeks.

- Elective: operation at a time to suit both patient and surgeon (e.g. cholecystectomy).

Further points arising form this report are:
- very few operations need to be performed at night (1987).
- trainees should not undertake operations without consultation with seniors (1987).
- there should be more consultant involvement in emergency operations (1991/2).
- surgeons operating laparoscopically should not hesitate to convert to an open procedure when necessary (1992/3).
- laparoscopic surgery may pose high risks for frail or elderly patients (1996/7).
- for airway management, fibreoptic laryngoscopy should be available in all anaesthetic departments, and junior surgeons should be competent at tracheostomy (1996/7).

Postoperative management

- continuity of care after operations is essential (1993/4).
- postoperative thromboembolism needs to be addressed: protocols are required (1991/2) and further research is needed (1993/4).
- fluid balance in elderly patients is of critical importance (1991/2).
- efforts should be made to increase the number of postmortem examinations (1990).
- clinicians and coroners should improve their working relationships (1993/4).

Administrative and general matters

- clinicians should audit results regularly and should check that coding is accurate (1987).
- more participation is required in clinical audit (1993/4) especially in gynaecology and ophthalmology (1994/5).
- audit of all deaths is important in anaesthetic departments (1996/7).
- protocols for common conditions should be more widely used, and should be audited (1993/4).
- information systems in the NHS should be considerably improved to provide accurate and timely information for clinical audit and quality assurance (1989, 1990).
- there is an urgent need to improve the quality of medical notes (1992/3, 1994/5), and their storage and retrieval (1991/2).
- in all hospitals admitting emergency surgical patients there should be 24 h operating rooms and critical care services, with sufficient

medical staff, including weekends and public holidays throughout the year (1995/6).

- anaesthetists and surgeons on for emergencies should be free from other commitments (1995/6).

- consultants and managers should plan emergency services together (1995/6).

- theatres, recovery, ICU, and HDU need to be on a single site wherever acute surgical care is delivered (1990).

- HDU/ICU facilities are inadequate and need to be increased (1994/5).

- more postmortem examinations should be done following death in hospital (1996/7).

Further reading

The NCEPOD reports are available from the Royal College of Surgeons of England, 35–43 Lincolns Inn Fields, London WC2A 3PN.

The panel of authors has included Buck N, Campling EA, Devlin HB, Gray AJG, Hoile RW, Ingram GS, Lunn JN, and Sherry KM.

The ASA classification of perioperative risk

Iain Wilson

The American Society of Anesthesiologists (ASA) score has been used for many years as an indicator of perioperative risk. A committee of the ASA originally conceived the score in 1941 as a method of standardizing physical status in hospital records for statistical studies in anaesthesia. A series of minor changes have been effected over the years and the current version of the classification completed in 1974, by the House of Delegates of the ASA is presented in Table 6.1. A patient is scored according to their physical fitness and the letter E added if the planned procedure is an emergency one.

Although the score is convenient and easy to use, it lacks scientific precision in its application. Anaesthetists may disagree about the

Table 6.1 ASA classification of physical status

Class	Physical status	Example
I	A normally healthy patient	A fit patient with an inguinal hernia
II	A patient with mild systemic disease	Essential hypertension, mild diabetes
III	A patient with severe systemic disease that is not incapacitating	Angina, moderate to severe pulmonary insufficiency
IV	A patient with an incapacitating systemic disease that is a constant threat to life	Advanced degrees of pulmonary disease, cardiac failure
V	A moribund patient who is not expected to survive for 24 h with or without operation	Ruptured aortic aneurysm, massive pulmonary embolism
E	Emergency cases are designated by the addition of 'E' to the classification number	

correct classification for certain patients. In addition, the risk of surgery and anaesthesia is dependent on other factors that are not considered by the score. These include age, weight, gender, and pregnancy. The grade of the surgeon and anaesthetist, facilities for postoperative care, and assistance for the surgical team are also not taken into account.

The score has been used in the NCEPOD study and is in widespread use in many surgical and anaesthetic audits. It has been shown that perioperative risk rises with the patient's ASA score. However, although it is useful, its limitations prevent it being more than a very approximate guide in individual patients. There are other, better prognostic scoring systems described in this book which deal with specific medical conditions.

Further reading

Buck N, Devlin HB, Lunn JN (1987). *The report of a confidential enquiry into perioperative deaths.* The Nuffield Provincial Hospitals' Trust and King's Fund, London.

Owens WD, Felts JA, Spitznagel EL (1978). ASA physical status classification. *Anesthesiology* 33:239–43.

Ruiz K, Aitkenhead AR (1990). Was CEPOD right? *Anaesthesia* 45:978–80.

Wolters U, Wolf T, Stutzer H, Schroder T (1996). ASA classification and perioperative variables as predictors of postoperative outcome. *British Journal of Anaesthesia* 77:217–22.

Preparing patients for elective and emergency surgery

Iain Wilson

Elective surgery

Elective surgery is performed at a time that is suitable to the patient and the hospital team. The surgeon will have explained the intended operation during the outpatient consultation and detailed some of the risks and benefits of the procedure. The time between the consultation and hospital admission varies from days to many months. Investigation and assessment of underlying medical problems are best dealt with at this stage, including referral to relevant specialists. Organization of this phase varies between hospitals and surgeons. Elective surgery in patients with chronic medical disorders should only be performed when the medical condition is optimized, and the risks minimized.

The patient should present for surgery requiring only routine admission procedures. Some hospitals operate a pre-admission clinic at which some of these tasks are performed.

The patient may arrive on the ward feeling stressed. Individuals cope with stress in different ways. Many people are ignorant of routine hospital procedures, so staff should make no assumptions about the patient's knowledge. The nursing staff will welcome the patient to the ward and discuss any necessary administrative details, including the next of kin and other relatives. They should answer some of the questions patients have, and communicate any relevant details to the medical staff.

- Obtain the history and examine the patient to detect any recent change in health since the outpatient consultation.
- Assess cardiovascular and respiratory fitness for surgery.
- If any previously unnoticed medical problem or history of anaesthetic problems arises, contact the relevant surgeon and anaesthetist, and make an appropriate plan to deal with it.
- Send off for routine investigations as detailed in Table 7.1. Before major surgery, blood should be grouped and saved or cross-matched according to local protocol. A guide is shown in Table 7.2.
- Request any other tests indicated by co-existent disease (e.g. coagulation screen with liver problems). See relevant sections in this book.

Consent should be obtained and relevant risks explained (Chapter 9). There is considerable variation in what patients wish to know. A patient

Table 7.1 Preoperative investigations

Urinalysis	All patients: for sugar, blood, protein
ECG	Age >50 years
	History of heart disease, hypertension or chronic lung disease
	A normal previous trace within 1 year is acceptable unless recent cardiac history
FBC	Age >40 years
	All females
	All major surgery
	Whenever anaemia suspected
Creatinine and electrolytes	Age >60 years
	All major surgery
	Diuretic drugs
	Suspected renal disease
Blood glucose	Diabetic patients
	Glycosuria
Sickle cell test	Black patients with unknown sickle status. If positive then haemoglobin electrophoresis should be performed
Pregnancy test	Whenever there is any chance of pregnancy
CXR	Not routine
	Acute cardiac or chest disease
	Chronic cardiac or chest disease worsened in last year
	Risk of pulmonary TB (recent arrival from developing world or immunocompromised)
	Malignant disease

Table 7.2 Suggested blood ordering schedule – refer to local protocols

Category	Procedure	Group and save or cross-match
General surgery	Oesophagectomy	2 units
	Oesophagogastrectomy	2 units
	Gastrectomy	G&S
	Cholecystecomy	G&S
	Liver resection	2 units
	Pancreatic surgery	2 units
	Small bowel resection	G&S
	Colectomy	G&S
	Rectum AP/anterior resection	2 units
	Laparotomy	G&S
	Mastectomy	G&S
	Splenectomy	G&S
	Thyroidectomy	G&S
Vascular surgery	Elective aortic reconstruction	2 units
	Emergency aortic reconstruction	6 units
	Carotid endarterectomy	G&S
	Distal reconstruction (fem-pop)	G&S
	Axillo-femoral bypass	G&S
	Amputation	G&S
Urology	Cystectomy	4 units
	Nephrectomy	3 units
	Open prostatectomy	2 units
	TURP	G&S
	Re-implantation of ureter	G&S
Transplantation	Renal	2 units
Thoracic	Thoracotomy	2 units
	Mediastinoscopy	G&S
Trauma	Major RTA	4 units
ENT/plastic surgery	Major head/neck reconstruction	2 units
	Free flaps	2 units
	Breast reduction	2 units
Orthopaedic surgery	Total hip replacement/revision	2 units/4 units
	Total knee replacement	G&S
	Total shoulder replacement	G&S
	Major spinal stabilisation	Obtain local advice
Maxillofacial	Bimaxillary osteotomy	2 units

with a tumour obstructing the bowel is very different from someone scheduled for total knee replacement. Take time to find out the questions that the patient doesn't like to ask at the start – they are often the most significant. If there are any questions that you cannot answer ask someone to help you. Refer questions about the anaesthetic to the anaesthetist.

- Ask if the patient objects to direct communication with his or her relatives. Confidentiality is paramount, and neither next of kin nor relatives have any right to information about a patient without their consent.
- If permitted by the patient, ask what the immediate family understands about the planned procedure and offer to speak to them.
- Record all your findings in the notes along with an account of the details given to the patient.
- Prescribe routine drugs and plan which ones should be omitted in consultation with the anaesthetist (see the relevant sections of this book). Ask about any allergies.
- Arrange anti-embolic precautions when necessary (Chapter 13).

The anaesthetist should always meet the patient before surgery. He or she will provide specific advice regarding perioperative prescribing, details of the planned anaesthetic and techniques of pain relief. Any other investigations required preoperatively will be requested and appropriate premedication prescribed.

Patients with significant chest disease, and all those having major surgery should meet the physiotherapist preoperatively (Chapter 21).

Emergency surgery

Patients facing emergency surgery are different from those scheduled for elective surgery. The underlying diagnosis may be unknown and the planned operation uncertain. Time to prepare the patient medically is usually limited, and there is often accompanying pain, anxiety, and distress to deal with. Many emergency procedures are in elderly patients who are frequently compromised by their underlying surgical condition and by pre-existing medical disease.

Emergency patients have a higher mortality and morbidity, particularly if there is associated hypovolaemia, cardiac disease, respiratory problems, or renal impairment. In the time available before operative intervention, any cardiovascular or respiratory compromise should be diagnosed and treated urgently. Early contact with the on-call anaesthetic team will produce a plan for the preoperative period. After discussion, delaying surgery is sometimes advisable to allow medical treatment to improve the patient, in other circumstances immediate surgery is required.

Preoperative care of emergency patients

- *History*: Obtain a history from the patient and/or relatives. Enquire specifically about current drug therapy and recent compliance. Has the patient any allergies or experienced any problems with a previous general anaesthetic?
- *Medical records*: Scan the hospital notes and laboratory records for evidence of significant medical disorders. Up to 50% of patients

with previous actual or suspected myocardial infarction will give an inaccurate history 5 years later. Patients may wrongly believe they have had an myocardial infarct when in fact they have not, and vice versa.

- *Examination*: Check for problems listed in Table 7.3. Specific management is detailed in different sections of this book.

- *Investigations*: Most patients will need routine haematology and biochemistry checked, and consideration given to cross-matching blood. Send these bloods as soon as possible. An ECG and CXR should be performed where there is reasonable suspicion of pathology. Perform pulse oximetry in those who are clinically dyspnoeic and check arterial blood gases.

- *Hypotension* is most commonly caused by hypovolaemia due to loss of blood or other fluids. Elderly shocked patients do not always develop a tachycardia. Patients with underlying hypertension may be 'hypotensive' with a systolic pressure of 100 mmHg.

- *Treat pain*. See Chapter 14, p. 54.

Table 7.3 Common medical problems in emergency surgical patients

Cardiovascular	Hypovolaemia/fluid deficits
	Sepsis syndrome
	Ischaemic heart disease
	Cardiac failure (acute or chronic)
	Uncontrolled atrial fibrillation (>100/min)
	Arrhythmias
	Uncontrolled hypertension
Respiratory	Hypoxia
	Lung atelectasis
	Consolidation
	Pulmonary oedema
	Diaphragmatic splinting (pain, or abdominal swelling)
	Inadequate cough
Blood	Anaemia
	Coagulopathy
Renal	Oliguria/anuria
CNS	Septic/toxic encephalopathy
	Pain/anxiety
	Confusion/depressed conscious level
Gastro-intestinal	Risk of aspiration
Metabolic	Fever/hypothermia
	Acidosis
	Hypo/hyperglycaemia
	Electrolyte imbalance, especially K^+ and Mg^{2+}

- *Fluid replacement* should be carried out urgently with regular, frequent reviews to assess the response to fluid loading. Large volumes of fluid should be given through a blood warmer. A urinary catheter should be inserted. Sometimes hypotension is caused by or worsened by cardiac failure or sepsis. If there is an inadequate response to fluid therapy, central venous pressure (CVP) monitoring will be needed. Avoid leaving the patient head down for long periods while establishing central access.

- *Shock*: Any patient with hypotension unresponsive to volume replacement is at serious risk and should be managed on the HDU/ICU. Alternatively, the patient may be transferred directly to theatre for management by the anaesthetic team. Hypotensive patients who are actively bleeding need life-saving surgery and theatre should be arranged urgently. Adequate stocks of cross-matched blood should be arranged. It is vital that blood supplies arrive in theatre at the same time as the patient, and in exsanguinating patients, uncrossmatched, group-compatible blood should be immediately obtained. (See also section on managing major haemorrhage on p. 253.)

- *Excessive fluid therapy*, which may result in pulmonary oedema or haemodilution, can usually be prevented by careful hourly fluid balance, regular review, and CVP monitoring.

- The *haemoglobin* (Hb) or haematocrit (Hct) should be regularly estimated. A portable Hb meter such as the Hemocue is the easiest method.

- Administer *oxygen* to hypotensive patients and to anyone with an oxygen saturation (SpO_2) of less than 95% on pulse oximetry. Clinical examination and a chest radiograph will usually determine the cause of hypoxia. In critically ill patients dyspnoea (p. 281) may due to metabolic acidosis. A lactic acidosis due to tissue hypoxia will often respond to general resuscitation, although other causes of acidosis should be looked for.

- *Metabolic correction*: Electrolytes should be corrected as effectively as time allows. Hypokalaemia and hypomagnesaemia may provoke cardiac arrhythmias. Control diabetes with an insulin and dextrose infusion.

- *Insert a nasogastric (n/g) tube* in patients presenting with intestinal obstruction to relieve gastric distension and reduce the risk of aspiration. Ensure that patients with a depressed conscious level have a clear airway, are receiving oxygen and are being nursed in the appropriate position, preferably in a high dependency area. In patients with a history of acid reflux give omeprazole 40 mg orally (or ranitidine 50 mg i/v if absorption is unlikely) as soon as possible before surgery.

- Decide on appropriate thromboembolic prophylaxis (see p. 48).

- Start antibiotics when indicated (see p. 74).

- *Communication*: Keep the patient and their family informed of your plans and obtain consent for any planned procedure. Discuss specific risks that are relevant to the operation or underlying medical condition. If an operation entails a risk of dying, ensure that this is understood. Do not assume that all patients, particularly elderly ones, wish to undergo surgery.

Day surgery

Iain Wilson

Over the past 20 years, day surgery has increased in popularity owing to changes in medical practice and developments in anaesthesia and surgery. It is often preferred by patients and is efficient in terms of hospital bed utilization and theatre throughput. The frequency and scope of day surgery is expected to rise considerably over the next two decades.

Patient selection

Careful selection of patients in surgical outpatients will prevent problems with unexpected cancellations or the need for postoperative admission due to medical problems. In general, patient selection should be based around the principles outlined in Table 8.1. Common medical factors leading to cancellation on the day of surgery are acute upper respiratory tract infections, uncontrolled hypertension, or fast atrial fibrillation.

After the patient has been selected for day surgery at the surgical outpatient clinic, the consent for the planned surgery should be signed, taking care that the procedure has been explained by a clinician capable of performing the procedure. Some preoperative investigations are best ordered at this stage. Most units give literature to the patient regarding their planned procedure and many employ a preoperative anaesthetic questionnaire to make the admission to hospital more efficient on the day of surgery. The questionnaire should be reviewed by the anaesthetist either prior to admission or on the day of surgery.

Table 8.1 Selection of patients for day surgery

Health status	Generally fit and healthy (ASA 1 or 2). Patients with significant cardiovascular or respiratory disease, insulin-dependent diabetics, or those with gross obesity are not suitable
Age	Patients should be less than 70 years: however, physiological fitness should be considered, rather than a strictly applied chronological age limit
Complexity of surgery	Operations lasting more than 45 min and those associated with a risk of significant postoperative pain, haemorrhage, or prolonged immobility should not be performed
Transport	All patients must be escorted home by a responsible, informed adult and be adequately supervised during their recovery at home for a minimum of 24 h
Social support	Patients must have suitable home conditions with adequate toilet facilities, and a telephone should be readily available for advice in an emergency
Geography	The patient should live within 1 h travelling distance from the hospital

Admission routine

On admission the patient's details, fitness for surgery, and scheduled operation should be checked. The medical staff should recheck consent. Check the results of preoperative investigations that have been performed. Confirm that the patient will not drive or operate machinery for 24 h following anaesthesia. Clinical evaluation should be limited to a check of the following:

- Has the patient's *physical condition* changed in any way from the outpatient assessment?
- Have any *new drugs* been prescribed?
- Has the patient suffered an *acute respiratory illness* in the previous 2 weeks?
- Is the patient's *blood pressure* outside the range 100/60–170/100?

If the answer to any of the above is yes, further assessment may be required.

Recommendations for investigations vary according to the age and fitness of the patient. Table 8.2 shows the scheme used in the Royal Devon and Exeter Hospital day surgery unit.

Premedication

Sedative premedication is not routine but may benefit the occasional particularly nervous person (temazepam 10–20 mg). Patients with symptoms of acid reflux should be treated with omeprazole 40 mg po 90 min before surgery.

Table 8.2 Preoperative investigations for patients undergoing day surgery

Urinalysis	All patients
ECG	Patients over the age of 60 years or when clinically indicated
Full blood count	If anaemia suspected
Creatinine and electrolytes	Patients on diuretics or those with possible renal disease
Blood glucose	All diabetic patients
Sickle test	All black patients who do not know their sickle status
Pregnancy test	Whenever there is any possibility of pregnancy

Anaesthesia

The emphasis is on rapid recovery to allow early ambulation with minimal postoperative pain, nausea, and vomiting. Local anaesthetic infiltration or nerve blocks and adequate doses of analgesics including NSAIDs may prevent significant postoperative pain. Severe pain may require treatment with opioid analgesics. Nausea and vomiting may also occur, most commonly in gynaecological patients. Advice on this problem is detailed on p. 64. Around 1% of day surgery patients require admission to hospital to deal effectively with these and other problems.

Discharge

Discharge from the day unit should be permitted when vital signs are stable, the patient is fully ambulant, and has passed urine. The patient should be orientated and their pain adequately controlled. A check should be made of the operative site prior to discharge. The arrangements for the patient's wound care and a further briefing to the carer made before the patient leaves. The discharge details should be reconfirmed, particularly that driving or working with machinery for 24 h following surgery is not permissible.

Further reading

Warner MA, Shields SE, Chute CG (1993). Major morbidity and mortality within 1 month of ambulatory surgery and anesthesia. *Journal of the American Medical Association* 270:1437–41.

Patient consent

Anthony Nicholls

Only a competent patient can give informed consent. If the patient is by virtue of acute illness temporarily incompetent, then the next of kin has no legal right to give consent for treatment or to withhold therapy. The doctor must act in the best interests of the patient. Furthermore, relatives cannot take decisions for a competent patient, but are perfectly entitled to help the patient and the doctor come to the appropriate decision. Competence is discussed below.

Consent may be implied for examination or simple investigation, but express consent (written or oral) is essential for any procedure that carries material risk. Material risks are defined as those to which a reasonable person in the patient's position would be likely to attach significance. Safe practice encourages patients to be advised of all possible risks, rather than those above a certain likelihood. The language of risk that might be employed is discussed below. Written consent is not necessary in law, but provides documentary evidence that consent has been obtained.

Informed consent

The components of informed consent include the following:

- a description of the proposed procedure
- a discussion of alternative therapeutic options
- mentioning possible complications and their likelihood

- balancing benefits against risks
- decision making by the patient.

Discussion of the proposed surgical procedure and the expected benefit for the patient will include brief details of immediate post-operative care and issues like pain relief and the placement of various tubes, lines and drains. It is common practice for ward nurses to expand upon this after the consent form has been signed. Consent can only be informed if the patient is aware of the risks of various complications including the risk of dying. Obtaining consent must respect the patient's right to self-determination. Some competent patients may prefer not to undergo surgery even when the risks may be greater by not operating. Provided the doctor is confident that the discussion about risks has been understood, the patient's wishes must be respected.

The right of self-determination

A competent adult has a fundamental right to give or withhold consent to treatment. Respect for autonomy is a moral imperative. Treatment without consent may lead to civil or even criminal litigation. It also constitutes serious professional misconduct.

Obtaining consent

Consent should be obtained in advance of an operation and before the use of sedation. Explanations about elective surgery can be given in an outpatient consultation, and the outline of the discussion recorded in the notes. **The person who discusses a procedure with a patient should either be the person who will carry out the procedure, or someone who is capable of doing so.** If the person records in the notes that the discussion has taken place (including a summary of major risks), the actual signing of the hospital consent form can be delegated to a junior doctor. The junior doctor should not take on the responsibility of full explanation of risks and benefits unless capable of the proposed operation, but must ensure that the discussion with an appropriate clinician has taken place.

The surgical team cannot give details of the anaesthetic planned. This should be left to the anaesthetist who will explain the details of the planned anaesthetic and gain consent for any specific details.

Information about risk

Discussion of risk with a patient depends partly upon the *inherent risk* of the procedure and partly upon the *perception of risk* by the individual concerned. Different individuals interpret the same risk differently; some people by nature accept risk whereas others are more cautious. The doctor must not only give information, but also listen to anxieties.

Patients who have underlying medical disorders will inevitable be at increased risk of perioperative complications, including, in many cases, increased mortality. Exact statistical quantification of the degree of excess risk compared with fit patients is not available save in a minority of cases. It is perfectly acceptable, for example, to explain to a patient that chronic bronchitis carries an increased risk of postoperative pneumonia without quantifying the exact risk.

Inherent risks

The language used to discuss risk will need to find common ground with the patient's experience. Terms like negligible, low, moderate, and high risk will be meaningless unless a numerical figure is attached to the description, along with an analogy from everyday life.

- *Negligible* risk is an adverse event occurring at a frequency below 1 per million – roughly the risk of dying from lightning strike.
- *Minimal* risk describes an event occurring in the range of 1 in 100 000 to 1 in a million – the risk of dying on the railways. Few surgical procedures involving general anaesthesia can realistically be said to have negligible or minimal risk in these terms.
- *Very low* risk, between 1 in 10 000 and 1 in 100 000, is the mortality of even the simplest and safest operations. This is the annual risk of dying of an accident at home or work.
- *Low* risk denotes a mortality between 1 in 1000 and 1 in 10 000. This is the annual risk of dying from a road traffic accident.
- *Moderate* risk, in public health terms, is in the range 1 in 100 to 1 in 1000. Many patients will be surprised that this is the risk of dying within the next year of natural causes for patients over 40.

Thus, most surgical risk discussions focus on the identification of high risk, the risk of an adverse event of greater than 1%. More than 1% of patients have diarrhoea after antibiotics, for example, and many minor complications of surgery are as frequent as this. 'Very high risk' would only be used to describe risks of greater than 5%.

Perception of risk

In describing the risk of a procedure, distinct classifications of risk perception need to be made explicit. This involves assessment of the risk/benefit ratio.

- Firstly, a risk may be *avoidable* or *unavoidable*. For example, an avoidable risk may entail modification of the patient's behaviour – losing weight or stopping smoking before elective surgery. On the other hand, unavoidable risk, such as a history of IHD, has to be accepted by the patient or the procedure will never be undertaken.
- Next, a risk may be *justifiable* or *unjustifiable*. Joint replacement for intractable pain in a patient with IHD will entail the patient balancing his or her perception and experience of pain against the finite

risk of morbidity and mortality from myocardial infarction. The patient assesses the gain and the doctor defines the risk. The patient will decide if the risk is justifiable.

- Thirdly, risks can be *acceptable* or *unacceptable*. A patient may believe that any risk is justifiable. The surgeon must then explain that the risk is unacceptable for non-life-threatening conditions, but may become acceptable if death is likely unless surgery is undertaken.

- Finally, there is the dimension of *seriousness*. This is not just the magnitude of risk in numerical terms but also the nature of the adverse event. Risks can range from trivial (haematoma, wound infection, venous thrombosis), through modest (pneumonia, myocardial infarction), to serious (permanent disability and death). It it always crucial in discussion about risk to distinguish between mortality and morbidity.

Competence

A competent adult is a person over 18 who has the capacity to make his own decisions. Capacity is defined in law as the ability to:

- comprehend and retain information
- believe information
- assess information and arrive at a choice.

Mental illness and learning difficulty are not alone grounds to deny that a patient is competent. The BMA and the Law Society have issued further guidance on assessing mental capacity. In order to demonstrate capacity an adult must be able to:

- understand in simple language what treatment is proposed and why it is proposed
- understand the benefits, risks, and alternatives
- understand the consequences of refusing the proposed treatment
- retain the information long enough to make a decision
- make a free choice.

A competent adult can refuse treatment even if the doctor feels that decision is unreasonable and not in his or her best interests.

There is no legal mechanism for any person to authorize consent to treatment on behalf of another adult, irrespective of the competence of that adult. Doctors must act in the best interests of incompetent patients. When deciding what is in the patient's best interests the doctor should consider

- the past feelings and wishes of the patient, if they can be ascertained
- the ability of the incompetent patient to participate in therapy and decision-making, however rudimentary
- the views of others (relatives, carers) about what the patient might wish, and what would be his or her best interests

• whether decision making can be achieved effectively without restricting the patient's freedom of action.

In an emergency, no consent is necessary for life-saving treatment of an unconscious patient. Good practice should include informing relatives what is proposed, but only necessary treatment should be undertaken without consent.

Advance statements (directives)

Advance statements have never been tested in UK courts, but recent judgements support their concept. When a situation falls within the full terms of a written advance statement, then a clinician should regard it as the wish of the patient. In general, advance statements seek to prohibit therapy to prolong life when a patient is both incompetent and terminally ill.

Restricted consent

Some patients may limit their consent to only part of their treatment, and specifically refuse other components of care. The refusal of Jehovah's Witnesses to allow blood transfusion is a typical example. despite the restriction this may place on optimal care, the doctor must accept it. All essential treatment must be provided, short of that specifically banned by the patient.

It is wise to interview such a patient in the presence of a witness. A religious adviser or counsellor is usually available at short notice in the case of refusal of a Jehovah's Witness to allow blood transfusion. The potential hazards and risks should be made clear, and the patient then be allowed to specify on the consent form the procedure(s) for which consent is not given. The interview should be documented in the patient's notes along with the precise nature of the restriction to consent.

Further reading

Calman K (1996). Understanding the language of risk. *Health Trends* **28**:82–8.

Gilberthorpe J (1997). *Consent to treatment.* The Medical Defence Union, London.

Information and consent for anaesthesia (1999). Association of Anaesthetists of Great Britain and Ireland.

Jones HJS, de Cossart L (1999). Risk scoring in surgical patients. *British Journal of Surgery* **86**:149–57.

Management of anaesthesia for Jehovah's Witnesses (1999). Association of Anaesthetists of Great Britain and Ireland.

Resuscitation decisions

Anthony Nicholls

'Do not resuscitate' (DNR) orders

Although patients undergoing elective surgery should automatically receive cardiopulmonary resuscitation (CPR) in the event of cardiac arrest, there are patients in hospital for whom resuscitation would be futile and inappropriate. All hospitals should have policies in place about withholding CPR from these patients, so called 'do not resuscitate' or DNR orders.

Doubts about the appropriateness of CPR may arise when a patient has major life-threatening complications, when a patient is extremely elderly or frail, when malignancy is the cause of admission, or when the underlying quality of life is poor. CPR in these circumstances may be wrong for the patient, offensive to relatives, and upsetting to medical and nursing staff. An explicit decision about CPR must be made in these patients and recorded in the notes. Relatives should be reassured that in the event of cardiac arrest the patient will be left undisturbed and in dignity.

It is wrong to assume that patients and their relatives need to be routinely included in making decisions about resuscitation. If CPR is deemed medically futile, there is no moral or legal obligation to offer treatment that is ineffective, even if patients or their relatives request it. On the other hand, there is a requirement to communicate information about a decision not to resuscitate, and in general, this should initially be to the next of kin. This will require time, compassion, simple explanation, and reasoning. Don't leave the relatives thinking they have to make a decision about resuscitation: aim to help them understand your reasoning, and listen to any of their anxieties, misconceptions, and unrealistic expectations. A doctor should not embark on such discussions without adequate training and experience.

Resuscitation of patients with life-threatening complications

Resuscitation of patients who suffer a cardiac arrest when receiving active treatment for shock, sepsis, or haemorrhage is often unsuccessful, and a full cardiac arrest procedure may be considered futile in these circumstances. The survival of such patients depends on effective management to prevent them deteriorating to the point of a cardiac arrest. If a decision is taken not to defibrillate or ventilate such patients, it must be recorded in the notes. Relatives should be informed of the grave situation and told that if the patient stops breathing or suffers cardiac arrest nothing further can be done. However, some patients in this category may have readily reversible pathology and CPR may be fully appropriate.

CPR in the elderly

Old age is not a bar to CPR. Although the chance of a successful outcome in extreme old age may be low, anaesthesia and recovery from surgery may be associated with life-threatening cardiac arrhythmias. The default position in this situation will normally be CPR. There may be some elderly patients who would prefer not to be resuscitated and if they raise the subject of resuscitation directly then open discussion is straightforward.

Cardiac arrest in patients with advanced malignancy

For patients with advanced malignancy, CPR is generally futile. Virtually no patients with advanced malignancy, be it localized or metastatic, survive resuscitation from cardiac arrest to be discharged from hospital. An exception may be perioperative cardiac rhythm disturbances, but in general, the value of resuscitation in this group should be carefully considered on surgical wards.

CPR in incompetent patients

Patients who are incompetent can never participate in decision-making. Incompetence may be permanent by virtue of brain disease, or temporary from severe illness such as sepsis, metabolic disturbance, or drugs. Decisions regarding resuscitation will hinge on the underlying surgical disease and its prognosis, the likelihood of the patient's becoming competent again, and an assessment of the patient's previous quality of life and anticipated future status. Relatives or carers are usually vital sources of information, but although they may express a view, they cannot legally or morally mandate a course of action that is deemed medically inappropriate.

Practical guidelines for resuscitation decisions

- Work within the guidelines in operation in your hospital.
- Form an opinion about resuscitation based on previous lifestyle, underlying disease prognosis, and acute physiological disturbances.
- If resuscitation is considered appropriate, take no further action: the default position is that CPR will be instituted in such patients.
- If you think the patient should not be for resuscitation, see if the nurses caring for the patient agree. If so, discuss your opinion with the consultant and record the decision in the medical notes together with your brief reasoning. Ensure that there is also a DNR order in the nursing record.
- Arrange as soon as possible to communicate your decision with the next of kin. Such a discussion should initially focus on the condition and prognosis of the patient. This leads on naturally to a reassurance that in case of cardiac arrest, nature would be left to take its course and the patient would be undisturbed at the end of their life. Do not ask relatives whether they wish resuscitation or not, but consider asking what they think their relative would wish. Communicate your considered medical opinion, leaving room for relatives to question you and clarify the decision. The language used to tackle this sort of discussion needs to be adapted to the comprehension of the relatives, and couched in sympathetic, reassuring tones.
- If the relatives are unable to accept a DNR order, or if the nurses on the ward disagree with your assessment, then seek the advice of the consultant.
- Review resuscitation decisions on each ward round, or whenever the patient's condition changes substantially, with your senior ward staff.

Further reading

British Medical Association (1999). *Decisions relating to cardiopulmonary resuscitation*. A statement from the BMA and RCN in association with the Resuscitation Council (UK). [Can be accessed from BMA website http://www.bma.org.uk]

Doyal L, Wilsher D (1993). Withholding cardiopulmonary resuscitation: proposals for formal guidelines. *British Medical Journal* 306:1593–6.

O'Keefe S, Ebell MH (1994). Prediction of failure to survive following in-hospital cardiopulmonary resuscitation: comparison of two predictive instruments. *Resuscitation* 28:21–5.

Stewart K (1995). Discussing cardiopulmonary resuscitation with patients and relatives. *Postgraduate Medical Journal* 71:585–9.

Wall JA, Palmer RN (1994). Resuscitation and patients' views. *British Medical Journal* 309:1442–3.

11

Preoperative optimization of high-risk patients

Julia Munn

Identification of high-risk patients

Recent work has suggested that critical attention to cardiovascular and respiratory function in the perioperative period improves postoperative outcome. Selected patients may benefit from assessment and manipulation of their cardiorespiratory systems by preoperative invasive monitoring and haemodynamic optimization in the HDU/ICU. The following risk factors identify those patients who may benefit:

- pre-existing severe cardiovascular disease
- pre-existing severe respiratory disease
- aortic surgery
- major surgery for malignancy (oesophagectomy, cystectomy, etc.)
- septic patients undergoing unplanned surgery
- haemodynamic instability due to an acute abdominal problem.

Preoperative care

Typical preoperative management of such high risk patients in the HDU/ICU may involve the following:

- insertion of a CVP or pulmonary artery catheter
- monitoring of pulmonary capillary wedge pressure, cardiac output, and urine output

- blood transfusion if anaemic
- oxygen if hypoxic
- infusion of colloid until target values for CVP, pulmonary capillary wedge pressure, urine output, and cardiac output are reached
- administration of an inotrope until O_2 delivery (product of cardiac output and arterial O_2 content) is optimized.

Mortality and postoperative complications may be reduced by this approach. Unfortunately most HDU/ICUs do not have the capacity to admit all such high-risk patients. However, simply monitoring fluid status more closely and replacing fluids more aggressively in emergency patients perioperatively may also improve outcome. Such measures do not need to be undertaken in the HDU/ICU but can be performed before surgery on the ward, in the anaesthetic room, or even the recovery room.

Elective or emergency patients who may benefit from a period of preoperative preparation in HDU/ICU should be discussed with the anaesthetists or the ICU team as early as possible. Local protocols for the care of such patients should be available.

Further reading

Boyd O, Grounds RM, Bennett ED (1993). A randomized clinical trial of the effect of deliberate perioperative increase of oxygen delivery on mortality in high-risk surgical patients. *Journal of the American Medical Association* 270:2699–707.

Sinclair S, James S, Singer M (1997). Intraoperative intravascular volume optimization and length of hospital stay after repair of proximal femur fracture: randomized controlled trial. *British Medical Journal* 315:909–12.

Wilson J, Woods I, Fawcett J, Whall R, Dibb W, Morris C, McManus E (1999). Reducing the risk of major elective surgery: randomised controlled trial of preoperative optimisation of oxygen delivery. *British Medical Journal* 318:1099–103.

12

Postoperative care after major surgery

Julia Munn and Iain Wilson

Principles of postoperative care following major surgery

The principles involved with looking after patients who have under-gone major surgery are the same whether the patient is on the ward, ICU, or HDU.

Who needs intensive care?

Major surgery in patients with chronic medical illnesses carries a high mortality. Some of this is unavoidable, but detection and correction of physiological abnormalities can reduce mortality and shorten length of hospital stay. If hypotension or hypoxia is untreated for several hours, complications such as myocardial infarction, renal failure, or even cardiac arrest may occur. Recognition of physiological deterior-ation requires frequent review of the patient. Once adverse signs are recognized, a downward trend may be often reversed by simple measures undertaken on a general ward. Other patients will need transfer to an HDU/ICU.

Patients who are admitted directly from theatre to HDU/ICU fall into two broad categories:

- *Planned admissions* either following major elective surgery where the nature of the surgery requires a high level of postoperative care, or in patients with serious underlying medical conditions.

- *Emergency admissions* following elective or emergency surgery which has resulted or will result in severe physiological derangement.

Planned ICU/HDU admissions should be booked in advance and the patient informed. A preoperative visit may be possible.

Postoperative management

The following aspects need consideration:

- oxygenation and ventilation
- analgesia
- body temperature
- fluid balance
- urine output
- blood loss and transfusion
- routine investigations
- feeding
- thromboprophylaxis
- antibiotics.

Oxygenation and ventilation

- *All patients require O_2 immediately postoperatively.* Pain and shivering increase O_2 consumption, and anaesthesia worsens ventilation/perfusion mismatch and depresses respiration. These effects are exaggerated by intrathoracic or upper abdominal surgery and after any prolonged operation. The elderly and smokers are particularly prone to becoming hypoxic postoperatively.
- *Hypoxia* is most hazardous in patients with ischaemic heart disease or cerebrovascular disease. Hypotension, hypovolaemia, or severe anaemia reduces O_2 delivery to tissues even further. Hypoxic episodes occur up to 72 h following major surgery, particularly during sleep. Give O_2 (40% by mask or 2 l/min by nasal cannulae) for at least 24–48 h in all patients at risk. Check oxygenation by measuring SpO_2.
- *Ventilation*: Patients who are admitted directly to ICU from theatre may remain intubated and ventilated after major surgery until they are re-warmed, pain-free, haemodynamically stable and adequately oxygenated. When breathing spontaneously, ventilation and oxygenation are improved by sitting the patient up in bed. Most patients feel more comfortable in this position.

Analgesia

Pain is unpleasant, unnecessary, impairs oxygenation, and delays recovery. The patient should be as pain-free as possible without depressing ventilation (see p. 54).

Temperature

- Patients lose heat during major surgery and may remain cold for many hours unless active re-warming measures are taken.
- Hypothermia causes vasoconstriction and shivering which feels unpleasant, increases oxygen demand, and increases cardiac afterload. The viability of free flaps will be threatened by vasoconstriction caused by hypothermia, pain, or hypovolaemia.
- Measures to maintain body temperature include an adequate ambient temperature, a reflective 'space' blanket or warm air blanket, and a fluid warmer for blood and for other fluids if rapid infusion is required.
- Patients should not leave recovery until their core temperature has recovered to $>36°C$.

Fluid balance

- Following major thoracic or abdominal surgery there is a continuing loss of fluid into the pleural or peritoneal cavity.
- Fluid requirements are assessed using a number of simple factors: aim for the following:
  - CVP 5–8 mmHg (8–10 cm H_2O)
  - heart rate <100/min
  - blood pressure within 20% of patient's preoperative value
  - core–peripheral temperature difference $<2°C$
  - urine output >0.5 ml/kg per h.
- Fluid deficits should normally be replaced with 0.9% saline. Estimate the initial rate of volume replacement, then reassess the patient using the above guidelines and adjust the rate of infusion. Once circulating volume has been restored, continue to infuse 0.9% saline and 5% dextrose in a ratio of 2:1. Add potassium according to losses and serial measurements of serum K.
- Colloids for fluid resuscitation: Colloids should not be used to replace simple crystalloid losses (diarrhoea, vomiting, ileus, enteric fistulae), but are indicated in complicated surgical cases with haemorrhage, sepsis, peritonitis, or shock. Albumin solutions are not indicated for hypovolaemia (see p. 251).

Urine output

- *Oliguria is common in the immediate postoperative phase* owing to the hormonal effects of the stress response. Persistent oliguria is often related to hypovolaemia.
- *If urine output is <0.5 ml/kg per h for more than 2–3 h* it may indicate poor renal perfusion. Oliguria in patients with pre-existing renal impairment should be managed very aggressively if worsening of renal function is to be prevented.

- *For optimum renal function the patient needs to be well-filled* (using CVP guidelines above) and have a near normal blood pressure. This can usually be achieved with close attention to fluid balance but it may be necessary to increase the blood pressure with inotropes or a vasoconstrictor on HDU/ICU.

- *Frusemide (furosemide) should not be given until these goals have been reached.* Persistent oliguria after major vascular or urological surgery needs further investigation to exclude a vascular cause or an obstructive uropathy. See p. 299 for further details.

- *NSAIDs may decrease urine output* temporarily for a few hours after administration. They should not be administered to patients who are oliguric, hypotensive, or hypovolaemic (see p. 298).

Blood loss and transfusion

- Haemoglobin levels will continue to fall after surgery when there is *continuing blood loss* (e.g. major orthopaedic surgery) or when there is haemodilution due to the administration of large volumes of clear fluid.

- Optimum O_2 delivery occurs with a *haemoglobin of 10 g/dl*, but fit patients will tolerate 8 g/dl. Transfusion should be considered earlier in patients with IHD, cerebrovascular disease, or hypoxia.

- *Use a fluid warmer when blood is infused rapidly.*

- *Do not give frusemide (furosemide) routinely with blood* unless the patient is overloaded or in cardiac failure.

- *Check a clotting screen after 6–8 units of blood.* Bank blood lacks clotting factors and platelets, so fresh frozen plasma (FFP) and platelets may need to be given. The usual indications for FFP and platelets are an INR >2 and platelets $< 50 \times 10^9/l$ respectively, although tighter control is advisable if the patient is still bleeding.

- If continuing haemorrhage is suspected, *drainage bottles must be reviewed frequently* although they cannot be relied on to detect bleeding.

- *Abdominal girth measurement is not a reliable method of detecting intra-abdominal bleeding*, as very large volumes of fluid can collect before there is an increase in girth – regular palpation is more sensitive.

- Immediately after a thoracotomy *chest drains should swing with respiration* in addition to draining blood-stained fluid – if not they may be blocked, kinked, or displaced so should be aspirated and radiographed and withdrawn or re-sited as necessary.

- See Chapter 37, p. 253 for further guidance on the management of major haemorrhage.

Routine investigations

- FBC, creatinine, and electrolytes: Check postoperatively if major fluid shifts in theatre and then daily until stable.
- Clotting screen: Immediately postoperatively if major transfusion.
- ECG:
  - all patients after major vascular surgery
  - those whose intra-operative course has been complicated by hypotension or hypoxia.
- CXR:
  - to check the position of CVP lines and other tubes (endo-tracheal, chest drains, n/g) inserted in theatre
  - following any thoracic procedure.

Feeding

There is a long tradition that patients remain nil-by-mouth following abdominal surgery, but there is increasing evidence that early feeding does not increase complications and may confer benefits in terms of speed of recovery. See Chapter 18.

Thromboprophylaxis

Start before surgery and continue postoperatively unless there are specific contraindications. See Chapter 13, p. 48.

Prophylactic antibiotics

See Chapter 17, p. 74.

Prophylaxis of venous thromboembolism

Bruce Campbell

The rationale for prophylaxis

Venous thromboembolism is a major cause of death and morbidity among surgical patients. Most deep vein thromboses (DVTs) produce no clinical signs, and most pulmonary emboli (PE) are caused by clinically silent DVTs. DVT may be followed by troublesome postphlebitic syndrome with leg swelling, lipodermatosclerosis, and ulceration.

There is now plentiful evidence from good randomized studies that prophylactic measures are effective in reducing (but not eliminating) the risk of thromboembolism. If a patient at risk develops DVT or PE and demonstrable prophylaxis was not used, then the responsible clinician may be successfully sued.

Risk factors

Risk factors for DVT include major abdominal and pelvic surgery and major orthopaedic and cardiovascular surgery. Patients having operations for major trauma and burns are at especially high risk. Operations lasting longer than 30 min confer a higher risk than shorter procedures. In addition, the following factors have been documented as predisposing to venous thromboembolism in surgical patients:

- previous DVT or PE
- thrombophilia or hyperviscosity
- pregnancy or puerperium
- hormone therapy (important with the contraceptive pill but less with HRT – see later)
- obesity
- malignancy
- heart failure
- immobility
- increasing age (clinically important over 40 years)
- use of a leg tourniquet during surgery
- inflammatory bowel disease
- varicose veins (in the context of major abdominal or pelvic surgery).

Depending on the nature of their illness, type of surgery, and co-existing risk factors, patients can be graded for their level of risk.

Special prophylactic measures are not generally necessary for low risk patients (those without any other risk factors having minor operations lasting <30 min; and patients <40 years having longer operations that are not abdominal, pelvic, cardiovascular, or neurological). Most other patients should receive some form of thromboembolism prophylaxis at the time of surgery.

High-risk patients can develop DVT or PE even without an operation. Patients with obvious risk factors should receive prophylaxis as soon as they are admitted to a surgical bed. Sick elderly patients admitted as emergencies, who have a period of observation and investigation followed by surgery, are at especially high risk.

Methods of prophylaxis

There have been large numbers of clinical trials on the effectiveness of different methods for prevention of DVT and PE in different kinds of surgery. Most have involved major abdominal and pelvic operations, and major joint replacements, which carry a particularly high risk of thromboembolism. The methods most commonly used are subcutaneous heparin and anti-embolism stockings. All surgical units should have explicit written policies for prophylaxis, so there is no doubt about what methods to use, and in precisely which patients.

General

General measures that seem sensible in the prophylaxis of DVT include:

- avoiding immobility, particularly by early mobilization after surgery
- avoidance of dehydration

- taking measures to cover the period of surgery. Most of the immobility takes place in this period and DVT formation may occur on the operating table. Prophylaxis given only postoperatively is not as effective
- the traditional nursing command 'uncross your legs' has no proven benefit.

Subcutaneous heparin

- *Low dose unfractionated heparin* (ordinary heparin injection) has been shown in many trials to reduce the risk of DVT from about 25% to 8%, and to halve the risk of PE in general surgical patients. Doses of 5000 U should be started about 2 h before operation (or on admission for sick patients) and given either 8 or 12 hourly thereafter. There is some evidence that 8 hourly dosage may be more effective than 12 hourly, and it is therefore advisable to prescribe 8 hourly heparin for patients at particularly high risk. The main risk of subcutaneous heparin is increased bleeding and haematoma formation. Heparin induced thrombocytopenia is a rare complication (incidence about 0.3%) and some authorities recommend monitoring the platelet count if heparin is given for more than about 5 days.
- *Low molecular weight heparin* (LMWH) is more convenient than unfractionated heparin, because it is given once daily. Daily doses of the LMWHs are: certoparin 3000 U, dalteparin 2500 U, enoxaparin 2000 U, and tinzaparin 3500 U. It is at least as effective as unfractionated heparin in general surgery, and is preferable for patients having hip or knee replacement. It is associated with slightly fewer bleeding complications than unfractionated heparin. The major disadvantage of LMWH is its greater cost.
- *Adjusted-dose heparin* is more effective than fixed low dose heparin in high-risk patients (e.g. hip replacement) but is seldom used because it is time consuming and complex to manage unfractionated heparin 8 hourly. It involves starting with 3500 U 48 h before operation, and adjusting the dose depending on the activated partial thromboplastin time.

Graduated compression stockings (anti-embolism stockings)

These stockings reduce the risk of leg DVT, but have not been proven to reduce proximal DVT or PE. Combination with subcutaneous heparin may be more effective than either method alone. Below-knee stockings are probably as effective as full length ones, and are more comfortable. Stockings should be fitted with care and the limbs checked regularly for pressure damage. Patients with legs of unusual shape may be unable to wear compression stockings. Stockings are best avoided if foot pulses are impalpable or if the patient has symptoms of peripheral vascular disease: if in doubt, check ankle systolic pressure index.

It is advisable to use stockings in patients having laparoscopic procedures, which cause venous stasis by increasing abdominal pressure during abdominal insufflation.

Intermittent pneumatic compression (IPC) devices

These involve compression of each leg for about 10 s every minute (35–40 mmHg). They are as effective as heparin in preventing leg DVT. Availability and use of these machines requires a hospital or unit policy.

Foot pumps are another mechanical means of prophylaxis. They work by emptying the plantar venous plexuses by rhythmical compression. Compression devices are used widely in plastic and orthopaedic surgery, where there may be concern about increased bleeding with anticoagulant drugs.

Warfarin

Warfarin has been shown to provide effective prophylaxis for patients having hip surgery (elective joint replacement or fractures) and gynaecological operations. It can be used either as a fixed low dose (2 mg/day) or as a monitored dose with a target prothrombin time (international normalized ratio, INR) of 2.0–3.0. Some trials have used postoperative warfarin only, to reduce bleeding complications, but it is probably best started the day before operation. 'Two-step' warfarin prophylaxis has also been described, giving a low dose for 2 weeks before operation, and then a higher monitored dose postoperatively.

Warfarin prophylaxis is most widely used in orthopaedic surgery. It may occasionally be appropriate for very high-risk general surgical patients.

Dextran

Intravenous dextran (dextran 70 and 40) is as effective as low dose heparin for preventing PE. It seems less effective in preventing DVT, except after hip fractures. Dextran has not become popular for prophylaxis because of the need for intravenous infusion, the risks of fluid overload, and anaphylaxis.

Aspirin

Aspirin may have some effect in reducing the risk of DVT and PE. However it is less useful in general surgery and it is less effective than other methods in orthopaedic practice.

Duration of anti-thrombotic prophylaxis

Ideally, prophylaxis should continue until the patient has returned to full activity. In practice, this usually means until discharge from hospital. Prophylaxis may need to be prolonged in some very high-risk patients, but patients remaining in hospital for largely social reasons may reasonably stop prophylaxis when they have become normally mobile.

Hormone therapy and prophylaxis for thromboembolism

The decision about stopping hormone treatment before operations is controversial, and is driven almost as much by medicolegal as by clinical considerations, so discussions should be recorded in the patient's notes. There should always be a written note of whether or not any woman facing surgery is on hormone treatment. With regard to the risk of DVT and PE, there are three main types of hormone therapy:

- *Oestrogen-containing contraceptive pills* (including those combined with progestogen): The risk of thromboembolism is significantly increased and is directly related to the oestrogen content. It is best to stop these pills for 4 weeks before major surgery, and until the first menses occurring at least 2 weeks after full mobilization. For minor and intermediate surgery there is a case for allowing women to continue on their pill, with clear advice on early mobilization, the use of other prophylactic measures, and thorough counselling (recorded in the notes). Each case should be judged on its merits, and the wishes of the patient taken into account. The need for alternative contraceptive precautions must be emphasized to any woman who is advised to stop the pill for surgery.

- *Progestogen-only contraceptive pills*: There is no evidence that the risk of DVT or PE is increased, but the general level of concern about 'thromboembolism and the pill' leads many surgeons to treat patients similarly to those on oestrogen-containing preparations. Again, individual discussion and decision making is important.

- *Hormone replacement therapy (HRT)*: Recent evidence has shown that there is a small but significant increase in the rate of venous thromboembolism in women on HRT. The risk is nevertheless very low and there are no good data on postoperative risk. Currently it seems reasonable to allow women to continue HRT at the time of surgery, but to ensure that prophylactic measures such as subcutaneous heparin are used.

Anaesthesia and anticoagulation

Central neural blockade (spinal or epidural anaesthesia) is contraindicated in fully anticoagulated patients owing to the small but serious risk of developing a haematoma within the spinal canal. The position of anticoagulants used as prophylaxis for DVT or PE is controversial. Anaesthetists vary in their practice and it is vital to work out a joint plan of DVT prophylaxis with the anaesthetic team, particularly with regard to preoperative heparin injections.

Further reading

Checketts MR, Wildsmith JAW (1999). Central nerve block and thromboprophylaxis – is there a problem? *British Journal of Anaesthesia* 82:164–7.

Clagett GP, Anderson FA, Heit J, Levine MN, Wheeler HB (1995). Prevention of venous thromboembolism. *Chest* 108:312–34S.

Thromboembolic Risk Factors (THRIFT) Consensus Group (1992). Risk of and prophylaxis for venous thromboembolism in hospital patients. *British Medical Journal* 305:567–74.

Wells PS, Lensing AWA, Hirsh J (1994). Graduated compression stockings in the prevention of venous thromboembolism: a meta-analysis. *Archives of Internal Medicine* 154:67–72.

The management of acute pain

David Conn and Julie Murdoch

Acute pain is often badly managed. This need not be so. Pain control can often be improved by a simple strategy:

- assess the pain
- treat with drugs and techniques with which you are familiar
- re-assess the pain after treatment and be prepared to adjust the treatment accordingly.

Good pain relief reduces postoperative complications such as chest infections, nausea and vomiting, DVT, and ileus.

General principles

- Patients who say that they are in pain invariably are. Listen to your patients and believe them.
- There are no physiological or behavioural patterns that can be used to prove that someone is fabricating pain.
- The same surgical operation may produce widely differing analgesia requirements in different patients.

- The same level of pain may be expressed in widely differing ways by different patients.
- Opioids given for acute pain do not produce drug addiction.
- Severe pain after surgery is preventable.
- Look for treatable causes of pain, but never withhold analgesia for fear of masking surgical signs.
- The correct dose of an opioid analgesic is 'enough and often enough'.
- The maximum benefit with fewest unwanted effects is often obtained by a combination of different drugs given by different routes (e.g. an opioid with an NSAID and a local anaesthetic).

Assessment of pain, analgesia, and sedation

- Scoring systems are used to assess pain and to measure the effectiveness of treatment. The pain score can be charted on the temperature chart or on a separate pain chart.
- A *visual analogue scale* (VAS) is a 10 cm line whose end-points are 0 (no pain) and 10 (the worst imaginable pain). The patient puts a mark on the line to represent their pain severity. This technique may be difficult to apply if the patient is in severe pain.
- A *verbal rating scale* (VRS) is simpler. The patient is asked if they have no pain, mild, moderate or severe pain and is scored 0 for no pain, 1 for mild pain, 2 for moderate pain, and 3 for severe pain.
- The patient should be assessed after gentle arousal. Sedation should be scored at the same time: 0 if awake, 1 if dozing intermittently, 2 if mostly sleeping, 3 if difficult to waken.
- A combination of the sedation score and the respiratory rate can be used to diagnose opioid overdose.
- A rate of < 8/min with a sedation score of 3 indicates overdose.
- A slow respiratory rate without over-sedation is acceptable, but does require extra vigilance.
- Intravenous naloxone should be titrated in increments of 200 μg until the over-sedation is reversed without reversing the analgesia. Naloxone may be shorter acting than the opioid, so continuing assessment is vital, as re-sedation can occur.

General principles of drug therapy

Know a limited number of drugs well and consider the following:

- Can the patient take *oral analgesics*?
- Do they need *i/v* administration for speed of onset?
- Can *local anaesthesia* better treat the pain, or be used in combination with systemic analgesics?
- Can *other methods* be used to help ease the pain, such as splinting of fractures, dressing of burns, reassurance?

Opioids

- *Weak opioids* (codeine, dihydrocodeine, dextropropoxyphene) have limited use on their own. They are best used in combination with paracetamol or aspirin. Codeine is a pro-drug and is relatively inactive until metabolized to morphine. Weak opioids cause nausea and constipation as often as strong opioids but without the benefit of potent analgesia.

- *Strong opioids* (morphine, diamorphine, pethidine, methadone, fentanyl) are all pure agonists, acting on similar receptors. All have similar unwanted effects including nausea, vomiting, sedation, itching, reduced gut motility, constipation, and respiratory depression.

Morphine

- Morphine is the drug of choice for postoperative analgesia. It is cheap and widely used.

- Treat severe acute or postoperative pain with i/v boluses of 2–3 mg every 3–5 min (1 mg bolus for the elderly and frail). The patient should be closely observed for at least 30 min thereafter.

- The i/m dose is 7.5 mg for 40–65 kg body weight or 10 mg for 65–100 kg. See Fig. 14.1.

- Rarely, morphine can cause anaphylactoid reactions, and bronchospasm. Avoid its use in those who are actively wheezy. Urticaria along the line of the vein is very common owing to local histamine release but does not indicate 'allergy'.

- Use morphine with caution in severe renal impairment. The metabolite morphine 6-glucuronide is active and long-acting. Repeated doses of morphine accumulate leading to excessive sedation and respiratory depression without analgesia.

- Oral morphine can be used if absorption can be guaranteed. The required dose of oral morphine is approximately 3–5 times the parenteral dose. Take care when giving oral morphine postoperatively: if there is delayed gastric emptying initially, overdose may occur when normal gastric emptying resumes. Do not combine morphine by different routes.

- Prescribe oral morphine 4 hourly regularly with a similar dose available to take 'as required' between each dose.

- If oral morphine is needed for more than a few days then use one of the slow-release preparations (MST, MXL, Morcap). All slow-release preparations are not the same. A change from one preparation to another requires care.

Diamorphine

- No real benefits over morphine.

- More lipid-soluble than morphine. 1.5–2 times as potent.
- Commonly used in palliative care because it can be prepared in high concentrations for s/c infusion.
- Useful in addition to local anaesthetic in epidural injections or infusions.

Pethidine

- Said to be better than morphine for colicky pain and pancreatic pain, but there is no evidence for this.
- The dose is 75–100 mg and may be increased to 150 mg if required.
- Shorter acting than morphine. Has a neurotoxic metabolite norpethidine which may accumulate with long-term use and can cause confusion, twitching, and in extreme situations grand mal seizures.
- Can be used for patients with true morphine allergy or significant asthma.
- Useful in addition to local anaesthetic in epidural injections or infusions, or for treatment of severe postoperative shivering.

Methadone

- Primarily used orally but can be used i/m or i/v.
- Has a variable half-life with a considerable risk of accumulation. This may take several days to occur.
- Carries the stigma of being a drug used in addiction, but is a very useful analgesic.
- Should only be used by those with experience in its use.

Fentanyl

- A very potent opioid used primarily in anaesthesia.
- Useful in PCA pumps if there is true allergy to morphine.
- Useful in addition to local anaesthetic in epidural injections or infusions.
- Available in transdermal formulations. The patches release 25, 50, or 75 μg/h, but are not licensed for postoperative pain. The drug can take a number of hours to reach maximum dosage and many hours to wear off after removal of the patch.

Tramadol

- Acts as an opioid receptor agonist. Also has an action on noradrenergic and serotonergic pathways.
- Not a controlled drug but shares opioid side effects such as nausea and vomiting.
- Useful in mild to moderate pain. Use 50–100 mg 4 hourly, maximum dose of 400 mg/24 h.

The partial agonists and agonist/antagonist groups

Partial agonists and agonist/antagonists, including drugs such as buprenorphine and nalbuphine, have little advantage over the pure agonists and therefore are not recommended.

Routes of opioid administration

i/m injection

- the traditional administration route, often on an 'as required' basis. In many cases this leads to grossly inadequate levels of pain relief.
- i/m analgesia is effective if given regularly according to an algorithm relating to time of last dose, pain score, sedation score, and respiratory rate. See Fig. 14.1.

i/v bolus injection

- Gives the fastest onset of analgesia, and repeated doses can be titrated against effect.
- Close supervision of the patient is required.

i/v infusion

- Often used where the patient is unable to use a PCA pump (see below).
- The time to steady state blood levels is 4–5 times the drug half-life. Morphine may take 10 h to reach the maximum blood level, so there is a danger of complications if nursing supervision is not adequate.
- Unsafe if the patient cannot be observed closely.

Epidural administration

- Opioids have around 10 times the potency when given epidurally as opposed to parenterally.
- Lipid-soluble opioids (e.g. fentanyl) have segmental effects whereas lipid-insoluble opioids (e.g. morphine) have a more generalized effect.
- Typically used in combination with local anaesthetic for synergistic effects.
- Can cause delayed respiratory depression, but this will respond to the opioid antagonist naloxone (200 μg intravenously repeated as required).

Patient-controlled administration (PCA)

Can give high quality pain management. It gives patients control over their own pain. Staff are not immediately needed to provide analgesia and patients receive more rapid pain relief. The success of PCA is dependent on several factors:

- patient suitability and preoperative education
- education of staff in the concepts of PCA and the use of equipment
- appropriate monitoring of the patient for effects and side-effects
- funding – PCA infusion pumps are expensive.

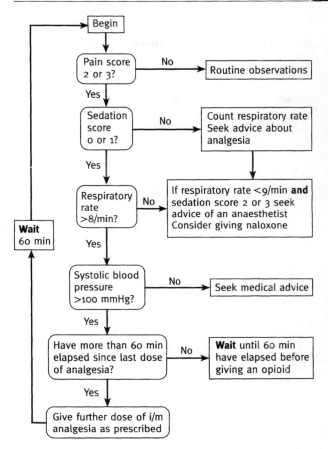

Fig. 14.1 Algorithm for i/m opioid administration. (Reproduced by kind permission of *Anaesthesia*).
Pain score: 0, no pain; 1, mild pain; 2, moderate pain; 3, severe pain.
Sedation score: 0, awake; 1, dozing intermittently; 2, mostly sleeping; 3, difficult to waken.
Morphine: weight 40–65 kg, 7.5 mg; weight 65–100 kg, 10 mg.
Naxolone: 200 μg i/v, as required.

Box 14.1 gives a typical PCA regime.

The bolus dose and lockout time can be altered to meet individual needs. Background infusions are rarely used, generally only if the patient was previously taking regular strong opioid analgesics such as MST.

Box 14.1 Typical PCA regime

> **Drug:** morphine
> **Concentration:** 1 mg/ml
> **Bolus dose:** 1 mg
> **Lockout time:** 5 min
>
> *Bolus dose:* the amount of drug given by the pump when the patient makes a successful demand.
> *Lockout time:* the amount of time in which the patient will gain only one successful demand from the pump. This is a safety feature.

The patient should have a dedicated i/v line for PCA or a one-way valve in the i/v fluid line (if piggybacked in the i/v line). This stops accidental accumulation of large amounts of opioid in the line that may then be flushed to the patient.

Non-steroidal anti-inflammatory drugs (NSAIDs)

- Have moderate analgesic potency and are anti-inflammatory. Effective after dental surgery and minor orthopaedic surgery. Reduce the requirement for opioids after major surgery. They all work in a similar way, so never prescribe two different NSAIDs at the same time.
- Recognized to increase the bleeding time, and may increase blood loss.
- Can be given by many routes: oral, i/m, i/v, rectal, topical. The oral route is preferred if available. I/m diclofenac should be avoided as it is painful and may lead to sterile abscess formation.

Contraindications to NSAIDs

- history of peptic ulceration
- renal impairment or oliguria
- hyperkalaemia
- renal transplantation
- anticoagulation or other coagulopathy
- severe liver dysfunction
- dehydration or hypovolaemia
- loop diuretic therapy
- history of exacerbation of asthma with NSAIDs.

Use NSAIDs **with caution** (risk of impaired renal function) in

- patients over 65
- diabetics who may have nephropathy and/or renal vascular disease

- patients with widespread vascular disease
- cardiac disease, hepatobiliary disease, major vascular surgery
- patients on ACE inhibitors, potassium-sparing diuretics, β-blockers, cyclosporin, or methotrexate.

Electrolytes and creatinine must be measured regularly and any deterioration in renal function or symptoms of gastric upset is an indication for stopping the NSAID.

Ibuprofen is safe and cheap. Longer-acting drugs (e.g. piroxicam) tend to have more unwanted effects. Cyclo-oxygenase 2 (COX-2) specific inhibitors (e.g. meloxicam) may be safer as they have less effect on the gastrointestinal tract and renal COX systems.

Prolonged courses of NSAIDs are more likely to cause unwanted effects than short perioperative courses. H_2 blockers (e.g. ranitidine) given with NSAIDs may protect against GI side-effects.

Local anaesthesia

Provides additional analgesia for all types of surgery. Can provide excellent analgesia with no effect on consciousness. A simple technique such as local infiltration into the wound edges at the end of a procedure will provide short-term analgesia. There is little excuse for not using it. Nerve, plexus, or regional blocks can be made to last many hours or days if catheter techniques are used.

Complications can occur:

- The commonest complications are related to the specific techniques, such as hypotension with epidural local anaesthetics due to sympathetic nerve block, and muscle weakness that accompanies any block of a major nerve.
- Systemic toxicity can occur from excessive dosage or accidental intravenous administration of local anaesthetics. This can range from mild confusion, through loss of consciousness, seizures, cardiac arrhythmias, and cardiac arrest.
- Accidental administration of the wrong drug can be a personal and medico-legal disaster. Great care must be taken when administering all drugs.

Epidural infusion of local anaesthetics

Local anaesthetic agents can be useful when used alone, but more commonly a mixture (e.g. bupivacaine 0.166% and diamorphine 0.1–0.2 mg/ml) is used. The drugs are synergistic in combination. Hypotension and respiratory depression are possible: patients should be nursed in an area where there is adequate supervision.

Management of this technique requires experience. Inadequate analgesia should be referred to the duty anaesthetist.

Reducing the risk of local anaesthetic toxicity

- Decide the concentration of the local anaesthetic that is required for the block to be performed. Calculate the total volume of drug that is allowed according to Table 14.1.
- Use the least toxic drug available.
- Use lower doses in frail patients or at the extremes of ages.
- Always inject the drug slowly (slower than 10 ml/min) and aspirate regularly looking for blood to indicate an accidental intravenous injection.
- Injection of a test dose of 2–3 ml of local anaesthetic containing adrenaline 1 : 200 000 will often (but not always) cause a significant tachycardia if accidental i/v injection occurs.
- Add adrenaline (epinephrine) to reduce the speed of absorption. This reduces the maximum blood concentration by about 50%. Use adrenaline at a concentration of 1 : 200 000, with a maximum dose of 200 μg (for an average sized adult). Take adrenaline 1 : 1000 (1 mg/ml, or 0.1 mg%.) and add 0.1 ml to each 20 ml of local anaesthetic. Better still, use premixed local anaesthetic with adrenaline. Adrenaline makes no difference to the toxicity of the local anaesthetic if it is injected i/v.

Table 14.1 Maximum safe local anaesthetic doses

Drug	Maximum for local infiltration	Maximum for plexus anaesthesia
Lidocaine (lignocaine)	3 mg/kg	4 mg/kg
Lidocaine (lignocaine) with adrenaline (epinephrine)	5 mg/kg	7 mg/kg
Bupivacaine	1.5 mg/kg	2 mg/kg
Bupivacaine with adrenaline (epinephrine)	2 mg/kg	3.5 mg/kg
Prilocaine	5 mg/kg	7 mg/kg
Prilocaine with adrenaline (epinephrine)	5 mg/kg	8 mg/kg

Entonox

A gas containing 50% nitrous oxide (N_2O) and 50% O_2; a potent analgesic that depends on self-administration by a co-operative patient. It is quick acting and short-lived when administration ceases. An ideal agent for pain of short duration.

- Self-administration safeguards the user from overdose – when the patient becomes drowsy the mask/mouthpiece falls from the face.
- Entonox can be used for procedures such as dressing change, removal of drains and sutures, application of traction and plaster of Paris, etc.

- Contraindications include pneumothorax, decompression sickness, intoxication, maxillofacial injuries, head injuries, severe bullous emphysema, and bowel obstruction.
- Success depends on patient and staff education and the availability of suitable equipment.

The acute pain team

An acute pain team exists in many hospitals. It is an invaluable source of help and information for the junior surgical staff. An anaesthetist usually heads the team, with a specialist nurse running the day-to-day service. If a pharmacist and surgeon are also involved, improvements in practice and the implementation of change is easier.

The aim of the team is to improve and maintain standards in the management of acute pain. It is their responsibility to:

- train and educate medical and nursing staff
- provide information for patients
- provide an advisory and trouble-shooting service for problems associated with acute pain management
- audit the effects (wanted and unwanted) of pain management practices.

Summary

To provide your patients with good pain relief you need to know how to assess pain, the drugs and techniques available, their effects (wanted and unwanted), your own limitations, and where to go for help if things are not going well.

Further reading

Gould TH, Crosby DL, Harmer M *et al.* (1992). Policy for controlling pain after surgery: effect of sequential changes in management. *British Medical Journal* 305:1187–93.

Harmer M, Davies KA (1998). The effect of education, assessment and a standardized prescription on postoperative pain management. *Anaesthesia* 53:424–30.

Report of the Working Party on Commission on the Provision of Surgical Services (1990). *Pain after surgery.* Royal College of Surgeons of England and the College of Anaesthetists.

Royal College of Anaesthetists (1998). *Guidelines for the use of non-steroidal anti-inflammatory drugs in the perioperative period.*

Postoperative nausea and vomiting (PONV)

David Conn

Frequency

Postoperative nausea and vomiting (PONV) is common. It may affect up to 35% of patients after day case surgery. Although rarely life-threatening, it is distressing and debilitating, and can lead to delays in returning to normal oral intake, delayed discharge from hospital, increased bleeding, wound dehiscence, and aspiration pneumonia. Although PONV is usually short-lived, many patients find it the most distressing part of their hospital stay.

Physiology

Nausea and vomiting is mediated through central and peripheral pathways, with a number of neurotransmitters involved.

- *Central structures* include the chemoreceptor trigger zone (CTZ) in the area postrema, which lies outside the blood–brain barrier. The nucleus of the tractus solitarius (NTS) and the vagal nuclei receive afferent impulses from the vagus nerve and interconnect with the CTZ. It is within the CTZ that the signal are modulated and then transferred to the vomiting centre. Serotonin, dopamine, and acetylcholine are all active transmitters in this area.

- *Peripheral structures* include the mechanoreceptors in the muscular wall of the distal stomach and proximal duodenum, and the chemoreceptors in the gut mucosa of the upper small bowel. Both serotonin and cholinergic pathways are involved.

- There are further connections to the *vomiting centre* from cranial nerves, the hypothalamus, the cortex, and the vestibular system.

- *Learned responses* are also important, such as a strong history of PONV, or motion sickness.

Risk factors

Type of surgery

- strabismus surgery
- pelvic surgery, especially gynaecological
- middle ear surgery
- bowel surgery.

Anaesthetic drugs

Factors increasing nausea
- opioids – reducing the use of opioids decreases PONV. Avoid opioid premedication.

Factors decreasing nausea
- non-steroidal anti-inflammatory drugs
- local anaesthetic blocks
- avoiding nitrous oxide in high-risk cases (this risks intraoperative awareness)
- the use of short-acting neuromuscular blocking agents avoiding the need for neostigmine reversal
- propofol.

Patient factors

- Women suffer more PONV than men, possibly owing to increased gonadotrophin levels especially in weeks 3 and 4 of the menstrual cycle.
- Children suffer more than adults.
- Obese patients are more at risk, possibly due to increased reflux, or increased deposition of fat-soluble anaesthetic agents.
- Past history of PONV or motion sickness.
- Pain and distress.
- Decreased gastric emptying, such as after trauma.

Management of PONV

- Treat high-risk patients with prophylactic anti-emetics.
- If practical avoid drugs that are particularly associated with PONV such as opioids.
- Avoid dehydration.
- Treat pain and distress.
- Give anti-emetics, possibly in combination.

Anti-emetics

As there are multiple pathways to the vomiting centre and many neurotransmitters, there are also many types of anti-emetics; none is perfect. Some drugs have multiple actions, so the following classification is pragmatic.

Anti-dopaminergic agents

- *Phenothiazines* such as prochlorperazine (12.5 mg i/m) are active against the emetic effect of opioids, but are sedative and short-acting and risk extrapyramidal side-effects. Do not give prochlorperazine intravenously.
- *Butyrophenones* such as droperidol (0.5–1.0 mg i/v) and haloperidol are neuroleptic agents and are powerful dopamine receptor antagonists. Droperidol in small doses (i.e. < 1 mg) is a useful anti-emetic. It can cause disturbing dysphoriant effects and can be sedative as well as causing extrapyramidal side effects, although this is less likely to be a problem with lower doses. Droperidol is often added to morphine for use in PCA pumps. Doses in the range of 2.5–5 mg are added to 50 mg morphine. Oversedation can be a problem.
- *Substituted butyrophenones* such as domperidone (10–20 mg po or 20–60 mg pr) do not cross the blood–brain barrier and therefore avoid some of the side-effects of droperidol. It is best given orally or rectally.
- *Substituted benzamides* such as metoclopramide (10 mg i/v, i/m, or po) are popular but relatively inactive in the postoperative period. Metoclopramide is active against the emetic effect of opioids, but has a high incidence of extrapyramidal side effects, especially in young women. (See treatment of oculogyric crisis below.)

Antihistamines

- *Cyclizine* 25–50 mg i/m or i/v is partially effective in PONV especially after middle ear surgery. Sedation can be a problem.

Anticholinergics

- *Hyoscine* (scopolamine) 0.3–0.6 mg i/m and atropine 0.3–0.6 mg i/m are useful for the treatment of motion sickness, opioid-induced vomiting, and PONV. Adverse effects (sedation, confusion, dry mouth) limit their use.

5HT$_3$-antagonists

Ondansetron is widely regarded as the anti-emetic with the lowest side-effect profile, particularly effective in chemotherapy-induced emesis. There is little evidence that it is better than any other anti-emetics for either prophylaxis or treatment of PONV. Ondansetron is poor for either prophylaxis or treatment of nausea. If given for protracted vomiting, the dose is 4 mg i/v. The cost of ondansetron prohibits its routine use.

In paediatric practice, where the extrapyramidal effects of the anti-dopaminergic drugs can be a serious problem, ondansetron is the drug of choice. The dose is 50–100 μg/kg by slow intravenous injection. Side-effects include headache, constipation, and altered liver enzymes.

Other drugs

- *Benzodiazepines* have been shown to decrease anticipatory vomiting before chemotherapy.
- *Cannabinoids* are available in the form of Nabilone. It was originally used for chemotherapy-induced emesis, but has been superseded by ondansetron.
- *Steroids* are used for reducing the emesis related to chemotherapy.
- *Ginger root* is used in some folk remedies, and is probably effective.

Special note

Avoid combinations of drugs with extrapyramidal effects, and avoid these drugs completely in patients with Parkinson's disease.

Other treatments

Acupuncture or acupressure is popular with some people. The classical point for treatment is PC 6 (neiguan), located proximal to the wrist crease between palmaris longus and flexor carpi radialis, which lies immediately above the median nerve. Other points are quoted but evidence for the effectiveness of acupuncture is lacking.

Treatment of oculogyric crisis

This extrapyramidal drug side-effect is occasionally seen after anti-dopaminergic drugs, especially in young women. Signs include muscle rigidity and involuntary jaw and/or eye movements. Treatment is with an anticholinergic agent such as procyclidine, 5–10 mg by slow i/v injection. The response is usually rapid.

Summary

Avoiding PONV

- Prophylaxis for high-risk patients with an anti-emetic of your choice.

- Alter the anaesthetic technique to avoid opioids, N_2O, and reversal of neuromuscular blockade if appropriate.
- Consider not treating pain too aggressively, as your patient may prefer mild pain and no PONV to total analgesia and PONV.
- Ensure adequate hydration, by the i/v route if necessary. Do not push oral fluids too early, especially if the patient is about to embark upon a car journey.

Treatment of the vomiting patient

- Look for causes such as ileus, too early return to oral intake, or too much or too little analgesia.
- Ensure adequate hydration; consider short-term i/v fluids.
- Give an anti-emetic, preferably i/v; if this is not successful give a different one. If the patient is a day case consider ondansetron in low dose.

Further reading

Strunin L, Rowbotham D, Miles A Eds. (1999). *The effective management of post-operative nausea and vomiting.* (UK Key Advances in Clinical Practice Series). London, UEL Centre for Health Services Research.

Tramèr MR, Phillips C, Reynolds DJM, McQuay HJ, Moore RA (1999). Cost-effectiveness of ondansetron for postoperative nausea and vomiting. *Anaesthesia* 54:226–35.

Watcha MF (1996). Nausea and vomiting: choice of drugs and treatment. *Current Opinion in Anaesthesiology* 9:300–5.

Fluid balance

Iain Wilson

Surgical patients require careful attention to their fluid balance. Several factors alter fluid and electrolyte requirements.

- Patients who are *nil-by-mouth* after major surgery cannot depend on thirst to regulate body fluids. They rely solely on i/v fluids to maintain their fluid balance.
- *Fluid shifts* after surgery result from sequestering of fluid in the operative site or other places such as the abdomen (e.g. ileus). These unseen losses are commonly known as 'third space' and consist of mainly extracellular fluid. In other situations, loss of plasma occurs across leaking capillary membranes.
- *Blood loss* is usually easy to estimate in theatre, but may be concealed in the pre- and postoperative phase. Indirect estimations of blood loss may be inaccurate.
- The *stress response* to surgery or critical illness causes hypersecretion of aldosterone and ADH and a general increase in sympathetic drive. This results in sodium and water retention.
- *Ascites and pleural effusions* may form.

General principles in i/v fluid therapy

The most critical aspect of fluid balance is to maintain circulating volume, ensuring adequate tissue blood flow and function.

Careful charting of fluid balance is important.

i/v fluid therapy may be considered as:

- *Maintenance fluid* to replace fluid that would normally have been ingested by the patient. It replaces insensible losses, urine, and bowel output. Requirements vary but a method of estimating maintenance requirements is shown in Box 16.1. When possible use bags of fluid with K^+ already added rather than add K^+ on the ward. Standard solutions contain either 20 or 40 mmol K^+/l (0.15 or 0.3%).

Box 16.1 Approximate normal maintenance requirements in adults

Water: 1.5 ml/kg per h of fluid (estimate lean body mass to avoid excess fluid in obese patients)
Na^+: 1–2 mmol/kg per day
K^+: 1 mmol/kg per day

Suitable regime for 70 kg adult
1000 ml 0.9% saline + KCl 20–40 mmol/l
1000 ml 5% dextrose + KCl 20–40 mmol/l
500 ml 5% dextrose

Increase by 10% per degree of pyrexia, also with excess sweating or hot climates

Decrease to 1 ml/kg per h if fluid restricted (head injuries, cardiac failure, etc.)

K^+ supplements unnecessary in first 24 h unless hypokalaemic preoperatively

- *Replacement fluid* replaces all abnormal losses, both seen and unseen. This includes blood, plasma, third space loss, output from drains, fistulae or nasogastric tubes and diarrhoea. A guide to replacement fluids is shown in Table 16.1. When writing a fluid regime, estimate the maintenance fluids and the replacement fluids and then prescribe these on a suitable fluid chart. If the patient is likely to require alteration of the regime later, do not write up fluids for more that a few hours so that someone has to review the patient clinically.

Table 16.1 Common fluid losses and suitable replacement options in surgical patients

Losses	Approximate content (mmol/l)		Suitable replacement fluid
	Na^+	K^+	
Blood	140	4	Hartmann's/0.9% saline/colloid/blood products
Plasma	140	4	Hartmann's/0.9% saline/colloid
Third space losses	140	4	Hartmann's/0.9% saline
NG losses	60	10	50:50 0.9% saline/0.15% KCl and 5% dextrose
Upper GI losses	110	5–10	0.9% saline (check K^+ regularly)
Diarrhoea	120	25	0.9% saline/0.15% KCl

Perioperative management

Elective surgery

Patients may drink clear fluids up to 2 h before surgery (check your local policy). Patients with chronic renal failure or obstructive jaundice require preoperative i/v fluids to maintain renal blood flow and urine output perioperatively – see specific sections of this book. Patients should not eat for at least 6 h before surgery.

- *Minor surgery*: Patients can usually drink when they are fully conscious. The anaesthetist may request a delay in drinking if the upper airway has been sprayed with local anaesthetic.

- *Intermediate surgery*: Take into account the nature of the surgery performed and the surgeon's protocols. Start i/v fluids if blood loss is >250 ml, or if normal fluid intake is likely to be delayed for more that 8 hours postoperatively.

- *Major surgery*: I/v fluids are routinely used during the operation and often for some days afterwards.

Anaesthetists usually supervise perioperative fluid balance and prescribe a postoperative regime. Different patients with different underlying medical conditions undergoing various types of surgery may all need different prescriptions. Some operations, for example total hip or knee joint replacement surgery, may be associated with heavier blood loss in the postoperative phase than during the surgery. Fluid regimes will need reviewing in these patients.

Following extensive surgery (e.g. oesophagectomy, abdominal aneurysm, thoracotomy) fluid requirement are difficult to predict as patients may require large volumes of i/v fluids to maintain the circulating volume. They may have very high third space losses and/or significant postoperative blood loss. Regular review of the patient, careful clinical monitoring and adjustment of the fluids is required. CVP monitoring (see p. 260) is common in this group of patients and should always be performed if assessment of fluid requirements proves difficult.

In most patients fluid balance can be satisfactorily managed by careful attention to clinical details as shown in Box 16.2. Trends are more important than single observations.

Box 16.2 Assessing and monitoring fluid balance in the surgical patient

Monitor clinical signs:	Pulse/BP/peripheral perfusion
	Urine output (>0.5 ml/kg per hour)
	CVP (8–10 cm H_2O, 5–8 mmHg)
Check losses:	Fluid chart (urine, drains, aspirates, etc.)

Emergency surgery

- Unprepared patients with underlying medical and metabolic problems are frequently complex in terms of i/v fluid therapy (see p. 25).

- Every emergency patient is different and needs a personalized approach!

- Many patients require resuscitation due to dehydration and hypovolaemia before theatre. Most of them will have had an inadequate fluid intake for several days and will also have sequestered fluid internally, worsening the situation. In addition, electrolyte abnormalities often coexist. Fluid depletion may be severe and take some hours to correct. The principle is to restore the circulating volume rapidly and then other deficits more slowly.

- Management of active bleeding often includes immediate surgery – see p. 253.

- When planning a regime, estimate the degree of hypovolaemia and give rapid i/v fluids to replace this. If the patient is going to theatre communicate with the anaesthetist as soon as is practical, so that an overall plan may be developed.

- When resuscitating the hypovolaemic patient estimate the haemoglobin regularly, either using a laboratory sample, or a portable device such as a Haemocue.

Problems with fluid balance

- *Patient needs more fluid than expected to keep BP stable.* Exclude surgical bleeding. If following major surgery, check the CVP. After major surgery this situation is usually due to the patient not retaining fluids within the vascular space. Careful clinical monitoring of the patients preferably on HDU/ICU is necessary. Early sepsis often presents as hypotension resistant to i/v fluids.

- *The patient is hyponatraemic.* Unless the Na$^+$ was abnormal preoperatively, hyponatraemia is usually due a relative excess of water (excess 5% dextrose or the TUR syndrome). Refer to p. 302.

- *The patient is very oedematous but is also hypovolaemic.* Many such patients are unable to maintain fluid within the vascular space. This may be due to hypoalbuminaemia or a capillary leak syndrome such as sepsis. The patient requires fluid to maintain circulating volume. The oedema is difficult to improve as the fluid is often sequestered in the peripheries and is only mobilized as the patient improves. The use of concentrated albumin solution with loop diuretics has not been shown to improve outcome and should be avoided. Heart failure (particularly right sided) worsens this tendency and the diagnosis should be considered.

- *What regime should be used in a patient with cardiac failure?* Give a restricted maintenance and prescribe replacement fluids according to losses. Monitor urine output and CVP with major surgery. Although these patients are at risk of worsening heart failure with overenthusiastic i/v fluid administration they will do equally badly if underfilled. Consider involving HDU/ICU as a pulmonary artery catheter may help.

- *The patient is passing a lot of urine.* Commonly this is normal if it occurs 2–3 days after surgery when the patient is mobilizing fluids that have been sequestered in the tissues. If the creatinine and serum Na^+ are normal, then this is the likely cause and no therapy is indicated. Typically, the polyuria settles after a few hours. However, other conditions may also present in this way (diabetes mellitus, diabetes insipidus, non-oliguric renal failure), and may need exclusion.

Prevention and management of infection in the surgical patient

Marina Morgan

Nosocomial (hospital acquired) infections are expensive, largely avoidable, and can have a high mortality. In origin, 42% are from the urinary tract, 24% surgical wound infections, 10% pneumonia, and 5% bacteraemia.

Infection control consists of basic commonsense measures to prevent or limit development and spread of infection between patients. The infection control team is made up of a doctor (usually a microbiologist) and an infection control nurse(s) who liaise with clinical staff to advise on prevention of cross-infection. Most hospitals publish local infection control and disinfection policies in a manual.

If you have a potentially infectious patient to deal with, seek the help and advice of the infection control team.

Infection control

Universal precautions against blood-borne viruses (BBV) are described in Chapter 19.

- Hand washing is the single most important measure to prevent cross-infection between patients – many organisms are easily carried on the hands of staff.
- Alcohol hand rub will suffice between patients if hands are not visibly soiled, but hands should be washed thoroughly before and after wearing gloves where needed, and gloves should be changed between patients.

Isolation of potentially infectious patients

- A side room, preferably with en-suite facilities, is recommended for 'skin contact' isolation or organisms spread via contact, air, or dust (e.g. MRSA).
- 'Enteric' precautions isolation: Patients with diarrhoea or vomiting can be highly infectious, spreading viruses or *Clostridium difficile* spores that contaminate the environment infecting other patients through ingestion.
- Staff should wear gloves and aprons while handling potentially infectious materials, and wash their hands thoroughly between patients.
- Patients transferred from foreign hospitals or hospitals known to have multiresistant organisms: Colonization with resistant organisms is highly likely if a trauma patient has been in a high-dependency area and subjected to multiple antibiotics. Screen on admission as per your local protocol – usually throat swab, nasal swab, wound swab, and urine will detect most multiresistant organisms. Isolate the patient until the status is known.

Antimicrobial prophylaxis

The aim is to administer antibiotics to treat contamination during surgery or other procedure before bacteria are able to invade host tissue (infection).

Endocarditis prophylaxis

This is indicated for patients with heart valve lesions, septal defects, patent ductus, prosthetic valves, or previous endocarditis. For full details consult the current BNF.

Table 17.1 gives details of prophylaxis for dental surgery, and Table 17.2 for GU, O&G, and GI procedures.

Splenectomy prophylaxis

Postsplenectomy, the incidence of serious sepsis is 0.5–1% per year, usually with encapsulated organisms e.g. *Pneumococcus, Meningococcus, Haemophilus* spp.

- Vaccinations: Pneumovax; Meningovax (covers groups A and C only); *Haemophilus influenzae* type B (HIB) – give 2–4 weeks prior

Table 17.1 Endocarditis prophylaxis for dental surgery

Condition	Prophylaxis
Structural heart lesion or prosthetic valve with no previous endocarditis	amoxycillin 3 g orally 1 h prior to the procedure
As above, allergic to penicillin	clindamycin 600 mg orally 1 h before procedure
Previous endocarditis or prosthetic valve and GA	amoxycillin 1 g i/v plus gentamicin 120 mg i/v at induction with amoxycillin 500 mg po 6 h later

Note: Endocarditis is commonly due to α-haemolytic streptococci from the mouth, hence clindamycin or amoxycillin is used.

Table 17.2 Endocarditis prophylaxis for GU, O&G, and GI procedures

Condition	Prophylaxis
Heart valve lesions, septal defects, patent ductus or prosthetic valve or patients who have had endocarditis	amoxycillin 1 g i/v plus gentamicin 120 mg i/v at induction, with amoxycillin 500 mg po 6 h later
As above, allergic to penicillin or received >1 dose of penicillin in the preceding month	vancomycin 1 g i/v over 100 min then i/v gentamicin 120 mg at induction or 15 min prior to procedure
	or
	teicoplanin 400 mg i/v plus gentamicin 120 mg i/v at induction or 15 min prior to procedure

to elective splenectomy for optimal results or within 48 h of surgery following emergency splenectomy.

- Antibiotics: amoxycillin 250 mg od or penicillin 250 mg bd (penicillin will not cover *Haemophilus*) or erythromycin 250 mg od.

Antibiotic prophylaxis after splenectomy should be offered:

- to children till they are 16 years of age
- to all asplenic/hyposplenic adults for 2 years
- lifelong if on long-term immunosuppression.

Warn patients to seek medical advice early or to begin prophylactic antibiotic therapy with a drug active against *pneumococcus*, *Haemophilus*, and *meningococcus* (e.g. co-amoxiclav) if they develop a RTI. Increased susceptibility to malaria and the need for prophylaxis should be stressed if a patient is considering foreign travel.

Animal bites or scratches in asplenic patients can be associated with septicaemias with unusual organisms carrying a high mortality such as *Capnocytophaga canimorsus* (also sensitive to co-amoxiclav), so patients must be warned of the risks of even trivial bites or scratches.

Surgical prophylaxis

Timing

- First dose within 30 min of surgery starting, and not more than 2 h before surgery, particularly with β-lactams.
- Normally 1 dose of antibiotics should suffice, lasting about 12 h from induction. Additional doses are necessary if the operation carries on for more than 4 h.

Soiling risk

Clean surgery (e.g. varicose veins)

- 1–2% risk of infection.
- No contamination from colonized or contaminated viscus or infected body cavity, hence normally no prophylaxis needed. The exception is prosthesis insertion (joint, vascular graft, stent, mesh etc.) or neurosurgery where infection (although rare) can be devastating.
- Need to cover staphylococci – hence cefuroxime 1.5 g or co-amoxiclav 1.2 g i/v is commonly used. Arterial surgeons are increasingly using prostheses impregnated with rifampicin.

Potentially contaminated surgery (e.g. cholecystectomy or a routine appendicectomy)

- <10% risk of infections e.g. with an open viscus but no spillage.

Contaminated surgery (e.g. rectal surgery)

- Has a high rate of infection (15–20%), so give gentamicin 3–5 mg/kg i/v and metronidazole 1 g pr, or cefuroxime 1.5 g i/v and metronidazole 500 mg i/v or 1 g pr on induction of anaesthesia (or preferably 2 h before).

'Dirty' surgery (e.g. perforation or devitalized tissue)

- Already heavily contaminated wound/pus/faecal contaminants.
- Needs maximal cover (see Table 17.3), started as soon as diagnosis made.
- Will need more than simple prophylaxis, with antibiotics continued for several days as therapy.

Clostridium difficile

- A common gut commensal in elderly patients.
- Spores survive in the hospital environment for weeks, and are resistant to disinfectants. Cross-infection occurs easily via the

Table 17.3 Choice of antimicrobial prophylaxis (note that local practice may differ)

Soiling risk	Operation	Bacterial prevalence	Antibiotics (usually single doses)
Clean	Head and neck	Oral streptococci/anaerobes/S. aureus	clindamycin 300 mg i/v or co-amoxiclav 1.2 g i/v
	Hysterectomy	S. aureus/anaerobes	co-amoxiclav 1.2 g i/v or cefuroxime 1.5 g i/v + metronidazole 1 g pr
	Cardiac/vascular surgery/amputation/vascular prosthesis	S. aureus/coagulase negative staphylococci	cefuroxime 1.5 g i/v or co-amoxiclav 1.2 g i/v or vancomycin 1 g i/v (over 2 h) if penicillin allergic
	Urinary catheterization/instrumentation	Previously uninfected urine/not catheterized	None necessary
		Change of catheter/recently catheterized	gentamicin 80 mg i/v or cefuroxime 1.5 g i/v or ciprofloxacin 500 mg orally
	Prosthetic joint insertion	Staphylococci (including coagulase negative)	cefuroxime 1.5 g i/v at induction or vancomycin 1 g i/v over 2 h (Some surgeons advocate antibiotics in the cement for revision surgery)
Potentially or actually contaminated	ERCP (significant sepsis occurs in 0.5–1%)	Gram negatives/Pseudomonas sp./Enterococci	ciprofloxacin 750 mg po stat (will not cover enterococci) or piperacillin 2 g i/v + gentamicin 160 mg i/v stat
	Cholecystectomy	Enterococci Gram negatives	cefuroxime 1.5 g i/v or co-amoxiclav 1.2 g i/v
	'Routine' appendicectomy	Anaerobes	metronidazole 1 g pr or 500 mg i/v stat
	Elective colorectal surgery	Coliforms/anaerobes/Pseudomonas sp./enterococci	gentamicin 3–5 mg/kg i/v stat at induction + metronidazole 500 mg i/v or cefuroxime 1.5 g i/v + metronidazole 500 mg i/v
'Dirty'	Often emergency, perforated viscus, peritonitis	Coliforms/anaerobes/Pseudomonas sp./enterococci	gentamicin 240 mg stat i/v + cefotaxime 2 g i/v + metronidazole 500 mg i/v or imipenem 500 mg–1 g i/v Continuation therapy will be necessary

ingestion of spores that later germinate into vegetative organisms, capable of toxin production.

- *C. difficile* toxin production results in gut endothelial damage producing a spectrum ranging from 'antibiotic associated diarrhoea' or, at worst 'pseudomembranous colitis'.
- Foul-smelling liquid stools with leucocytes is typical.

Management of suspected *C. difficile* infection

All patients in hospital with offensive diarrhoea should be isolated, and a stool sent for toxin testing. Some conditions predispose to *C. difficile* infection:

- recent antibiotics
- chemotherapy
- immunosuppression
- diabetes.

Table17.4 suggests management strategies for proven *C. difficile* infection. It may be useful to add Phillips brewers yeast 1–2 tablets tds empirically to antibiotic therapy for the above high-risk patients, since it possibly binds the *C. difficile* toxins. Bio/live yoghurt consumption can be encouraged to replace normal gut flora.

Table 17.4 Management of proven *C. difficile* infection

Microbiology	Symptoms	Drug therapy	Other management
C. difficile toxin +ve	Mild diarrhoea	Stop prescribing the causative antibiotics if possible. Oral metronidazole 400 mg tds if not too unwell	Isolate in side room with with 'enteric precautions' barrier nursing till 24 h after diarrhoea settled. Do not use antiperistaltic agents – risk of perforation
	Severe symptoms or peritonism	Vancomycin 125 mg qds orally + i/v metronidazole 500 mg tds	Surgical referral No need to measure serum levels with oral vancomycin
	Relapsing infection	Pulsed therapy using vancomycin or metronidazole (2 days on, 2 days off, 2 days on and repeat)	This kills the resistant spores that germinate into vegetative forms during the 2 days off treatment
No diarrhoea but C. difficile toxin +ve			No treatment needed No need to isolate

Multiresistant organisms

Methicillin-resistant *Staphylococcus aureus* (MRSA)

- Resistant to flucloxacillin (equivalent to methicillin tested in the laboratory).
- Hence resistant to all β-lactams, cephalosporins, and carbapenems by the same mechanism.
- To date, glycopeptides (vancomycin and teicoplanin) still cover MRSA, although vancomycin-resistant *S. aureus* (VRSA) has been reported.
- Epidemic MRSA (EMRSA) are typically resistant to many other antibiotics.
- Each hospital has its own policy which you should consult.
- Usually screening swabs to check for MRSA carriage are done, together with CSUs, tracheostomy swabs etc. whenever it is suspected. Where appropriate, decolonization with a combination of topical disinfectants, nasal mupirocin, antiseptic gargles, etc. may be attempted.
- Patients are usually barrier nursed in isolation where possible, until three consecutive negative sets of swabs can be taken as clear. Some hospitals have so much MRSA in non-acute wards (where patients are far likelier to be colonized and not actually infected) that the management is less proscriptive. However, on a surgical ward aggressive management coupled with emphasis on good infection control precautions – especially hand washing – is vital.

Vancomycin-resistant enterococci (VRE)

- Group D β-haemolytic streptococci ('enterococci') are low-grade pathogens.
- They are resistant to aminoglycosides and cephalosporins.
- *Enterococcus faecium* is far more resistant than *E. faecalis*, being resistant to antibiotics such as ampicillin, trimethoprim, rifampicin, and imipenem that often cover *E. faecalis*.
- VRE are increasing in incidence but usually only cause actual infection in transplant/immunocompromised patients.
- In 1992, 10% of enterococci in ICUs in the USA were VRE.
- Type A resistance (high level vancomycin-resistance) resistant to vancomycin and teicoplanin.
- Type B vancomycin-resistant, teicoplanin sensitive.
- Type C low level ('constitutive') resistance to vancomycin, but sensitive to teicoplanin, e.g. *E. gallinarum/casseliflavus*.

Epidemiology

- Many patients arrive in hospital with VRE (gut carriage). VRE can colonize the gut for more than 6 months. Selective pressure (antibiotics to which enterococci are resistant, e.g. cephalosporins) encourages proliferation. Uncontrolled multiplication and diarrhoea results in dissemination thus creating an environmental reservoir.
- VRE can survive high pH and temperatures, thus living in the environment (e.g. mattresses etc.) for long periods.
- The mainstay of infection control for VRE is barrier nursing in a side room, and good hand-washing. If infected then treat with whatever antibiotic will work, e.g. streptogramins, bacitracin, tetracycline. Discuss treatment with a microbiologist.

Prescribing antibiotics

- Consult your hospital formulary for local protocols. The following is intended only as a general guide.
- Review the need for i/v antibiotics after 2 days therapy.
- If a patient develops diarrhoea on any antibiotic, think of *C. difficile* infection. Discuss with microbiologist (see p. 79).
- If patient remains unwell on an antibiotic, discuss with microbiologist and consider changing.

Penicillin allergy

- How 'allergic'? What happens (e.g. diarrhoea with antibiotics is not an allergy).
- What type of rash ?i/v or oral penicillin.
- You may find your patient was OK with ampicillin given 'accidentally' in the recent past. Check charts because they may well have had a penicillin without any problems. This further strengthens the case against patient being genuinely penicillin allergic.
- If penicillin allergy is only a rash, cephalosporins may be used with care. There is 2–5% cross-sensitivity in practice.
- If true anaphylactic allergy, don't use any β-lactams (i.e. no penicillin, cephalosporins or carbapenems, e.g. imipenem). Table 17.5 gives alternatives for truly allergic patients. **Discuss options with microbiologist.**

Other issues

- Therapeutic monitoring of antibiotics may be indicated in certain situations. See Table 17.6.
- Figure 17.1 shows typical antibiotic spectra.

Table 17.5 Antibiotics for typical surgical situations with alternatives for truly penicillin-allergic patients

Site	Expected organisms	Normally would use	Alternative
Skin or wound infection	Staphylococci Streptococci	flucloxacillin penicillin	clindamycin or vancomycin
Urine infection No catheter in situ	Gram –ves	trimethoprim or cephradine or co-amoxiclav	trimethoprim or ciprofloxacin
Catheter-associated	Gram –ves including Pseudomonas	gentamicin + cefotaxime	gentamicin (1 dose) + either ciprofloxacin po or aztreonam i/v if very unwell
Gut sepsis (faecal peritonitis)	Coliforms Pseudomonas Anaerobes	cefuroxime + metronidazole or imipenem + metronidazole	gentamicin + ciprofloxacin + metronidazole or gentamicin + aztreonam + metronidazole
Chest infection	S. pneumoniae H. influenzae	amoxycillin or co-amoxiclav or cefaclor	clarithromycin or levofloxacin or doxycycline
	Gram –ve infection post op	cefotaxime or imipenem	ciprofloxacin + gentamicin or aztreonam + gentamicin
Pressure sores Amputations	Anaerobes	co-amoxiclav or penicillin + flucloxacillin + metronidazole	metronidazole ± clindamycin

- Fig. 17.2 suggests antibiotic cover for gut sepsis and peritonitis. For the worst case scenario, when faecal peritonitis is present, all these organisms need covering. Hence empirical treatment may be:
  gentamicin + ampicillin + metronidazole, or
  cefotaxime + metronidazole (+ gentamicin to cover *Pseudomonas* sp.), or
  ciprofloxacin + piperacillin + metronidazole (favoured by some for biliary-related sepsis) or
- (single agent) imipenem, meropenem, or piperacillin/tazobactam (Tazocin) (β-lactamase stable).

  Note: β-lactamase-producing organisms such as *Bacteroides fragilis* and some coliforms will inactivate ampicillin or piperacillin. 'Beefing them up' with β-lactamase stable clavulanic acid (to form co-amoxiclav) or tazobactam (to form tazocin) respectively extends the coverage considerably.

Table 17.6 Therapeutic monitoring of antibiotic levels

Antibiotic	Regimen	Levels
Gentamicin	Septicaemia: 3–5 mg/kg stat i/v	No need to measure after a stat dose
	Once daily gentamicin 3–5 mg/kg i/v	A pre-dose level before 2nd dose given (about 20–24 h after first dose) to ensure adequate excretion If < 1 mg/l continue same dose If > 1 mg/l increase dosage interval between doses If > 2 mg/l discuss with microbiologist
	Endocarditis treatment Streptococcal: 40–60 mg i/v bd with high dose penicillin)	Pre- and 1 h post-dose starting around the 3rd dose aim pre < 1 mg/l post 3–5 mg/l Send pre- and post-dose samples together to lab
	tds regimen, e.g. 80 mg tds i/v (generally now superseded by single daily dosing)	Pre- and 1 h post-dose aim pre < 2 mg/l post 5–10 mg/l Send pre- and post-dose samples together to lab
Vancomycin	Oral (for *C. difficile* only) 125 mg qds	Not absorbed: no need to measure levels
	1 g i/v bd	Take pre-dose level just before 3rd dose and post-dose level 2 h after infusion aim pre 5–10 mg/l post 20–40 mg/l
	Severe renal impairment: 1 g stat dose i/v	Take random level 24–48 h later. Give further dose when level < 10 mg/l
Netilmicin	4 mg/kg /day	Pre < 2 mg/l Post 5–12 mg/l
Amikacin	bd i/v 15 mg/kg/day in 2 divided doses	Pre < 10 mg/l Post < 30 mg/l
Teicoplanin	400 mg od i/v	Pre < 10 mg/l Post 30–40 mg/l Levels measured to ensure effective dosage

Once settled on a regimen, re-check levels twice weekly. Monitor renal function by the serum creatinine, and if deteriorating, re-check levels more often. Serum samples are either sent to the microbiology or biochemistry lab, depending on local practice.

- Table 17.7 shows initial antibiotic treatment of the septicaemic patient.

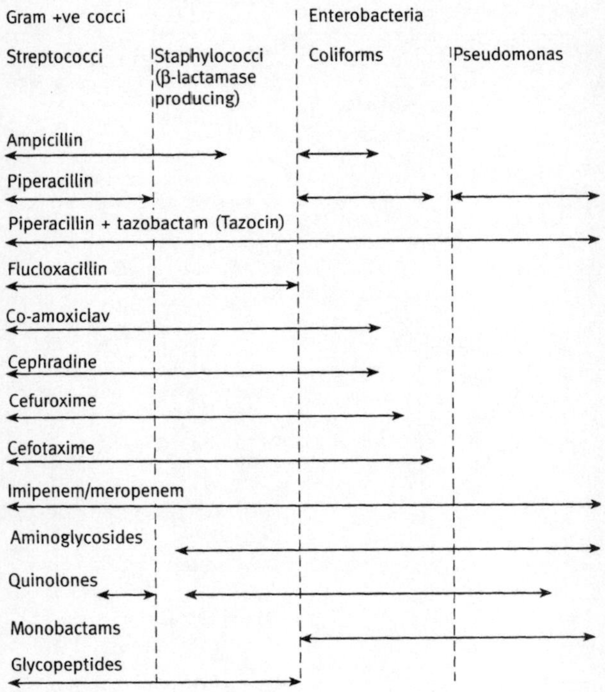

Fig. 17.1 Typical antibiotic spectra.

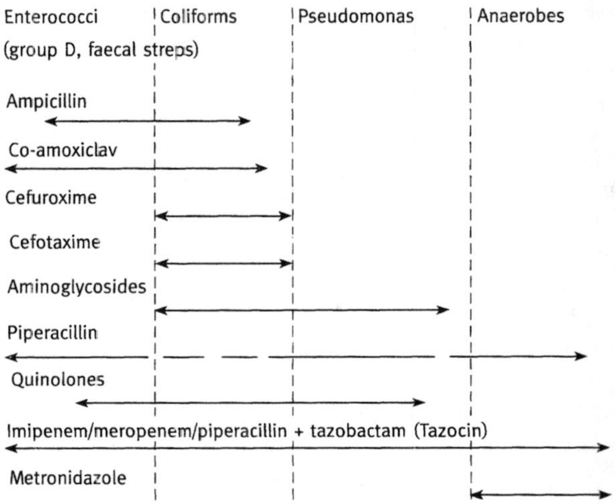

Fig. 17.2 Antibiotic cover for gut sepsis and peritonitis.

Table 17.7 Antibiotic treatment of the septicaemic patient

Signs	Organisms	Antibiotics	Comments
Skin generally red ± confluent or peeling rash ± diarrhoea ± confused	S. aureus Group A streptococcus	flucloxacillin 1–2 g qds i/v or clindamycin 450–900 mg qds i/v	Discuss with medical microbiologist
Catheter in situ or recently catheterized	Coliforms + Pseudomonas sp	gentamicin 3–5 mg/kg i/v + cefotaxime 2 g tds i/v	
Rampant cellulitis, blistering and dusky purple patches (necrotizing fasciitis)	Group A streptococcus	imipenem 500 mg qds i/v + clindamycin 450 mg–1.2 g qds i/v	Urgent plastic surgery opinion
Black blisters, foul smelling 'gas gangrene'	Clostridium perfringens	imipenem 500 mg qds i/v + clindamycin 1.2 g qds i/v + metronidazole 500 mg qds i/v	Consider hyperbaric oxygen therapy to stop toxin production
TPN/CVP line infection	Staphylococci If TPN line consider fungal infection	vancomycin 1 g bd i/v add fluconazole 400 mg i/v od if fungus likely or proven	Discuss with microbiologist re Gram –ve cover
No obvious focus	Anything!	gentamicin 3–5 mg/kg stat i/v + cefotaxime 2 g tds i/v + metronidazole 500 mg tds i/v	Discuss with microbiologist
Community-acquired pneumonia	Streptococcus pneumoniae	cefotaxime 2 g tds or ampicillin 1gm qds i/v	Add macrolide or ciprofloxacin if Legionella sp. or 'atypical infection' suspected
Hospital-acquired pneumonia ± recent anaesthetic	Gram –ves	gentamicin 3–5 mg/kg i/v + cefotaxime 2 g tds i/v or imipenem 500 mg qds i/v or ceftazidime 1–2 g tds i/v	

Nutritional support

Will Woodward

Many surgical patients are undernourished and at risk of developing overt nutritional deficiency. Undernutrition is associated with increases in the risk of postoperative infection, the length of hospital stay and mortality. Patients at particular risk are those who are:

- already *undernourished* on admission to hospital (elderly, unsupported, poor, self-caring, chronically infected, alcoholic, anorexic, nauseated, or vomiting owing to disease process, e.g. upper GI cancer)
- presenting acutely with *sepsis* (e.g. emergency surgery for bowel perforation, urological sepsis)
- with major *trauma*
- with *burns*.

Appropriate nutritional support can reduce mortality in severe illness, increase the rate of recovery and reduce complications.

Basic principles

Nutritional management begins as you take the history and examine the patient. Nutritional status, risk, and need for intervention are based on simple clinical assessment without special tests or formulae.

Develop a threefold approach to nutritional requirements:

- recognize and understand the problem of nutrition
- refer early when necessary to the ward dietician or hospital nutritional support team; nutritional support is more cost-effective and has a lower incidence of major complications when managed by such a team
- reassess your patient regularly, monitoring the effects of the nutritional intervention.

Physiology of nutrition in surgical patients

- During starvation of a healthy patient, endogenous fuels are utilized to meet daily energy requirements.
- Liver and muscle glycogen stores are meagre – approximately 150 g – and are exhausted within 24 h.
- After this, structural protein and lipid are mobilized. During each of the first few days of starvation, around 75 g of protein from skeletal muscle and around 160 g of adipose tissue are broken down, providing 1800 kcal (7.5 MJ).
- Amino acids are converted to glucose for obligate glucose-using tissues such as the central nervous system. Nitrogenous residues are lost from the body, resulting in an initial negative nitrogen balance of about 12 g/day.
- Adaptive processes in health result in an increasing reliance on lipid stores, reducing gluconeogenesis from protein (nitrogen sparing). After 1 week of fasting, daily nitrogen loss is more than halved.
- Injury, major surgery, or serious illness results in a different response to starvation. Energy requirements increase dramatically and the body switches from 'structural support' to 'energy generation': hypercatabolism.
- The nitrogen-conserving response is rapidly overwhelmed, with a marked increase in skeletal muscle protein breakdown, whole body protein turnover, and a net nitrogen-losing state. This may rise as high as 35 g/day in severe sepsis or burns.
- A daily nitrogen loss at this rate will result in a loss of >50% of body cell mass over 2.5 weeks.
- Nutritional physiology in surgical patients can be summarized as follows:
    - The sick surgical or trauma patient has a markedly increased energy requirement.
    - Food intake is reduced.
    - Utilization of available energy sources is impaired.
    - A gross imbalance between energy supply and demand may develop rapidly.

Nutritional assessment

Clinical

Clinical information from the admission clerking is sufficient to determine the need for nutritional intervention.

A nutritional assessment tool (e.g. BAPEN) may be recorded during the nursing admission procedure. This stratifies the patient into low, moderate and high risk of nutritional deficiency according to five readily observable parameters as shown in Table 18.1.

- *Low risk* patients require review weekly or if there is a change in their clinical course.

- *Moderate risk* patients require advice with food choice, assistance with eating and a record of food intake; the ward dietician should keep them under review.

- *High-risk* patients should be referred to the dietician or nutritional support team for detailed assessment of the level of nutritional support to be offered. Typical interventions include nasogastric, percutaneous endoscopic gastrostomy (PEG) or jejunostomy tube siting, TPN prescribing, and line insertion.

A treatment algorithm is shown in Fig. 18.1, but anthropometry and biochemical calculations are beyond the scope of this book.

Table 18.1 Preliminary assessment of nutritional status/risk of elderly patients

Assessment parameter	Low risk	Moderate risk	High risk
Body weight for height	Normal BMI[a] (20–25)	Underweight but stable	Severely underweight or actively losing weight
Appetite	Good: eats all meals	Poor: eats part of meals	Eats very little; or i/v only; or NBM for > 2 days
Ability to eat	Fully independent	Needs help choosing menu; some feeding or swallowing difficulty	Dependent on others for feeding or severe swallowing difficulty
Psychological state	Fully alert	Mildly confused	Disorientated or depressed
Skin condition	Healthy	Dry or flaky	Broken or with pressure sores

From *Standards and guidelines for nutritional support of patients in hospital*, British Association of Parenteral and Enteral Nutrition, May 1998.
[a] Body mass index = wt (kg)/ht^2 (m).

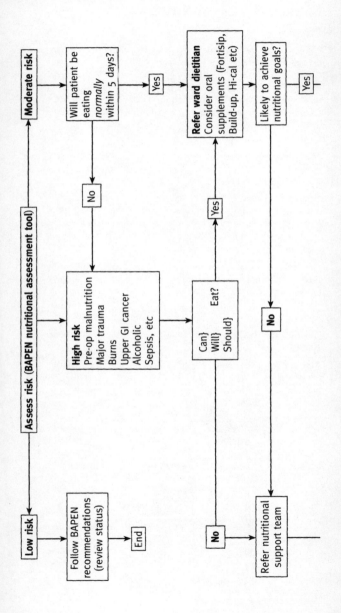

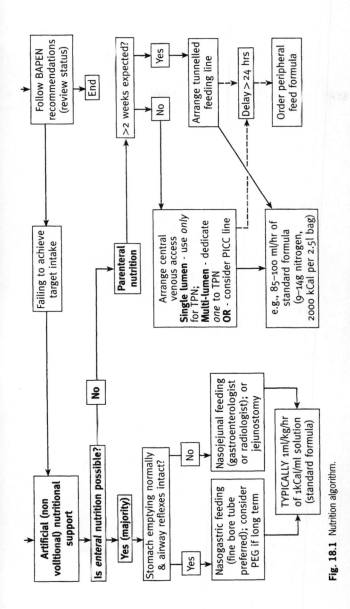

Fig. 18.1 Nutrition algorithm.

Laboratory assessment

- *Serum albumin*: A normal albumin on admission to hospital indicates good nutritional status. It is a sensitive but non-specific nutritional marker, a level <35 g/l being associated with increasing morbidity, longer hospital stay, higher costs, greater use of antibiotics, greater duration of mechanical ventilation, and increased mortality. However, the albumin level falls rapidly following surgery with large fluid shifts and is not a reliable marker of nutritional status at that time.
- *Haematological indices*: Hb, lymphocyte count, haematinics, and biochemical variables have some value in further quantifying general nutritional status or identifying areas of specific nutritional deficiency.

Nutritional intervention

The majority of patients undergoing surgery regain their ability to eat normally within a few days and do not require specialized nutritional support. However, undernourished patients, those facing a long delay in return to normal food intake (> 5 days) or those with specific problems such as sepsis, burns, or major trauma will require close nutritional support. The vast majority of these patients will be able to be fed enterally. TPN will be required for only a few.

Always consider enteral feeding if at all achievable. Resist the temptation to resort to TPN by default and encourage your consultant to consider an enteral option first! Enteral nutrition:

- supports and promotes gut function
- protects the gut from breakdown of its barrier function
- reduces the risk of Gram-negative sepsis
- has a lower rate of serious complications than parenteral nutrition
- is technically easier to manage
- is approximately one tenth the cost of parenteral nutrition.

The concept of bowel rest following anastomotic bowel surgery and pancreatitis is outmoded. Enteral feeding of both these groups of patients may be both feasible and beneficial.

Enteral nutritional support

Consider the appropriate site to deliver the feed:

- Is the stomach emptying adequately?
- Is there evidence of significant gastro-oesophageal reflux or impaired airway protective reflexes?
- Decide whether gastric (via n/g tube or percutaneous endoscopic gastrostomy – PEG); or postgastric (nasoduodenal, nasojejunal, or feeding jejunostomy tubes) would be best.

- Gastric stasis is common perioperatively, but not always accompanied by small-bowel ileus. These patients can be fed via the small bowel, even when gastric aspirates are significant. Jejunal feeding reduces the risk of aspiration in those with reflux or unprotected airways.
- Restoration of gastric emptying may be promoted by prokinetic drugs such as metoclopramide (10 mg i/v 8 hourly), cisapride (10 mg n/g 6 hourly – caution with arrhythmias), and erythromycin (150 mg i/v as needed).

n/g feeding is technically simplest as the tube can be sited on the general ward. Percutaneous and transnasal distal techniques need an appropriately trained surgeon, gastroenterologist, or radiologist, except where a tube has been inserted in theatre. The perioperative insertion of a feeding jejunostomy or nasoenteral feeding tubes during upper GI surgery (e.g. oesophagogastrectomy) is strongly recommended.

Aspiration pneumonia, feed-associated diarrhoea, and tube dislodgement are the main complications of the enteral feeding route.

Parenteral nutritional support

TPN is a complex treatment that is often inappropriately used. Most hospitals have recommended TPN regimes and many have a clinical team which run the service locally. Liaise closely with these experts when considering the use of TPN. It should never be given in situations where it will only be used for 1–2 days.

Parenteral nutrition is usually indicated in the following circumstances:

- when concern exists about distal bowel anastomosis
- severe exacerbations of inflammatory bowel disease
- high-output proximal small-bowel stomas
- enterocutaneous fistulae
- critical illness states where the alimentary tract globally fails to function.

Partial parenteral nutrition (and possibly TPN) can be given by peripheral venous access for a limited duration, but central venous access is necessary in most patients. The siting of feeding lines should be organized by a nutrition team who provide a dedicated service. Should parenteral nutrition be required when there will be a long wait before an appropriate central line can be sited, e.g. at a weekend, an appropriate feed can be supplied by the pharmacy for peripheral venous administration.

The major complication of TPN is infection. However, line-related sepsis is not inevitable, and both TPN and other therapy may be safely delivered for a week or more via a non-tunnelled multi-lumen central line with a dedicated delivery port if aseptic precautions are meticulously adhered to.

Recent evidence suggests that peripherally inserted central catheters (PICC lines) may have an acceptably low incidence of infective and thrombotic complications over medium-term use.

For intravenous feeding over the longer term (greater than 2 weeks duration) subcutaneously tunnelled central lines are often sited. This should be at the recommendation of the nutrition service and performed in theatre by experienced personnel.

Combined feeding

Most patients recovering from serious illness cannot tolerate full alimentary feed immediately and it is advisable to build up the volume towards target over a few days with TPN being maintained and weaned down commensurately.

Nutritional requirements

Energy

Most patients should receive a maximum of 25 kcal/kg per day – approximately 2000 kcal (8.4 MJ) in a 75 kg individual. (Protein calories are not included in calculating energy requirement.) This is provided in standard feed formulae as 1 kcal/ml with approximately 70% as glucose and 30% as lipid (long-chain triglyceride).

- Enteral or parenteral feed should therefore be prescribed at 75–100 ml/h in the majority of patients.
- Avoid excess calories that can lead to hyperglycaemia, increased risk of infection, increased carbon dioxide production, and fatty change in the liver.
- The maximum glucose oxidation rate in health is 4 mg/kg per min. In severe illness, the body may not be able to assimilate or utilize the energy supplied.

Nitrogen

Requirements are 0.15–0.25 g/kg per day of estimated lean body mass (ideal weight). The higher value relates to extreme catabolic states such as burns and sepsis where profound negative nitrogen balance develops very rapidly.

Although nitrogen input may be calculated using formulae for nitrogen balance and urinary nitrogen output (see nutritional monitoring below), in practice such calculations are rarely performed.

- Standard amino acid solutions contain 6–12 g nitrogen/l. TPN mixtures typically contain either 9 g or 14 g nitrogen/2.5 l bag, as amino acid and oligopeptide solutions.
- 1 g nitrogen equates to 6.25 g protein.
- An excessive nitrogen load may precipitate or worsen renal and hepatic impairment.

Water

Feed volume should be included in the patient's total fluid requirement.

Other nutrients

Vitamins (water- and fat-soluble), minerals (e.g. phosphate), electrolytes, and at least seven trace elements including iron are now added routinely to feed solutions either in manufacture or at the pharmacy stage. Many of these compounds are now recognized to be essential in the prevention of specific nutritional deficiencies that may have a profound effect on recovery from surgery.

Do not concern yourself too much with the minutiae of feed composition but liaise closely with your nutrition team or pharmacy.

Nutritional supplements

- Some nutrients non-essential in health are now recognized to become essential in severe illness.
- Arginine and glutamine are important in immune function, metabolic regulation, gut protection, and alternative substrate provision. They both become severely depleted early in serious illness. Supplementation with these amino acids improves immune response and reduces length of hospital stay.
- Omega-3 polyunsaturated fatty acids (eicosapentaenoic acid, docosahexanoic acid) and ribonucleic acid may have beneficial effects on organ function and particularly immunity independent of their general nutritional value. These compounds have been incorporated into new, expensive feed formulae. The benefits are not yet fully evaluated.

Nutritional monitoring

Clinical

Weight

- daily weight changes reflect fluid balance
- rapid weight gain results from fluid accumulation and may lead to overload
- early weight loss may simply reflect diuresis: malnutrition is characterized by an expanded ECF which reverts to normal as nutrition improves
- strict fluid input/output measurement should be maintained throughout any nutritional intervention episode plus an estimate of insensible losses.

Signs of infection

- fever
- local signs at site (PEG or CVP line)

- hyperalimentation can cause pyrexia independently of the presence of sepsis.

Rehabilitation
- muscle strength (objective/subjective)
- mobility
- well-being
- appetite.

Laboratory

Blood
- haematology
    - FBC (for Hb and white cell count – evidence of infection) – every 3rd day
    - INR (hepatic synthetic function) – every 3rd day
    - B_{12}, folate, iron parameters – baseline then fortnightly
- biochemistry
    - U&E, glucose – at least once daily
    - LFTs, albumin – every 3rd day
    - Ca^{2+}, Mg^{2+}, PO_4^-, – every 3rd day
    - trace metals – zinc, copper, selenium, and others – baseline, then if indicated
    - CRP for infection if indicated.

Urine
- 24 h collection for urinary electrolytes and urea – every 3rd day
- nitrogen input should equal or exceed losses to maintain or promote positive balance
- all clinical and laboratory measurements should be entered on a flow chart kept at the patient's bedside.

Box 18.1 Nitrogen loss

Urinary nitrogen output (g) = [24 h urinary urea (mmol) × 0.035] + [24 h urine protein (g) /6.35]

Total nitrogen loss (g) = [Urinary nitrogen (as above)]
+ [Change in blood urea × body weight (kg) × 0.017]
+ [Sweat loss:1.6 g/day (norinothermia) + 0.8 g/day/°C of fever]
+ [Stool loss: 2–4 g/l (if not measured)]

Universal precautions against blood-borne viruses

John Searle

The problem

Blood-borne viruses (BBVs) can be transmitted from infected patients to health care workers and may cause serious illnesses, some of which are fatal. The prevalence in the population of the viruses which are particularly important in the UK are given in Table 19.1.

Transmission of BBVs to health care workers is well documented. The commonest cause is by blood-to-blood contact by a 'sharps' injury (usually a hollow needle). The risk of transmission by contamination of broken skin or mucous membranes with infected blood is rare but it does occur.

The seroconversion rate following percutaneous inoculation is as follows:

- HIV: 1 in 300

- HBV: 1 in 3 if source patient is 'e' antigen positive and contact is not immune. (This has declined greatly in recent years owing to the

Table19.1 Blood-borne viral prevalence

Virus	Prevalence
Human immunodeficiency virus (HIV)	0.21% in women attending antenatal clinics in London (20 times that elsewhere in the UK) Over one half of all cases of AIDS in Britain occur in London
Hepatitis B virus (HBV)	Annual incidence of new cases is approximately 100 for England and Wales. Prevalence is much higher, and subject to regional variation
Hepatitis C virus (HCV)	1:2000 new blood donors (routine screening for HCV antibody)
Hepatitis D virus (delta agent) (HDV)	Unknown, but it can only occur in those positive for HBV

widespread vaccination of health care workers, which provides protection in up to 90% of recipients.)
- HCV: 1 in 3 to 1 in 10 (estimates vary).

General protection against BBVs

It is not practically possible to identify all those patients who are infected with BBVs. The only safe way to proceed is to treat all patients as if they were infected. It is essential therefore that you:

- *Ensure that you are effectively vaccinated against HBV.* About 10% of people fail to respond to a primary course of vaccine. Your response to vaccination must therefore always be checked. Immunization is not a substitute for good infection control practice since it provides no protection against infection with other BBVs.

- *Adopt universal precautions against transmission of infection:*
  - Wash hands between each patient contact, and both before and after wearing gloves.
  - Change gloves between patients.
  - Cover existing cuts, scratches and skin abrasions with a waterproof dressing while you are working in the hospital.
  - Wear gloves when contact with blood or blood-stained body fluids is anticipated, such as inserting peripheral venous, central venous and arterial cannulae, inserting or removing airways or tracheal tubes, examining orifices or wounds. If there may be substantial spillage of blood (as in trauma cases or surgical operations), you should also wear impermeable gowns or aprons and eye protection.
  - Avoid open footwear if blood may be spilt or sharps used.
  - Needles which have been in contact with a patient must not be re-sheathed. Dispose of sharps in the appropriate container.

- If you spill blood or bloodstained fluids you must let the person in charge of the ward or department know straightaway so that surfaces and floors can be decontaminated.

• *If you do sustain a sharps injury,* immediately wash the wound liberally with soap and water but without scrubbing. Encourage free bleeding of a puncture wound. Report the exposure promptly to the hospital infection control officer so that you can be given the correct advice about what to do. It may be appropriate to test the source patient for evidence of BBV infection, but this should only be done after seeking their fully informed consent. Most hospitals have a policy to deal with this type of accident. A senior ward or theatre nurse will know where the relevant documentation is.

Additional measures to reduce risks during surgical procedures

The highest rate of occupational exposure is in O&G practice. Most percutaneous injuries are caused by sharp suture needles, 20% caused by operator to the assistant. The rate of injury varies from 4% in orthopaedic procedures to 21% for vaginal hysterectomy. Glove perforation is common, and often unnoticed.

The following measures are advisable to minimize percutaneous exposure:

• Limit the number of personnel working simultaneously in an open wound or body cavity.
• Avoid passing sharp instruments hand to hand – use a 'neutral zone' such as a tray or identified area in the operative field. Where this cannot be done, sharps should be handled with great care.
• Remove sharps immediately from operative field as soon as used.
• Avoid using fingers for retraction or holding tissues.
• Use instruments to handle needles and remove scalpel blades.
• Direct needles and blades away from non-dominant hand or assistant's hand.
• Remove sharp needles before tying sutures.
• Electrocautery and stapling devices reduce sharps usage.
• Consider double gloving (half size larger innermost) for high-risk procedures.
• Rescrub and reglove as soon as is practical after glove puncture.
• Change gloves routinely at intervals in long procedures.
• Wear boots rather than shoes or clogs.
• Remove footwear on leaving theatre.
• Use protective eyewear or face shields if blood splatter or aerosol is likely.

The infected doctor

BBVs may also be transmitted from health workers to patients. If you have any reason to believe that you may be infected with a BBV you have a duty of care to inform your employer and take whatever professional and occupational advice is given to you.

Further reading

Department of Health (1998). *Guidance for clinical health care workers: protection against infection with blood-borne viruses.* Recommendations of the Expert Advisory Group on AIDS and the Advisory Group on Hepatitis. UK Health Departments.

20

Medical causes of acute abdominal pain

Anthony Nicholls

Patients admitted to surgical wards with acute abdominal pain may have a medical cause for their pain.

Table 20.1 lists the medical causes that mimic surgical pathology together with diagnostic features.

Table 20.1 Medical causes of acute abdominal pain

Cause	Diagnostic clues
Cardio-thoracic pathology	
Myocardial infarction	Previous history. ECG. Cardiac enzymes
Pericarditis	Aggravation by posture and/or respiration. Pericardial rub
	ECG – ST elevation in multiple leads
Pneumonia	Fever. CXR
Pneumothorax	CXR
Pulmonary embolism	ECG. Hypoxia on blood gas analysis. Hypotension
Endocrine	
Diabetic ketoacidosis	Blood sugar, blood pH, urine ketones
Adrenal insufficiency	Hypotension, hyponatraemia, hyperkalemia
Haematological	
Sickle cell crisis	History, ethnicity, blood film, sickle test
Acute leukaemia	Blood count and film
Drug-induced	
Lead toxicity	Very rare
Opioid withdrawal	History
Metabolic	
Acidosis	May be diabetic ketoacidosis, lactic acidosis or any other cause of acidosis. Gastric dilatation may be severe
Porphyria	Very rare. Recurrent pain

Table 20.1 *Continued*

Cause	Diagnostic clues
Metabolic	
Familial Mediterranean fever	Family history, recurrent symptoms, ethnicity. *Very rare*
Hyperlipidaemia	Xanthomas, xanthelasma. Serum lipids
Nervous system	
Herpes zoster	Distribution of pain. Wait for the vesicles
Nerve root compression	Distribution of pain. Aggravation by spinal movement

21

Principles of physiotherapy

Julia Gamlen

Respiratory care

Preoperative assessment

Patients undergoing major surgery and those with pre-existing pulmonary disease are seen prior to their operation. The preoperative assessment aims to identify pre-existing and potential problems and introduce the patient to the physiotherapy team.

Relevant data is taken from the medical notes. Factors are identified which may lead to postoperative complications:

- smoking
- obesity
- immobility
- pre-existing pulmonary disease
- old age
- poor nutritional status
- cardiovascular disease.

Instruction in breathing techniques and wound support is given. Analgesia is discussed – the patient must have sufficient pain relief to allow them to breathe deeply, move, and cough postoperatively. The patient is informed of any specific exercise plan and their expected progress.

When indicated, pre-existing pulmonary disease is treated. This is especially important in the emergency setting. For example, there may be a few hours to optimize a chronic bronchitic patient before a laparotomy.

Effects of surgery

These are most marked in upper abdominal and thoracic surgery:

- decreased ability to perform forced expiratory manoeuvres
- decreased lung volume, particularly at the lung bases
- decreased mucociliary clearance.

These physiological changes are due to:

- general anaesthesia
- recumbency/immobility
- incisional pain which inhibits deep breathing, moving, and coughing
- drying of the upper airway.

Postoperative care

Patients are usually assessed the day after surgery, although treatment sometimes starts the same day. Problems are usually diagnosed by regular assessment of patients at risk. Check for increased respiratory rate, abnormal breath sounds on lung auscultation, reduced SpO_2, or unexplained fever. Request a CXR and blood gases whenever significant chest problems are suspected. Respiratory problems may also be due to other underlying problems (e.g. cardiac, renal, metabolic, neurological), which require different management.

Postoperatively the patient is often compromised by factors beyond their control such as underlying medical problems, weakness, and poor nutritional status. Their rehabilitation is adapted accordingly. The physiotherapist may request analgesia if pain is preventing the patient from co-operating with treatment. An important part of the physiotherapist's role is motivating and supporting patients (and carers) who are afraid, dependent, and have low morale. Care is required to ensure that treatment is not more exhausting than the problem!

Common postoperative respiratory problems

- *Atelectasis*: Collapse of anything from a few alveoli to the whole lung. May be treated by mobilization, positioning, breathing exercises and positive pressure techniques.
- *Sputum retention*: Treated by increasing humidification/hydration, breathing exercises, manual techniques, positive pressure techniques, mobilization, and nasopharyngeal or tracheal suction.
- *Consolidation*: Replacement of air in the distal airways and alveoli by fluid or solid material. Often associated with infection. Treat by positioning, increasing humidification, positive pressure techniques, and encouraging expectoration.
- *Bronchospasm*: Manage with bronchodilators, positioning, and other management described on p. 283.

- *Respiratory failure*: Hypoxaemia and increased work of breathing requires oxygen therapy, positioning, and sometimes assisted ventilation.

Specific physiotherapy techniques

- Breathing exercises (e.g. breathing control): the active cycle of breathing techniques increase expansion and mobilize secretions.
- Manual techniques (e.g. chest shaking, vibrations, and percussion) augment expiratory flow rate and mobilize secretions.
- Thoracic mobilization to improve biomechanics.
- Positioning for postural drainage, V/Q match, or to facilitate cough.
- Suction via nasopharynx or orally in the self-ventilating patient where non-invasive measures have failed. Use of a nasopharyngeal airway or mini-tracheostomy may be recommended by the physiotherapist.

Specific physiotherapy adjuncts

- Positive pressure techniques, e.g. positive expiratory pressure mask (PEP), intermittent positive pressure breathing (IPPB), periodic continuous positive airways pressure (CPAP) increase lung volumes and mobilize secretions.
- Incentive spirometry increases tidal volume. The patient is motivated by visual feedback.
- Non-invasive positive pressure ventilation (NIPPV) used in some centres to deliver inspiratory pressure support and positive end expiratory pressure.
- Humidifiers are used to ensure adequate mucociliary function, e.g. heated water bath, cold water humidifiers, ultrasonic nebulizer, saline nebulizers. Selection depends on degree of humidification needed and oxygen delivery device.
- Pain relief (e.g. Entonox inhalation, see p. 62) can facilitate physiotherapy techniques when poorly controlled pain is a limiting factor. Transcutaneous electrical nerve stimulation (TENS) is occasionally useful.

On-call respiratory physiotherapy

The on-call physiotherapy service varies from 24 h cover by specialist respiratory physiotherapists to no out-of-hours cover. Where a service exists, it is set up to treat acute respiratory problems that may deteriorate before the next working day.

Indications

- General (with deteriorating oxygenation)
  - sputum retention

   – atelectasis
   – consolidation.
- Specific
   – aspiration
   – rib fractures.
- Specialized (some units may provide a wider scope of practice than others)
   – induced sputum (e.g. for the diagnosis of PCP in HIV +ve patients)
   – NIPPV
   – CPAP.

Non-indications
- acute bronchospasm
- inhaled foreign body
- pulmonary oedema (except in centres where CPAP is administered).

Contacting the on-call physiotherapist

The doctor who has assessed the patient should contact the physiotherapist. This may establish whether physiotherapy will help the patient. Different treatment options may be discussed.

The therapist may request that the patient is positioned in a particular way or given certain medication prior to treatment.

Mobilization

Physiotherapists are often asked to 'mobilize' patients – to help get them out of bed, walk, and regain their independence. Many of these patients can be identified preoperatively, either by virtue of the surgical procedure (major joint replacement, spinal surgery, thoracotomy, prolonged stay in HDU/ICU), or by pre-existing medical disorders (arthritis, neuromuscular disease, cerebrovascular disease, obesity, depression, anxiety and, often, simply old age). The planned programme of physiotherapy (and its benefits) should be explained to such patients before surgery.

Rehabilitation is the overall process of maximizing the patient's potential for independence. For most surgical patients this is a straightforward process. Others require a team approach due to underlying medical problems, the nature of the surgery, or its complications.

If local guidelines for rehabilitation after specialist surgery exist, then these should be followed: many units will have clear procedures after joint replacement, for example. The general principles for any patient are outlined below.

Active mobilization
- Bed rest is associated with increased morbidity and mortality: venous thrombosis, pressure sores, loss of muscle tone, loss of

postural reflexes. Early active mobilization of patients helps prevent this.

- Most patients are encouraged and assisted out of bed on the first postoperative day. Limiting factors are major surgical procedures, pain, and cardiovascular instability. If sitting out is well tolerated the patient is encouraged to continue mobilizing at his or her own pace.
- Functional activities such as rolling, sitting, and standing are facilitated by the physiotherapist as soon as can be tolerated by the patient.
- Moving and handling in the early stages can be problematic with obese or immobile patients. The physiotherapist will advise on safe handling techniques and on the use of aids (sliding sheets, hoists). Along with the ward nursing team, who also have considerable expertise in this area, a plan should be developed to prevent injury to the patient or staff caring for them.
- The physiotherapist usually assesses mobility (transfers in and out of bed, walking, stairs) and provides appropriate support such as walking aids (frames, crutches, sticks), supervision or full assistance.
- If the patient is unable to leave the bedside, an alternative form of exercise is recommended (e.g. walking on the spot, static bike).

Passive movements

The physiotherapist will organize a treatment programme for incapacitated patients depending on the individual's status and response to intervention. This may include:

- positioning of the limbs or splinting to prevent peripheral nerve injury
- passive movements performed on thoracic and peripheral joints to maintain range of movement.

As the patient's status improves, movements progress from passive to active assisted to active.

Specialist teams

Specialist skills are required to provide optimal care for patients with specific problems such as CVE, head injuries, burns, fractures, and spinal injuries. In some cases, this will involve transfer to a specialist centre.

Further reading

Clinical practice guidelines (1996). Association of Chartered Physiotherapists in Respiratory Care.

Hough A (1993). *Physiotherapy in respiratory care*. London: Chapman and Hall.

Webber B, Pryor J. Eds (1995). *Physiotherapy for respiratory and cardiac problems*. London: Churchill Livingstone.

Palliative care

Jim Gilbert

Palliative care is often needed on surgical wards for those with progressive advanced cancer and limited prognosis. Competent palliative care can be practised outside a hospice, and is based on four basic principles:

- *Symptom control*: Quality of life depends on good symptom control, both physical and psychological.
- *Communication*: Open and sensitive communication should extend to patients, informal carers, and professional colleagues.
- *Autonomy*: Respect the patient's autonomy and choice (e.g. over place of care, treatment options).
- *Support for relatives and friends*: Care must take account of not only the patient with terminal disease but also those who will be bereaved.

Specialist palliative care by a multi-professional team is required by those with more complex or persistent problems. Such services usually encompass hospital-based palliative care support teams, home care services working alongside primary care teams, inpatient hospices, and bereavement services. Most patients referred to specialist palliative care services from surgical wards will have cancer, but some may not. Referral should be made on the basis of need rather than diagnosis.

The place of major surgery in advanced incurable progressive disease

Major surgery should normally be avoided towards the end of life. The decision to offer surgery usually depends on the likelihood (or otherwise) of controlling symptoms satisfactorily without surgery.

For instance, unstable, pathological fracture of a long bone may cause pain resistant to medical management so surgery may be justified even in very advanced disease. In contrast, low, multiple-site intestinal obstruction in advanced malignancy is probably better managed medically, with subcutaneous anticholinergics, analgesics, and anti-emetics, than by surgery.

The final decision should reflect the attitude, beliefs, and values of the patient.

Always bear in mind the possibility that the problem is coincident with rather than caused by the primary disease.

Symptom control

Pain

- Many patients will already be on opioids preoperatively.
- Continue preoperative opioid analgesia perioperatively and post-operatively unless the surgical management will relieve the pain for which the opioids were prescribed.
- The predicted daily dose of subcutaneous morphine postoperatively will be approximately one third of the previous oral dose. This may guide the initial strength of postoperative prescribing. Initially intravenous PCA can be used.
- If PCA is not used, prescribe i/m or s/c bolus opioids for break-through or postoperative pain in doses of approximately one sixth of the preoperative 24 h oral dose.
- Review opioid prescribing frequently if surgery is likely to have removed or reduced the source of pain.
- Review the benefit/burden equation of preoperative medication. Antihypertensive drugs and lipid-lowering agents may not be necessary; anticoagulants and metformin may be dangerous in advanced disease.

Fluid management

- Standard supportive perioperative management may not be appropriate in advanced disease where there is no expectation of recovery. Standard n/g aspiration and intravenous infusion (drip and suck) may be burdensome and restrictive if intestinal obstruction/peristaltic failure cannot be reversed.
- Patients with immobility and cachexia require very little extra fluid. Not only is much less fluid lost in such circumstances, but catabolism produces more endogenous water and fluid requirements may be only a few hundred ml per day.
- Subcutaneous or intravenous fluids may be unnecessary even in those who drink little or whose urine output is low if malignant disease is advanced and incurable.

Bowel obstruction

- Obstructive symptoms may be functional rather than mechanical, so in a significant minority of cases spontaneous remission occurs.
- If abdominal pain is thought to be due to colic, both pro-kinetic drugs (metoclopramide, domperidone, cisapride) and bulking or stimulant laxatives should be discontinued.
- Treat persistent colic with subcutaneous hyoscine butylbromide (Buscopan) infusion 20–60 mg/24 h (sometimes more).
- Treat continuous abdominal pain with subcutaneous diamorphine. Add 20–400 mg diamorphine to 5 ml water and infuse at 0.2 ml/h.
- Treat persistent nausea with an anti-emetic active at the chemo-receptor trigger zone (haloperidol 5 mg/24 h, levomepromazine (formerly methotrimeprazine) 12.5–200 mg/24 h).
- Dexamethasone has second line anti-emetic activity and is used in some centres in intestinal obstruction, but the evidence for benefit is poor.
- Octreotide has anti-secretory and bowel relaxant effects, but is expensive and is best used by specialists when conventional therapy fails.

Communication

Sensitive, effective communication with patients and those close to them is often the key factor in maintaining a sense of control and meaning towards the end of life. The starting point is always active, unhurried listening to the patient's story. Only in this way can important misunderstandings be avoided, and assumptions minimized.

If you do not feel able to handle communication with dying patients, ask for someone to help you or rehearse the strategy of your interview with the nursing staff beforehand. They will often have more insights into the patient's state of mind and more experience in dealing with cancer sufferers.

Preparation

- Ask a nurse to be with you when you talk to the patient. Continuity of communication and support can then be offered when you leave.
- Introduce yourself by name and by role.
- Indicate in outline what information you already have, and its source, e.g. from family doctor, previous hospital notes.
- Whenever possible, sit down. This brings you to a similar level to the patient and indicates that you are not imminently about to walk away.
- Ask the patient if they wish anyone who happens to be with them to stay while you talk. Never assume that the person of similar age and opposite sex sitting by the bed is the patient's spouse.

Diagnosis

- Be prepared to explain the patient's problem in general terms, e.g. 'a blockage in the bowel causing pain and sickness'.

- Do not feel it is necessary to use the word cancer or even tumour, but be prepared to give a realistic assessment of what may be achieved, e.g. 'we expect to be able to control your pain and vomiting, but unfortunately this is not an illness that we can cure'.

- If the patient asks directly if they have cancer, share their anxiety if the diagnosis is likely, but not proven. Be honest but gentle if the diagnosis is confirmed.

Management options

- Recognize that while some people will want full explanations and options for treatment, for others these details may be burdensome. Sometimes it will be right to be explicit, but let the patient guide you as to how much to say: e.g. 'Some people want to know all the ins and outs of the problem, whereas others would rather leave decisions largely to the doctors and nurses. Which sort of person are you?'

- Give a realistic assessment of the consequences of each option. Avoid coercing people towards a particular decision by exaggerating either risks or benefits of different approaches. Take care not to offer options that are clearly against the patient's best interests, or that you are not prepared to undertake.

- Be clear about what a successful outcome to a proposed operation would be. Take care to put this in the context of progressive, incurable disease. Success might, for instance, be presented as the possibility of controlling symptoms better without extending life expectancy.

Prognosis

- Even those who do not ask will have the question 'how long have I got' in their minds. Despite the fact that as doctors we cannot know the answer, patients should not be made to feel this is a silly question. Neither should patients ever be left without hope, nor with the suggestion that 'there is nothing more that can be done for you'.

- Any mention of a specific time, even if heavily qualified, is likely to be remembered as 'the doctor gave me 6 months to live'.

- Those who persist in requesting an estimated time should be asked to reflect on how their health has changed recently over an appropriate period, perhaps a month or 6 months.

- Explore what particular reasons there may be for wanting an estimated survival time. Particular personal or business arrangements may be relevant, for instance, or information to be passed on to family living away.

- Recognize that the best answer for some people asking 'how long have I got' involves a description of how things might be when death is approaching, i.e. not so much 'when' as 'how will I die'?
- Do not be so evasive over prognosis as to fail to acknowledge the tragedy of a significantly shortened life.

Family and other informal carers

- Although close involvement and sensitive communication with those close to the patient are often crucial, a number of safeguards must be borne in mind.
- Neither next of kin or other family members, nor the closest of friends, can legally take health care decisions on behalf of the patient.
- Information about the patient should be shared only with those who the patient wants to know.
- Any information given to family or friends before the patient jeopardizes patient autonomy and risks harmful collusion, for instance 'you mustn't tell her – it would kill her'.
- If collusion has already been embarked upon, it is often possible to find a balance between becoming part of it (and therefore aggravating the situation) and direct confrontation. Although this may require specialist skills, often an approach involving a refusal to lie to the patient coupled with reassurance that information will not be forced upon them is successful.

Denial

Although denial is a very common reaction to first diagnosis, it is a continuing problem in only a very few people. Denial is clearly a problem when persistent and when it jeopardizes coping mechanisms. For instance, secrets or lack of satisfactory communication may mar a previously close and sharing relationship. Simple reluctance to use the word cancer or to speak openly of dying should not be regarded as denial. Often, there is a tacit but clear acknowledgement of failing health and the lack of a medical remedy. Managing true denial requires some specialist skills, but can be approached by encouraging recognition of the patient's capabilities today, compared with a few weeks or months ago.

Anger

Not infrequently patients and those close to them will direct anger at medical staff at the time of receiving bad news. It is important to avoid taking such anger personally and to avoid becoming angry or defensive in return. It may help to reconcile oneself in advance to the idea that receiving anger in such circumstances may be a legitimate part of a doctor's job.

Further reading

Baines M *et al.* (1985). Medical management of intestinal obstruction in patients with advanced malignant disease: a clinical and pathological study. *Lancet* 2:990–3.

Buckman R (1993). Communication in palliative care: a practical guide. In Doyle D, Hanks GWC, Macdonald N, eds. *Oxford textbook of palliative medicine.* Oxford: Oxford University Press, 47–61.

Twycross R (1997). *Symptom management in advanced cancer,* 2nd ed. Oxford: Radcliffe Medical Press.

Teamwork on the surgical ward

Alison Authers

Understanding how to work in a team will help you with the demands of your job. As you establish your role and appreciate that of others, your confidence and job satisfaction will increase.

The basics

- Be at the right place at the right time for lists and ward rounds. Late arrival can cost you your confidence.

- Make a good impression on your colleagues. Most of them will notice.

- Do the basics well: sloppiness is never tolerated. An efficient junior doctor attracts support from all areas when it is needed. Efficiency can carry you through the inevitable difficult times, which are usually not your fault.

- Patients value effort, and even in the fast turnover of surgical wards they still have time to observe and respond to efficiency.

- You will find you work better when people thank you, remember to do the same.

Local guidelines and protocols

- Does the ward have any guidelines to help new staff? On some wards junior doctors update an informal book of guidelines for junior staff when they leave, so the information will be current. Ideally, your predecessor will hand over to you, or there may be an overlap between old and new staff. New staff gain much help and comfort from some written information, and you should update it when you leave, even if it is just a handwritten list of things you wish someone had told you when you started.

- Ask about specific ward or unit policies. The nurses will know where they are. A policy on the management of diabetic patients pre- and postoperatively, or on prophylactic anticoagulation will save you a lot of time and phone calls. There will be other guidelines on more general, but no less important matters, such as hospital policies on confidentiality or resuscitation.

Nurses

Don't underestimate time spent talking things through with ward nurses, especially when starting with a new firm. Find someone who is established within the team and don't forget that he or she will be used to new staff. Wards can be very transient places, and nurses will be keen to help you along as it makes for a smoother running department. Ward nurses can be very supportive towards a house surgeon or SHO who works well within the team, and can be powerful allies.

Other ward staff

- Check how the ward receptionist/clerk does the filing. Results need to be scanned by you and action taken before the result goes in the notes. Sign your initials on each lab report when you have acted on it: it can then be filed in the notes. Most established staff have their own system, so adopt the system used on the ward rather than imposing your own.

- The ward pharmacist is a vital team member for help with complex prescribing, drug interactions, dose modification in renal or hepatic disease, and parenteral nutrition.

- Physiotherapists are often linked to wards. Meet them and ask how and when they work.

- Phlebotomists usually work to set timetables. Find out the deadlines for blood taking and the results service. Obtain your security number to access the ward computer.

Hospital departments

Get to know the staff in key hospital departments: MLSOs in the labs (don't call them lab technicians!), radiographers, theatre staff, pharmacists. A personal approach to specific individuals always helps. If you help make their life easier by legible, timely requests, they will usually reciprocate.

Discharge planning

Discharge planning starts at admission, sometimes earlier with elective cases. Although delays in discharging patients can occur while waiting for community facilities, it is hard to justify blocked beds due to poor planning. A team approach helps. The nursing assessment on admission should highlight potential problems, and further issues picked up during the admission (or pre-admission) clerking can be referred on in good time to allow plans to be made.

Some discharges can be very complicated, particularly after a long admission that changes a patient's lifestyle (e.g. colostomy, amputation). An intricate package of care may need implementing, involving various teams and agencies (district nursing, community occupational therapist or physiotherapist, stoma therapist). Ward doctors and nurses will need to work closely and plan early to coordinate a safe and appropriate discharge.

Nurses normally arrange the practicalities of discharge, but the medical input relates to assessing the likely prognosis, time-scale, and potential for rehabilitation. Transport, dressings, drain and suture removal, follow-up appointments, and postoperative advice are all normally familiar to surgical nurses. Timely prescribing of discharge medication, communication with the general practitioner, arrangements for histology and other test results needs input from the houseman and SHO.

The role of the patient and his or her carers is central. Most patients and families wish to make their own discharge plans; the earlier information is given on the likely length of hospital stay, the easier it is to plan for home, or at least recognize the difficulties.

Coping with death and failure

Coping with crises and death is a personal issue and different for everyone, but do not underestimate how much it may upset you, particularly if you are tired and busy. How you deal with it will depend on your own beliefs and coping strategies, and, of course, on the circumstances. After the practicalities, find time to talk it over with other members of the team and share their reactions.

Perhaps even more difficult is the giving of bad news, or talking to a patient or relative afterwards. This may be a painful experience and it helps to observe others experienced in this role. Learn from good practice whenever you see it, and then adapt it if necessary for your own use. Use words with which you are comfortable, and note how some experts handle these difficult situations by seeming to make endless time to listen and talk, even when they have very little. The right words and simple kindness can make a lasting impression and give tremendous comfort to patients and relatives, long after the event.

Allow time for yourself

Finding time for yourself between meeting all the demands of what sometimes feels like the entire hospital takes considerable skill and perseverance. Hopefully your consultant will take time to talk to his or her new junior staff, individually, about looking after themselves. Depending on the job and the rota this may not be too difficult, but generally it is a hard balancing act. Make time for eating and sleeping, and try not to allow practicalities of the job get in the way of common sense. Let your colleagues help you if they will, and plan your holidays carefully and selfishly. They will recharge you and help you enjoy what is a demanding but fulfilling job.

Care of surgical patients with chronic medical disorders

This section describes practical steps for assessing and minimising risk in patients with underlying chronic medical disorders. Each Chapter addresses the basic features of the condition, points to look for in history and examination, relevant investigations to define risk, and a guide to safe perioperative prescribing. Special points of relevance for anaesthesia are addressed, and the preparation of patients for both elective and emergency surgery is dealt with.

Cardiovascular disorders

John Dean and Richard Telford

Cardiac risks

Cardiac disease is the commonest cause of morbidity and mortality among surgical patients, increasing the risk of perioperative death by 25–50%. Careful preoperative assessment and perioperative monitoring are crucial to minimize mortality. Accurate information about risk must be given to patients before they give consent to surgery. Despite the increased risks, intervention by way of coronary artery bypass grafting or angioplasty is only rarely necessary to reduce the risk of surgery. Perioperative risks are determined by the combined effects of the underlying cardiac disease (Table 24.1) and the type of surgery planned (Table 24.2).

Table 24.1 highlights the important perioperative cardiac risk factors.

Ischaemic heart disease (IHD)

In 50% of patients with IHD the first manifestation of disease is myocardial infarction: critical coronary artery disease may exist with no symptoms.

Table 24.1 Clinical predictors of increased perioperative cardiac risk

Cardiac problem	Major risk	Intermediate risk	Minor risk
Ischaemic heart disease	Recent (< 1 month) myocardial infarction Unstable angina	Past history of myocardial infarction Mild stable angina	Abnormal ECG (LV hypertrophy, left bundle branch block, ST segment and T-wave abnormalities)
Heart failure	Decompensated heart failure (i.e. LV dysfunction with pulmonary and/or peripheral oedema)	Compensated heart failure (i.e. LV dysfunction optimally treated)	Poor exercise capacity
Arrhythmia	Malignant ventricular arrhythmia Supraventricular arrhythmia with rapid ventricular rate Profound bradycardia (heart block)		Abnormal cardiac rhythm (e.g. AF)
Other	Severe valvular disease	Diabetes	Past history of stroke Uncontrolled systemic hypertension Advanced age

Table 24.2 Surgery-specific risk

Risk level	Type of surgery
High	Major emergency surgery, particularly in elderly patients Aortic or major vascular surgery Prolonged procedures with major fluid shifts or blood loss
Intermediate	Carotid endarterectomy Head and neck surgery Intraperitoneal or intrathoracic procedures Orthopaedic surgery Prostate surgery
Low	Endoscopic procedures Cataract surgery Superficial surgery Breast surgery

Risks

Management is aimed at assessing and reducing the risk of the four main complications that may befall patients with IHD perioperatively: acute myocardial infarction (ami), acute myocardial ischaemia without infarction (unstable angina), arrhythmia, and acute LV dysfunction ('heart failure').

Acute myocardial infarction (AMI)

- Any patient with coronary artery disease is at risk of AMI.
- Risk correlates poorly with the severity of the underlying cardiac disease: patients with only trivial stenoses can develop plaque rupture leading to thrombotic occlusion and AMI.
- Risk increases with age, diabetes, hypertension, renal disease, male sex.
- Risk relates to the nature and length of surgery undertaken (Table 24.2).
- 60% of patients with peripheral vascular surgery have coexistent coronary disease although they may be asymptomatic. 20% have triple vessel coronary artery disease.
- Treatment of AMI hinges on reopening the occluded vessel. Thrombolysis is effective, but is contra-indicated after major surgery, and may cause significant bleeding even after minor surgery. Consideration should be given to immediate primary angioplasty if this is available.

Acute myocardial ischaemia without infarction (unstable angina)

- More likely to occur in patients with severe coronary arterial stenoses.
- Coronary blood flow occurs predominantly during diastole and is driven by the gradient between the diastolic arterial pressure and the ventricular end diastolic pressure. A fall in arterial blood pressure may cause a critical reduction in coronary blood flow through a stenosed artery leading to myocardial ischaemia. This in turn will lead to a rise in ventricular end diastolic pressure and a further fall in arterial pressure resulting in further ischaemia. A downward spiral ensues and measures to increase coronary blood flow by vasodilatation may be counterproductive, simply resulting in a further fall in perfusion pressure.
- Coronary vasospasm is another potential cause of acute myocardial ischaemia during surgery and is almost invariably seen in patients with coronary artery disease. Spasm is rare in patients with normal coronary arteries. Many anaesthetic agents are vasodilatory so spasm in normal vessels is unlikely during anaesthesia.

Arrhythmia

- Both brady- and tachy-arrhythmia may arise in patients with IHD.
- The cause is either acute myocardial ischaemia or scarring as a consequence of previous infarction.
- All patients with known IHD should have a preoperative 12-lead ECG.

- Postoperative management of serious arrhythmias should take place in an area capable of central ECG monitoring (ICU or CCU).

Acute LV dysfunction ('heart failure')

- Patients with compromised LV function because of previous infarction may decompensate perioperatively (i.e. develop breathlessness and overt pulmonary oedema).
- Clinical presentation is either a low output state and/or pulmonary oedema.
- Pulmonary oedema may be exacerbated by over-enthusiastic use of i/v fluids in an attempt to restore systemic blood pressure that has fallen because of pump failure.

Clinical features of IHD

History

History is the most important determinant of cardiovascular risk. The principal focus should be on the patient's functional capacity. Active patients who have an exercise capacity of 4 or more metabolic equivalents (METs) (i.e. can climb one flight of stairs without stopping or walk up hills) have a low risk. Those with a sedentary lifestyle may have occult coronary disease that may only be revealed by formal exercise testing.

Identify any past history of myocardial infarction, heart failure (dyspnoea and oedema), symptomatic arrhythmias (palpitations and syncope) and angina. The risk factors for IHD should be recorded along with any associated diseases such as hypertension, diabetes, peripheral vascular disease, renal disease, and chronic lung disease. With established heart disease, particular attention should be given to any recent change in symptoms. Pain at rest is a sinister feature, suggesting unstable angina, but is rare in the absence of any effort-related symptoms and casts doubt on the diagnosis of myocardial ischaemia.

Patients who have had coronary bypass surgery within 5 years and have had no recent change in symptoms do not pose a higher than average risk for surgery. Whether coronary balloon angioplasty confers the same protection remains to be proven.

Physical examination

- Look for pallor, cyanosis (either central or peripheral), breathlessness on minimal exertion, obesity or poor nutritional status, tremor and/or anxiety.
- Measure the blood pressure yourself.
- Assess the arterial pulse (rate, rhythm, volume and character), the jugular venous pressure (JVP), and precordial pulsations, particularly the character of the apex beat.
- Check the peripheral pulses and note any carotid bruits.
- Abdominal examination should include assessment of liver size and palpation of the aorta to identify aneurysmal dilatation.

- The presence of peripheral oedema is a poor indicator of congestive heart failure unless the JVP is elevated.
- Heart sounds provide clues to the presence of underlying cardiac disease. The presence of a third heart sound at the apex implies a diseased LV, but its absence is not a reliable indicator of good ventricular function.

Special investigations

Electrocardiography

- Request a preoperative electrocardiogram (ECG) in all patients aged over 50 years scheduled for inpatient surgery, and in all patients with significant risk factors, peripheral vascular disease, or undergoing very major surgery irrespective of age.
- Compare it with previous traces: new changes may require further investigation.
- Q-waves suggest previous infarction.
- ST segment and T-wave changes may indicate myocardial ischaemia or heart muscle disease.
- Conduction abnormalities such as bundle branch block may predispose to bradycardia or arrhythmias such as AF. Investigation by 24 h ECG monitoring should be reserved for those with blackouts or a history of significant palpitations.
- Many modern ECG machines report the tracing. The computer software tends to err on the side of caution, so a 'normal' report is usually sound, but minor abnormalities may be reported in an alarming fashion.

Stress testing

- Exercise treadmill ECG may be used to assess perioperative cardiovascular risk.
- The best indicator of significant myocardial ischaemia during an exercise test is ST segment depression.
- Chest pain, a fall in systolic blood pressure, the development of ventricular arrhythmias, and a poor effort capacity may also be due to myocardial ischaemia.
- The predictive value of a positive exercise test is poor, but a normal exercise test correlates very strongly with freedom from perioperative cardiac complications.
- Pharmacological stress testing is indicated for patients who are unable to exercise (arthritis, peripheral vascular disease, pulmonary disease) and those with a resting ECG which would make assessment of ST segment changes impossible (left bundle branch block, LV hypertrophy). This technique utilizes agents such as dipyridamole, adenosine, and dobutamine. The effect of stress is assessed by radionuclide scanning (looking for reversible myocardial perfusion

defects) or echocardiography (looking for reversible wall motion abnormalities).
- Pharmacological stress testing is more expensive and complicated to perform than exercise testing and has not been shown to be of any greater value in predicting adverse cardiac events perioperatively.

Cardiac catheterization and coronary arteriography
- May be required for patients with a positive stress test as a prelude to coronary revascularization.
- Patients should not be subjected to coronary revascularization simply to 'get them through' an elective operation, although this may be considered in highly selected cases.
- Coronary arteriography may identify high-risk patients who should be advised against non-essential elective surgery.
- Decisions with regards to coronary intervention depend on age, symptoms, LV function, and coronary anatomy: principles that apply to all patients, whether or not undergoing surgery.
- Coronary artery bypass surgery improves survival for patients with left main stem disease or triple vessel disease with impaired LV function. No comparable data exist for angioplasty.

Summary of recommendations for patients with cardiac disease scheduled for non-cardiac surgery

Table 24.3 summarizes patients who should be referred for a cardiac assessment prior to surgery.

Patients over the age of 75 years may not be suitable for coronary artery bypass grafting, although changes to their medical therapy may improve their cardiac status.

Table 24.3 Indications for preoperative cardiac assessment

	Cardiac risk				
	Major	Intermediate		Minor	
Exercise tolerance	Any	<4 MET	≥4 MET	<4 MET	≥4 MET
Surgery risk					
High	Refer	Refer	Refer	Refer	Operate
Intermediate	Refer	Refer	Operate	Operate	Operate
Low	Refer	Operate	Operate	Operate	Operate

Risk groups as defined in Table 24.1, surgical risk as defined in Table 24.2.
Refer means refer to cardiologist; **operate** means go ahead with planned surgery.

Myocardial infarction
Risks
- Increased risk of postoperative death after any surgical procedure.

- The risk is highest immediately after infarction and declines rapidly to a plateau at 3–6 months.
- Elective surgery should be postponed for 3–6 months after AMI.

Assessment

- The risk of future coronary events in most infarct survivors aged less than 75 years is usually assessed by exercise testing in the convalescent phase of infarction. Those with positive tests usually proceed to coronary arteriography and intervention when appropriate.
- Patients with a history of infarction, and who suffer continuing angina or dyspnoea, should normally be referred to a cardiologist before elective surgery if they have not been screened previously. (See Tables 24.1, 24.2, and 24.3.)

Perioperative care

Urgent or emergency surgery will need to take into account the increased risk that infarction imposes. The intensive care unit should be alerted to the presence of these patients and measures should be taken to minimize such risk by:

- ECG monitoring looking for arrhythmias and ST segment shifts
- haemodynamic monitoring with strict attention to fluid balance
- invasive arterial, central venous and pulmonary arterial pressure monitoring in very high risk cases (see section on optimization p. 41)
- close liaison with cardiologists
- optimizing drug therapy with β-blockers and ACE inhibitors.

Drugs

There are no large trials evaluating the use of cardiac drugs in reducing surgical risk. Only β-blockers have been shown to be of value in small trials and should be considered in all patients with known coronary disease where there are no specific contraindications such as asthma or heart failure (see Table 24.4).

- Aspirin reduces the risk of arterial thrombosis but increases the risk of postoperative bleeding. For some procedures (e.g. neurosurgery), aspirin may need to be stopped 10 days beforehand, but this is unnecessary routinely.
- β-blockers reduce heart rate, blood pressure, and myocardial contractility. This in turn leads to reduced myocardial oxygen consumption. β-blockers have been shown to confer a survival advantage when given after acute myocardial infarction. Abrupt withdrawal should be avoided; this may result in a rebound tachycardia and precipitate acute ischaemia.
- Ca^{2+} antagonists may be used to treat angina or hypertension. There is currently a question mark over the use of dihydropyridine Ca^{2+} channel blockers (nifedipine group), particularly short-acting

Table 24.4 Perioperative prescribing in ischaemic heart disease

	Aspirin	β-blockers	Ca²⁺ antagonists	Nitrates	ACE inhibitors[b]
Continue therapy: i/v if unable to absorb from gut		✓[a]		✓[a,c]	
Give normal preoperative dose; resume when stable postoperatively		✓	✓	✓	
Omit preoperative dose if nil-by-mouth; resume when stable postoperatively	✓				

[a] In high risk cases.
[b] See note in text. Check with anaesthetist.
[c] Or transdermal.

preparations, which have been implicated in increasing the risk of AMI. Continue nifedipine in stable patients, but convert to the long-acting preparation Adalat LA if the patient is on plain nifedipine capsules or tablets. ('Sustained release' nifedipine is not long-acting and has largely been superseded by other agents.)

- Nitrates are useful in treating the acute attack of angina when given sublingually and may be given intravenously for perioperative ischaemia. Long-acting preparations (oral or topical) are often taken by angina sufferers, but there needs to be a nitrate free period to prevent tolerance developing.

- ACE inhibitors have been shown to improve survival in patients with LV dysfunction due to ischaemic disease or dilated cardiomyopathy. They can cause profound, long-lasting hypotension in critically ill patients. Stop ACE inhibitors in emergency patients at risk of hypotension, but continue them in elective cases after checking with the anaesthetist. Caution may be required when restarting ACE inhibitors in view of the first dose hypotensive effect of most of these agents in hypovolaemic patients.

Heart muscle disease and heart failure

'Heart failure' is a term used to describe patients with a variety of symptoms and signs due to impaired ventricular function. The presentation may be acute, with low cardiac output (which in its extreme form is known as cardiogenic shock) or pulmonary oedema 'acute LVF'. In chronic, or congestive heart failure (CCF) the principle features are those of peripheral oedema and a raised venous pressure.

Table 24.5 Causes of heart failure

IHD	Chronic infarction
	Local aneurysm
	'Stunned' myocardium
Dilated cardiomyopathy	Idiopathic
	Alcohol
	Myocarditis
	Familial
Hypertension	
Drugs	β-blockers
	Ca^{2+} channel blockers
	Anti-arrhythmic agents
Others	Septicaemia
	Hypertrophic cardiomyopathy
	Restrictive cardiomyopathy
	Thyrotoxicosis or hypothyroidism
	Chronic persistent tachycardia
	Heavy metal poisoning
	Haemochromatosis

Table 24.5 lists the common causes of heart failure. Similar features may arise in patients with normal cardiac function in the setting of over-transfusion or renal disease, but this is not strictly 'heart failure'.

Treatment

- Diuretics, either thiazide or loop diuretics (sometimes both), to reduce circulating volume and produce some vasodilatation, and thereby relieve symptoms of peripheral or pulmonary congestion.
- Vasodilators, particularly ACE inhibitors (or the new angiotensin-II receptor antagonists such as losartan) and nitrates.
- Inotropes such as digoxin.
- Anticoagulation to reduce the risk of venous and arterial thromboembolism.
- Anti-arrhythmic agents such as amiodarone and digoxin.
- β-blockers have been shown to have beneficial effects in controlling heart rates and are occasionally used in selected cases under careful supervision.

Right heart failure and cor pulmonale

Occasionally the right ventricle may fail in the presence of a normal LV. This is most commonly due to chronic lung disease such as emphysema, but may be due to chronic pulmonary thromboembolic disease, primary pulmonary hypertension, or right ventricular cardiomyopathy. When right heart failure arises as a result of pulmonary hypertension it is termed cor pulmonale. Perioperatively, any rise in pulmonary vascular resistance (hypoxia, hypercarbia, acidosis) will worsen right heart failure and should be managed appropriately.

Acute right ventricular failure may complicate inferior myocardial infarction, and presents with low blood pressure and a high systemic venous pressure but clear lung fields. Treatment is aimed at increasing circulating volume with i/v fluids in an attempt to increase LV filling, not reducing it with diuretics. The diagnosis is made on enzyme rises and ECG changes and the condition may be confused with pulmonary thromboembolism.

Cardiomyopathy

Three forms of cardiomyopathy are identified: dilated, hypertrophic, and restrictive. Each form has a distinct pathophysiology, and treatment strategies are different.

Dilated cardiomyopathy

In the early stages there may be little or no increase in LV cavity size, simply impaired LV systolic function. This may be recognized by reduced amplitude of wall motion on echocardiography. At cardiac catheterization there is impairment of LV function with normal coronary arteries. Features include:

- ECG is invariably abnormal with non-specific features of LV disease.
- CXR showing an enlarged cardiac silhouette with pulmonary venous congestion and pleural effusions.
- The three main problems are heart failure, arrhythmia (particularly AF and ventricular tachycardia, rarely bradycardia), and thromboembolic disease from left atrial or LV thrombus.

  Treatment is with:
- diuretics and ACE inhibitors
- vasodilators (nitrates, α-blockers) and inotropes (particularly digoxin) may prove helpful in advanced cases
- many patients are given prophylactic warfarin
- anti-arrhythmics are reserved for those with evidence of arrhythmia.

Hypertrophic obstructive cardiomyopathy (HOCM)

- A genetic disorder characterized by excessive cardiac muscle mass which may obstruct the outflow of blood from the LV.
- Patients with HOCM rarely present with classical 'heart failure'. There is a wide spectrum of disease severity, some have unrestricted exercise capacity, but severe cases suffer breathlessness, angina, fatigue, and dizziness. Syncope is a sinister feature needing urgent investigation.
- Examination: pulse character normal or with a sharp upstroke (distinguishing it from aortic valve stenosis); apex beat heaving and/or double; often a harsh systolic murmur.

Table 24.6 Perioperative prescribing in heart failure

	Diuretics	Digoxin	Nitrates	ACE inhibitors
Continue therapy: i/v if unable to absorb from gut	✓a	✓ (in AF)	✓ (or transdermal)a	
Give normal preoperative dose; resume when stable postoperatively		✓ (in sinus rhythm)	✓	
Omit preoperative dose if nil-by-mouth; resume when stable postoperatively				b

a In high risk cases.
b Check with anaesthetist.

- The ECG is invariably abnormal, showing evidence of LV hypertrophy. Echocardiography is usually diagnostic (asymmetric LV hypertrophy, premature aortic valve closure, anterior systolic motion of the mitral valve, LV outflow tract gradient). Exercise testing and ambulatory ECG monitoring may be needed.
- Treatment includes β-blockers and Ca²⁺ antagonists such as verapamil. **Diuretics and vasodilators are contraindicated.** Some patients benefit from dual chamber pacing. More rarely, muscle from the interventricular septum can be surgically excised.
- Patients with severe HOCM need special perioperative attention. The vasodilator action of some anaesthetic agents and hypovolaemia will increase the gradient across the outflow tract and may lead to circulatory collapse. Strict attention to fluid balance is necessary.

Restrictive cardiomyopathy

- Due to infiltrative diseases such as amyloid. Rare.
- Echocardiography reveals normal or mildly impaired systolic function but profound diastolic dysfunction.
- Patients are often refractory to conventional medication, but may be very sensitive to the effects of diuretics.
- The condition needs to be distinguished from constrictive pericarditis which may be 'cured' by pericardiectomy.

Implications of chronic heart failure for surgery and anaesthesia

Patients compromised by heart failure are unable to respond to the stresses of the perioperative period. This increases the risk of surgery and anaesthesia, particularly in the setting of major surgery or emergency procedures. Surgery performed on patients with acute, untreated heart failure has a very high mortality.

Optimal medical therapy of heart failure involves balancing volume status, vasodilatation, and inotropic drugs and also ensuring that blood pressure is not symptomatically low. Perioperatively this balance may be upset by the following factors:

- general anaesthesia may cause vasodilatation and hypotension
- perioperative dehydration may lower blood pressure
- excess postoperative fluids may provoke pulmonary oedema
- increases in systemic vascular resistance (pain, hypertension) may result in acute heart failure
- patients with pulmonary hypertension and cor pulmonale may develop critical hypotension if volume depletion and vasodilatation are excessive.

Perioperative care in chronic heart failure

- Early discussion of all cases with anaesthetist and possibly cardiologist. For elective major surgery these patients are best reviewed by a cardiologist before admission for surgery. An echocardiogram will give an indication of the condition of the LV. Perioperative risks increase with the degree of ventricular impairment.

- Minor surgery is often best performed under local anaesthesia.

- Major surgery in patients compromised by heart failure (unable to climb stairs without symptoms) is high risk, particularly in an emergency setting. Consider whether non-operative treatment could be appropriate.

- HDU/ICU should be considered perioperatively if major surgery is planned. In some centres these patients receive optimization of their cardiovascular indices (p. 41).

- Close postoperative monitoring of blood pressure, fluid intake, urine output, SpO_2.

- Perioperative hypotension may be difficult to diagnose and treat. It should be managed in the HDU/ICU. It may be caused by hypovolaemia, cardiac failure, vasodilated state or any of the problems described on p. 250. Ask the ICU team for assessment and help.

- Fluid balance is critical. A central line is usually required with major surgery. Selected patients may benefit from a Swan–Ganz catheter; the anaesthetist will advise. Every patient is different and all need regular review postoperatively. Restricting fluids rather than prescribing diuretics is often appropriate in the immediate postoperative period.

- Renal perfusion is frequently compromised and the risk of renal failure with major surgery is increased. Oliguria is a frequent problem and should be managed as p. 299.

Cardiac arrhythmias

This section deals with the perioperative care of patients with pre-existing cardiac rhythm disorders. The management of a new arrhythmia presenting for the first time perioperatively and requiring emergency treatment is discussed on p. 274.

Tachycardias

Tachyarrhythmias are classified according to the site of origin within the heart: atrial, junctional or atrioventricular (AV) nodal, and ventricular.

Atrial arrhythmias
- *Atrial fibrillation* (AF):
  - *Epidemiology*: AF affects up to 5% of the population at some stage in their lives. It may be paroxysmal or persistent. The incidence increases sharply with age. Common causes include ischaemia, myocardial or pericardial disease, mitral valve disease, and thyrotoxicosis.
  - *Risks*: May precipitate cardiac failure if LV function is compromised. Systemic thromboembolism can occur if blood clots within the fibrillating atria: stroke risk ~4%/year.
  - *Clinical features*: Arterial pulse irregular with variable volume. In untreated AF heart rate is usually fast (130–200/min). Not all beats may be palpable peripherally, so assess heart rate by auscultation. Diagnosis confirmed by ECG: absence of regular P-waves, irregular baseline (f-waves), totally irregular QRS intervals.
  - *Preoperative investigation*: Echocardiography should be performed in those with significant angina or exertional dyspnoea. The purpose is to assess LV function, measure left atrial size, exclude significant mitral valve disease, and exclude pericardial effusion or constriction. Thyrotoxicosis should be excluded. Measure plasma digoxin levels if patient is taking 375 μg or more daily, or has possible side-effects (nausea is commonest).
  - *Treatment goals*: Attempts are normally made to restore and sustain sinus rhythm for recent onset or paroxysmal AF. Otherwise, the goals are control of the ventricular rate (60–100/min) and prevention of complications, particularly thrombo-embolism.
- *Atrial flutter*: Closely related to AF. Some patients may develop both arrhythmias. Typically a paroxysmal arrhythmia, so patients presenting for surgery may be on chronic prophylactic therapy. Many patients with this disorder have normal LV function, but this cannot be assumed.
- *Atrial tachycardia*: Due to an ectopic focus in either atrium. May resemble atrial flutter. Radio-frequency ablation is an increasingly popular treatment for this rhythm disturbance.

- *Atrial premature beats*: A benign finding. Require no special treatment unless shown to predispose to atrial tachy-arrhythmia.

Treatment of atrial arrhythmias

- *Cardioversion*: Patients with recent onset AF should normally have DC cardioversion attempted before surgery. This may entail a period of anticoagulation and anti-arrhythmic therapy. Refer to cardiologist. Some patients requiring emergency surgery may benefit from cardioversion and anti-arrhythmic therapy before undergoing surgery – see p. 275.

- *Digoxin* is typically used for persistent AF. Average maintenance dose is 250 μg/day according to age, size, renal function, serum K^+ and co-administration of other drugs (β-blockers, Ca^{2+} antagonists). Can be given by slow i/v infusion if oral therapy interrupted.

- *β-blockers or Ca^{2+} channel blockers* are often used for rate control in AF, but caution required if LV function is compromised.

- *Amiodarone* can be safely used in patients with impaired LV function, but has the potential for serious adverse side effects so would not be the drug of first choice for chronic therapy.

- *AV node ablation* with pacemaker implantation is sometimes used for patients refractory to drug therapy.

- *Anticoagulation* is frequently used in AF to reduce the risk of thromboembolism. Risk rises with age, left atrial size, and the degree of LV dysfunction. Patients with other atrial arrhythmias are not usually anticoagulated.

Table 24.7 Perioperative prescribing of anti-arrhythmic drugs

	Digoxin	β-blockers	Ca^{2+} antagonists	Amiodarone	Flecainide/ Propafenone (class 1c agents)
Continue therapy: i/v if unable to absorb from gut	✓[a]	✓[a]		✓	✓[b]
Give normal dose preoperative; resume when stable postoperative		✓	✓		✓

[a] In high risk cases.
[b] If prophylaxis of VT or VF.

Junctional tachycardia

The term SVT (supraventricular tachycardia) is sometimes used loosely for arrhythmias arising from (or involving) the AV node. Junctional (or AV nodal) tachycardia is a more precise term. Commonly the disorder arises from an abnormal pathway within or adjacent to the AV node, or an accessory AV pathway as in the Wolff–Parkinson–White (WPW) syndrome. Patients presenting for surgery on chronic anti-arrhythmic therapy for SVT will normally have been investigated to distinguish these disorders.

- *History:* Patients may give a history of paroxysmal tachycardia, occasionally associated with chest pain, breathlessness, or syncope. Young patients including children are often affected and the heart is usually structurally normal.
- *Investigations:* The ECG may be normal or may show evidence of pre-excitation in the WPW syndrome (short PR interval and a δ-wave).
- *Treatment:* AV nodal blocking agents such as β-blockers, Ca^{2+} channel blockers, or other anti-arrhythmic agents such as flecainide, propafenone, or amiodarone may control symptoms. Digoxin is best avoided unless the diagnosis is certain because this drug facilitates conduction through the AV accessory pathway in WPW syndrome.
- *Perioperative risks:* AF in the presence of an accessory AV pathway may allow very rapid ventricular conduction, which can degenerate to ventricular fibrillation. Symptomatic patients with a pre-excited ECG (δ-wave) should be referred for further investigation prior to elective surgery. Radio-frequency catheter ablation of the abnormal pathway is a popular alternative to chronic drug therapy for patients with junctional tachycardias.

Ventricular arrhythmias

- Ventricular premature beats (VPBs) or extrasystoles ('ectopics'):
  - *Clinical features:* Extremely common, increase with age, but may be associated with underlying cardiac disease. Symptoms are very variable. Some are asymptomatic, others complain of an erratic bumping in the chest at rest or during stress. Dizziness and breathlessness are due to associated anxiety. The terms bigemini, trigemini, etc. are often used to describe patterns of premature beating but are meaningless in this context and are best avoided.
  - *Risks:* In the absence of structural heart disease, ventricular ectopics are benign. VPBs are associated with increased mortality in those with significant heart disease, but anti-arrhythmic drugs do not improve survival (possibly adverse impact).
  - *Perioperative management:* Patients presenting for surgery who have very frequent VPBs and an abnormal ECG may have underlying heart disease. The heart disease itself is what may confer increased risk, not the VPBs themselves.

- Ventricular tachycardia (VT):
  - *Risks*: VT is a serious, life-threatening arrhythmia. There is usually some degree of ventricular disease, most commonly a history of myocardial infarction or cardiomyopathy. Patients with a history of VT should be carefully monitored in the perioperative period as the arrhythmia can be triggered by hypoxia, fluid loss (hypotension), fluid overload (pulmonary oedema), and electrolyte imbalance (K^+, Ca^{2+}, Mg^{2+}).
  - *Perioperative prescribing*: Patients with a history of VT will usually be on some form of anti-arrhythmic therapy. Therapy should be continued orally up to the point of surgery and should be given parenterally when the patient is nil-by-mouth.
  - *Automatic implantable cardioverter defibrillators* (AICDs) are becoming more common. These devices are capable of detecting and treating ventricular tachy-arrhythmias by pacing or shock therapy. **The AICD should be switched off during surgery** since electrical noise, particularly when electrocautery is used, may be interpreted by the AICD as an arrhythmia and result in an inappropriate discharge – refer to cardiologist for advice.

Bradycardias

- *Causes*: Disease in the sinus node, AV node, or autonomic hypersensitivity.
- *Clinical features*: Severe bradycardia causes syncope, but patients with chronic stable bradycardia may simply have fatigue, breathlessness, and angina. There may be features of congestive heart failure. When bradycardia is intermittent there may be no abnormality on examination or on the resting ECG, but symptoms and ECG changes may be provoked by manoeuvres such as carotid sinus massage or tilt table testing. Sinus node disease may result in sustained sinus bradycardia or periods of profound bradycardia due to sinus arrest.
- *Risks*: Surgery and anaesthesia may exacerbate a tendency to bradycardia due to vagal stimulation. Elderly patients presenting for surgery with unexplained episodes of syncope need investigation preoperatively by 24 h ECG monitoring ('Holter monitor'). Patients with heart block of various types may suffer cardiac standstill under anaesthesia if they give a history of syncope (see below).

Heart block

- Due to AV nodal disease. The incidence rises sharply with age.
- First degree AV block is prolongation of the PR interval without resting bradycardia. A frequent and often benign finding. In the absence of symptoms needs no further investigation or treatment.
- Second or third degree AV block is electrical dissociation between atria and ventricles leading to bradycardia. Long-term treatment is

by insertion of a permanent pacemaker. In an emergency temporary trans-venous pacing may be necessary prior to surgery.

- An incidental ECG finding of bundle branch block, bifasicular block (right bundle branch block and left anterior or posterior hemiblock), or trifasicular block (bifasicular block with 1st degree AV block) does not require pacing. The insertion of a temporary pacemaker electrode is not without risk and in the absence of symptoms of syncope, the risk of this procedure outweighs the risk of unexpected bradycardia.

Cardiac pacemakers

- A preoperative ECG and details of the patient's latest cardiological review should confirm that the pacemaker is functioning correctly.

- Special precautions are necessary for patients with permanent pacemakers when using electrocautery. A demand pacemaker may sense the electromagnetic signals and 'switch off' during diathermy leading to asystole for as long as the signal continues.

- The pacemaker electrode may act as an aerial and lead to heating at the site of contact with the endocardium.

- The use of bipolar diathermy avoids both of these problems. When conventional diathermy is required the indifferent pole ('plate') should be positioned such that current does not pass through the chest. Short bursts of diathermy are preferred.

- If pacemaker dysfunction does occur, a magnet may be applied over it, which will switch it to the fixed rate mode for as long as the magnet is left in position.

- The risk of endocarditis with pacemakers is very low and prophylaxis is not usually necessary.

- Pacemaker lead dislodgement by central lines or Swan–Ganz catheters is extremely unlikely in systems more than 4 weeks old.

Valve disease

Valve disease is found in 4% of patients over 65. The treatment of severe valve disease is usually surgical. Medical therapy often has little to offer. Surgical care of patients with valve disease may entail delicate balancing of risks and precise anaesthetic care.

Principles of anaesthesia and surgery in patients with valve disease

- The timing of valve surgery in relation to elective non-cardiac surgery is uncertain, but any patient who fulfils the accepted criteria for valve surgery should normally have this done beforehand.

- For emergency surgery, valve replacement is impractical.

- Volume depletion or vasodilatation may lead to drastically reduced cardiac output.

- Volume overload or vasoconstriction increases the risk of pulmonary oedema.
- Perioperative haemodynamic monitoring is essential.
- Antibiotic prophylaxis against infective endocarditis must be used in procedures likely to produce bacteraemia: the BNF contains the latest recommendations, but see p. 76.

Assessment of a new murmur

Any cardiac murmur may represent valve disease, but the intensity of a murmur is a poor guide to severity. Patients with severe aortic stenosis may have no murmur at all, simply a low volume, slow-rising pulse. Even the detection of trivial valve lesions should be documented since these patients may be at risk of endocarditis should perioperative bacteraemia occur. In general, any patient with a new murmur should be referred for echocardiography preoperatively, particularly if the murmur is diastolic, if there are symptoms suggestive of heart disease, or major surgery is planned.

Clinical assessment

- Breathlessness is the single most important symptom of significant valve disease.
- Left ventricular disease frequently leads to heart failure with functional mitral regurgitation.
- Syncope and/or angina are features of severe aortic stenosis.
- Blood pressure: Systolic pressure is low in severe aortic stenosis and diastolic pressure low in severe aortic regurgitation.

Investigations

- ECG: LV hypertrophy is typical in severe aortic valve disease.
- CXR may reveal cardiac enlargement, and possibly pulmonary congestion.
- Echocardiography should be performed whenever clinical features and simple investigations raise the possibility of significant valvular disease.

Aortic valve disease

Aortic stenosis

incidence rises with age. Commonly due to calcification of a bicuspid valve; rheumatic valve disease is much rarer. Elective surgery should always be deferred until full cardiological assessment. Emergency surgery may need to be done despite greater risks.

Clinical features:

- Symptoms of breathlessness, angina, and effort syncope or pre-syncope appear late in the disease process.

- Patients with symptomatic aortic stenosis have a grave prognosis (as low as 50% 1 year survival) without valve replacement surgery.
- The most important physical sign is a slow rising pulse character (best felt at the carotid or brachial artery). There is usually evidence of LV hypertrophy with a heaving or hyperdynamic apex beat and a harsh ejection systolic murmur that radiates to the carotid arteries. A high systolic pressure is unusual in severe aortic stenosis.

Investigations:
- ECG will show evidence of LV hypertrophy and possibly conduction abnormalities such as heart block associated with the calcific process.
- Echocardiography confirms the diagnosis and is capable of estimating the pressure gradient across the valve (< 40 mmHg mild, 40–80 mmHg moderate, > 80 mmHg severe). However, as cardiac output falls, the gradient falls, so pressure gradients are only an accurate assessment when there is well preserved LV function.

Implications for surgery:
- The greater the pressure gradient across the valve, the higher the perioperative mortality for any procedure. Patients with severe stenosis have an appallingly high mortality without valve replacement, so emergency surgery in such patients may be inappropriate. Balloon valvuloplasty has been suggested to reduce risk, but has largely been abandoned.
- Patients with aortic stenosis have a fixed cardiac output, so vasodilatation simply results in a fall in blood pressure. This in turn may reduce coronary perfusion pressure leading to a further fall in blood pressure, and so on in a rapid downward spiral.
- Strict attention to fluid balance is essential, excessive transfusion will readily result in pulmonary oedema and under-replacement of loss will rapidly lead to a fall in blood pressure.

Aortic regurgitation
Perioperative risk is lower than for aortic stenosis.

Clinical features:
- Symptoms of breathlessness due to pulmonary venous congestion arise at an advanced stage.
- The pulse has a sharp, unsustained character with a wide pulse pressure. The apex beat is displaced and hyperkinetic. A third heart sound is common, and a high-pitched early diastolic murmur is heard. The diastolic blood pressure falls in proportion to the severity of aortic regurgitation.

Investigations:
- ECG shows changes of LV hypertrophy, the CXR an enlarged cardiac silhouette.
- Echocardiography establishes the diagnosis and allows assessment of the severity of the leak and LV function.

Implications for surgery:

- In contrast to aortic stenosis, patients with aortic regurgitation tolerate vasodilatation well. This lowers arterial impedance and reduces the degree of regurgitation.
- Vasoconstriction will have a deleterious effect and should be avoided.

Mixed aortic valve disease

Most patients with aortic stenosis will have some degree of aortic regurgitation, and most patients with aortic regurgitation will have an ejection systolic flow murmur. This is sometimes referred to as mixed aortic valve disease, but it is important to determine which of the two valve lesions is predominant, both clinically and by echocardiography.

Mitral valve disease

Mitral stenosis

Incidence is declining in the Northern Hemisphere due to a decline in the incidence of rheumatic fever, which accounts for virtually all adult cases. More common in patients from developing countries.

Clinical features:

- Insidious decline in effort capacity over many years.
- Intercurrent crises, due to the development of AF or thrombo-embolic complications.
- Rarely dysphagia due to oesophageal compression from the enlarged left atrium.
- Physical signs are an irregular pulse (if in established AF), a tapping apex beat (corresponding to a loud first heart sound), a right ventricular heave, a mid to late low pitched diastolic murmur, and an opening snap.

Investigations:

- ECG: evidence of left atrial enlargement 'P-mitrale' (if in sinus rhythm) or AF, right ventricular hypertrophy, and/or right bundle branch block.
- CXR: left atrial enlargement (a straight left heart border, double right heart border, and splaying of the carina).
- Echocardiography to assess the severity of the stenosis by estimating the cross-sectional area of the valve orifice (>2 cm^2 mild, $1–2$ cm^2 moderate, <1 cm^2 severe).

Implications for surgery:

- Patients with mitral stenosis tolerate volume overload poorly and this may precipitate pulmonary oedema.
- An abrupt change from sinus rhythm to AF may have a similar effect due to sudden loss of atrial contraction. The ventricular rate in AF is critical. Rapid rates reduce the diastolic filling period; since rapid ventricular filling is impossible through a stenosed mitral valve this will lead to a fall in cardiac output and pulmonary oedema.

- Treatment of acute AF in mitral stenosis is aimed at rapidly slow-ing the heart rate. This is best achieved by i/v β-blockade (e.g. esmolol 500 μg/kg per min loading dose for 1 min, followed by 50–300 μg/kg per min infusion according to response). The nega-tive inotropic effects of β-blockers are irrelevant in this setting since ventricular function is usually normal. DC cardioversion should also be considered. Continuing prophylaxis with amio-darone may be necessary.

- Patients with mitral stenosis and AF are at high risk of arterial thromboembolism and are normally anticoagulated with warfarin. See details below for perioperative care.

- Treatment of severe valve disease is by valvotomy or valve replace-ment. This should be undertaken before elective surgical procedures.

- Percutaneous balloon valvotomy may be appropriate in the emerg-ency setting.

Mitral regurgitation

Much more common than stenosis. It is seen in a variety of clinical settings (ischaemic heart disease, dilated and hypertrophic cardio-myopathy, floppy mitral valve, rheumatic heart disease, etc.). In clin-ical practice, many patients with mitral regurgitation have papillary muscle dysfunction as part of their LV disease rather than primary valvular disease. The risks and management of these patients is as for the underlying LV dysfunction.

Clinical features:
- Evidence of a volume overloaded LV (displaced apex, third heart sound). Pansystolic murmur at the apex radiating to the axilla.

Investigations:
- ECG: Look for evidence of old myocardial infarction or LV hypertrophy.
- CXR: Look for cardiac enlargement and pulmonary congestion.
- Echocardiogram: Gives a guide to LV function and the severity of mitral regurgitation.
- Electrolytes and creatinine: Many patients will be taking diuretics.

Implications for surgery:
- Patients usually tolerate non-cardiac surgery well unless the leak is severe.
- Vasodilatation helps to encourage forward flow from the LV and reduce the regurgitant volume.
- Vasoconstriction and fluid overload should be avoided.

Tricuspid and pulmonary valve disease

These lesions are less commonly encountered. They are usually secondary to other problems that determine the risks and prognosis.

Tricuspid regurgitation

- Rarely due to structural valve disease.
- Usually occurs as a result of chronic LV or mitral valve disease. May persist after successful mitral valve surgery.
- JVP will be very high with a dominant systolic or V-wave. Liver is usually enlarged and pulsatile. The pansystolic murmur at the left sternal border varies with respiration.
- Attempts to lower the venous pressure by diuresis are futile and will simply result in a low output state and the venous pressure will still be high.
- Surgical and anaesthetic risks are the risks of congestive heart failure.

Tricuspid or pulmonary stenosis

Usually due to rheumatic or congenital disease. When severe, a reduction in right-sided filling pressures due to venodilatation or volume depletion will lead to a drop in cardiac output.

Pulmonary regurgitation

Usually occurs secondary to chronic pulmonary hypertension and it is this rather than the valve leak which gives rise to problems.

Hypertension

One in seven patients is hypertensive. Major complications of untreated hypertension are:

- coronary artery disease: angina, myocardial infarction
- LV failure
- cerebrovascular disease: stroke
- renal impairment.

Implications for surgery and anaesthesia

- Antihypertensive drugs exaggerate hypotension from hypovolaemia.
- β-blockers attenuate tachycardia in response to hypovolaemia.
- ACE inhibitors may increase the risk of postoperative renal failure in high risk patients (aortic disease, pre-existing renal impairment, diabetes, jaundice).
- Hypertensive patients have a greatly increased incidence of coronary artery disease.
- Patients with untreated or poorly controlled hypertension respond to agents affecting vascular tone with exaggerated swings in blood pressure. Stimuli altering vascular tone result in much greater swings in blood pressure in the hypertensive than in a normotensive patient. The blood pressure chart may look 'alpine' in appearance.

- There is an increased risk of MI, stroke, and renal impairment.

Causes

- 95% are essential hypertensives with no cause found.
- Alcohol consumption and obesity are important aggravating factors.
- Identifiable causes include renal disease, endocrine disease, and rarities such as coarctation of the aorta.
- Pre-eclampsia is a common cause of hypertension, but its management in relation to surgery (operative delivery) is beyond the scope of this book.

Preoperative preparation

- Patients are frequently hypertensive on admission to hospital. The blood pressure should be re-measured several times to get an accurate assessment. Automatic blood pressure monitors with a print-out are an easy and accurate way of doing this. If necessary, some mild sedation may help anxious patients.
- Cancellation of an uncontrolled hypertensive is reasonable (see below), providing a true estimation of blood pressure has been obtained.

Grades of hypertension

- Patients with severe diastolic hypertension (115 mmHg or greater) should be started on medication or have existing treatment optimized. Elective surgery should be deferred if possible to allow the benefits of treatment to accrue (at least 4 weeks).
- Moderately hypertensive patients (diastolic pressure 100–115 mmHg) should have their operation deferred if possible and be treated, or their treatment optimized, especially if there is evidence of target organ damage.
- Mild hypertensives (diastolic pressure <100 mmHg) may benefit from the addition of a β-blocker with their premedication – the anaesthetist will decide on this. Clonidine may be considered if β-blockers are contraindicated.
- Continue therapy. All patients on anti-hypertensive medication must remain on treatment during the perioperative period unless compromised by bleeding or sepsis. In such cases, stop the drug until cardiovascular stability is restored.

Postoperative care

- Careful monitoring is required. Try to minimize haemodynamic instability. Resume oral therapy as soon as the patient is stable.
- The treatment of uncontrolled hypertension in the postoperative period is dealt with in Chapter 32, p. 271.

Adults with congenital heart disease

Congenital heart disease occurs in 8/1000 live births. Adults with congenital heart disease may have totally uncorrected, palliated, or corrected lesions.

Uncorrected disease

Such patients have developed physiological changes that have made surgical correction impossible (e.g. irreversible severe pulmonary hypertension associated with a large ventricular septal defect). They have a limited life expectancy and are likely to be severely incapacitated. Perioperative mortality is high even with minor surgical interventions. They are best cared for in specialist cardiac centres.

Palliated disease

These patients have had a palliative operation that has not returned the anatomy to normal. Examples include the Senning or Mustard procedure for transposition of the great vessels or the Fontan procedure for various single ventricle anomalies (e.g. hypoplastic left heart syndrome, tricuspid valve or pulmonary artery atresia). They usually have some limitation of functional capacity.

Care of such patients requires a detailed understanding of the palliative procedure and its haemodynamic consequences. Even the most trivial of surgical procedures is best undertaken in a specialist cardiac centre, but if this is impractical, there should be discussion with the centre that undertook the initial cardiac surgery.

Corrected disease

These patients have a congenital defect that has either resolved spontaneously or has been completely corrected. If they have a normal functional capacity they can be treated normally. Remember that there may be associated non-cardiac abnormalities that might affect perioperative management.

Endocarditis prophylaxis

Required for all patients with congenital heart disease having dental or general surgery except:

- isolated secundum atrial septal defect repaired without a patch more than 6 months previously
- patent ductus arteriosus ligated and divided more than 6 months previously.

Chronic anticoagulant therapy

Warfarin is most commonly used but some patients may be taking phenindione or nicoumalone. These agents are monitored by measuring the ratio of the patient's prothrombin time to a laboratory control (international normalized ratio or INR). The dose required to achieve the same INR varies considerably from patient to patient according to age, size, and liver function. The main indications for chronic anticoagulation, the recommended INR and duration of therapy are shown in Table 24.8. Many patients presenting for surgery will be on chronic anticoagulant therapy.

Table 24.8 Chronic oral anticoagulation (BNF recommendations, updated according to the British Society for Haematology)

Indication	Target INR[a]	Duration of therapy
Low risk		
Prophylaxis of DVT	2	Until mobile after surgery
Medium risk		
Proximal DVT	2.5	6 months
Pulmonary embolism	2.5	6 months
Calf vein thrombosis: non-surgical	2.5	3 months
Calf vein thrombosis: postsurgical	2.5	6 weeks
Recurrence of thromboembolism off warfarin	2.5	At least 6 months
Chronic atrial fibrillation (any cause)	2.5	Permanent
Mitral stenosis with embolism	2.5	Permanent
Cardiomyopathy	2.5	Permanent
Myocardial infarction with mural thrombus	2.5	3 months
Symptomatic inherited thrombophilia	2.5	Permanent
Cardioversion	2.5	3 weeks before to 4 weeks after
High risk		
Recurrent thrombo-embolism on warfarin	3.5	Permanent
Mechanical prosthetic heart valves	3.5	Permanent
Antiphospholipid syndrome	3.5	Permanent

[a] Aim is ±0.5 INR units of target.

Managing anticoagulation in the perioperative period

Elective surgery
Preoperative care:
- Stop anticoagulation or perform surgery with the INR <2.5.
- If major bleeding risk, stop anticoagulation at least 3 days before surgery or reverse anticoagulation with low-dose vitamin K (see Table 24.9).
- Short-term risk of thromboembolism in patients with mechanical heart valves is very small when no anticoagulants are given (8 per 100 patient-years).

Table 24.9 Recommendations for management of bleeding and excessive anticoagulation (British Society for Haematology 1998)

INR 3.0–6.0, target 2.5 INR 4.0–6.0, target 3.5	Reduce or stop warfarin Restart warfarin when INR <5.0
INR 6.0–8.0, no bleeding	Stop warfarin Restart when INR <5.0
INR >8.0, no bleeding	Stop warfarin Restart warfarin when INR <5.0 If other risk factors for bleeding give vitamin K 0.5–2.5 mg po
Major bleeding Emergency surgery, INR >2.5	Stop warfarin Give prothrombin complex concentrate 50 U/kg or FFP 15 ml/kg Give vitamin K 5 mg po or i/v

- If anticoagulation has to be continued, reduce INR to <2.5 and start heparin.
- For minor surgery, oral anticoagulants should be stopped or the dose adjusted to achieve a target INR of approximately 2.0 on the day of surgery. Check INR preoperatively and if <2.5 proceed to surgery. If INR >2.5, surgeon must decide if surgery is safe.
- For major surgery, stop oral anticoagulants at least 3 days before surgery, monitor INR, and start heparin once the INR below the lower limit of the target range (e.g. <2.0 for a target INR of 2.5) (see below).
- Once warfarin is stopped it takes on average 4 days for the INR to reach 1.5.

Perioperative care:

- Low- and medium-risk patients need thrombo-prophylaxis once the INR is <2.0. This is usually subcutaneous unfractionated heparin 5000 U bd, but weight-adjusted low-molecular-weight heparin is more predictable in its anti-thrombotic effect and has an equally low risk of bleeding complications. Subcutaneous heparin can be started preoperatively.
- For patients at high risk of thromboembolism (e.g. mechanical heart valve), a continuous infusion of heparin can be given, with a loading dose of 5000 U followed by a continuous infusion of 1000–2000 U/h adjusted according to the APTR.
- Certain surgical procedures (e.g. neurosurgery) demand very low or no anticoagulant activity. Even with mechanical heart valves, the risk of thrombosis is very low even if warfarin is stopped for up to 7 days.

Restarting warfarin:

- Resume oral anticoagulants as soon as the patient can take tablets.

- If vitamin K has been given, then there will be a 48–72 h delay in achieving therapeutic anticoagulation.
- The standard loading regimen is 10 mg on 2 successive days, but this needs to be adjusted taking into account the patient's usual chronic warfarin dosage. For example, a patient taking 1 mg of warfarin daily will need a much lower loading dose, perhaps 4 mg twice, whereas a patient on 10 mg warfarin daily will need as much as 20 mg twice.
- Before restarting warfarin check that the patient still needs this treatment; occasionally the indications for anticoagulation are not secure or the treatment has been continued for longer than originally intended.

Urgent or emergency surgery
Preoperative preparation:
- These patients, including those with life-threatening haemorrhage, will need to have the effects rapidly reversed.
- According to the INR, give vitamin K (phytomenadione) with prothrombin complex concentrate (factors II, VII, IX, X) or FFP as in Table 24.9. Recheck the INR and repeat as necessary.
- In view of the risks associated with blood products it is unacceptable to reverse the effects of oral anticoagulants for the sake of expediency; moreover, giving vitamin K increases the difficulty in re-establishing stable chronic anticoagulation, so these measures should only be taken in an emergency.

Perioperative and subsequent care are as for elective surgery.

Previous venous thromboembolism
Previous DVT or PE puts the patient at increased risk of recurrence during surgery. The factors known to further increase the likelihood of a DVT are given in Table 24.10.

Prophylaxis should be given to those at high risk. This is discussed further on p. 48.

Table 24.10 Factors predisposing to DVT

Endothelial injury	Hypercoagulability	Stasis
Indwelling venous lines	Hereditary thrombophilia	Hip surgery
Irritant injection	Malignancy	Gynaecological surgery
Sepsis	Blood dyscrasia	Obesity
Thrombophlebitis obliterans	Oral contraception	Post partum
	Dehydration	Prolonged bed rest during chronic illness before surgery
	Idiopathic	Varicose thrombophlebitis

Further reading

Guidelines for perioperative cardiovascular evaluation for noncardiac surgery (1996). *Circulation* **93**:1286–1317.

Haemostasis and Thrombosis Taskforce for the British Committee for Standards in Haematology of the British Society for Haematology (1998). *British Journal of Haematology* **101**:374–87.

Mangano DT, Layug EL, Wallace A *et al.* for the Multicenter Study of Perioperative Ischemia Research Group (1996). Effect of atenolol on mortality and cardiovascular morbidity after noncardiac surgery. *New England Journal of Medicine* **335**:1713–20.

Turner M, Haywood G (1998). Preoperative assessment of cardiac risk for non-cardiac surgery. *Journal of the Royal College of Physicians of London* **32**:545–7.

Respiratory disorders

Chris Sheldon and Iain Wilson

General principles for surgical patients

Upper abdominal operations are associated with pulmonary complications in 20–40% of a general surgical population. The incidence with lower abdominal surgery is 2–5%. Following general anaesthesia for upper abdominal or thoracic surgery, there is a reduction in lung volumes, shallow respiration, and a reluctance and inability to cough effectively. These changes often result in inadequate basal air entry and sputum retention, which may be complicated by atelectasis and/or infection. Effective postoperative analgesia and physiotherapy may reduce their severity.

Patients with underlying respiratory disease are at increased risk of developing problems during and after surgery. Complications are minimized if the underlying condition is optimally controlled preoperatively. All patients benefit from a review of their medical therapy, early mobilization, and routine pre- and postoperative chest physiotherapy. Advice from a respiratory physician may be helpful for some situations.

Respiratory tract infections (RTIs) and elective surgery

- Patients who have RTIs producing fever and cough, with or without chest signs on auscultation, should not undergo elective surgery under general anaesthesia owing to the increased risk of pulmonary complications postoperatively.
- Patients with simple coryza are not at significantly increased risk of developing postoperative pulmonary problems unless they have pre-existing respiratory disease or are having major abdominal or thoracic surgery. Most elective surgery can be performed in these patients.

Smoking

Perioperative risk

- Smokers, both active and passive, are known to be at increased risk of developing perioperative respiratory problems.
- Cigarette smoke contains nicotine, a highly addictive substance, and at least 4700 other chemical compounds of which 43 are known to be carcinogenic. Long-term smoking is associated with serious underlying problems such as COPD, lung neoplasm, ischaemic heart disease, and vascular disorders.

Pathophysiology

In the respiratory tract of smokers, mucus is produced in greater quantities yet cleared less efficiently owing to impaired mucociliary clearance. The airways are hyper-reactive and there is impairment of both cell-mediated and humoral immunity. These changes make smokers more susceptible to respiratory events during anaesthesia and also to postoperative atelectasis or pneumonia, particularly after abdominal or thoracic surgery. Co-existing obesity increases these risks.

Risk reduction

- At least 8 weeks abstinence from smoking is required to decrease morbidity from respiratory complications to a rate similar to non-smokers.
- Smokers unwilling to stop preoperatively will still benefit by refraining from smoking for 12 h before surgery. During this time the effects of nicotine (activation of the sympatho-adrenergic system with raised coronary vascular resistance) will wear off. The level of carboxyhaemoglobin, which may reach 5–15% in heavy smokers, will also fall. Raised carboxyhaemoglobin (COHb) levels cause a reduction in O_2 carriage by the blood, and are not detected by most pulse oximeters.

Asthma

Asthma implies reversible airflow obstruction due to constriction of smooth muscle in the airways. Bronchial wall inflammation is a fundamental component of asthma and results in mucus hypersecretion and epithelial damage as well as an increased tendency for airways to constrict. Bronchoconstriction may be triggered by a number of different mechanisms.

Symptoms of asthma are most frequently a combination of shortness of breath, wheeze, cough, and sputum production. The presence of childhood symptoms, cough which wakes the patient at night, diurnal variation, specific trigger factors (especially allergic), absence of smoking history, and response to previous treatment may all be helpful in differentiating asthma from COPD.

Preoperative care

- Patients and doctors frequently underestimate the severity of asthma, especially if it is longstanding.
- Assess exercise tolerance (e.g. breathless when climbing stairs, walking on flat, or undressing) and general activity levels.
- Examination is often unremarkable but patients may have a hyperinflated chest and wheeze: there is little correlation between the presence or absence of wheeze heard with a stethoscope and the severity of underlying asthma.
- A single peak flow reading can be helpful but serial measurements are much more enlightening. When the peak flow is reduced the response to bronchodilators should be measured.
- Spirometry will give a more accurate assessment and is easy to perform. Results of peak flow and spirometry are compared with predicted values based on age, sex, and height (Fig. 25.1).
- Blood gases are usually only necessary in severe cases (breathless on minimal exertion).

Anaesthetists should be informed about patients with severe asthma (poorly controlled, frequent hospital admissions, previous HDU/ICU admission) prior to the list as they may wish to consider options such as additional medication or steroid cover. In general patients with mild asthma (peak flow >80% predicted and minimal symptoms) require little extra treatment prior to surgery.

Before surgery

- Emphasize the need for good compliance with treatment prior to surgery. Give this advice when an operation is first decided upon. Consider doubling dose of inhaled steroids 1 week prior to surgery if there is evidence of poor control of asthma (>20% variability in peak flow rate). If control is very poor, consider review by a chest

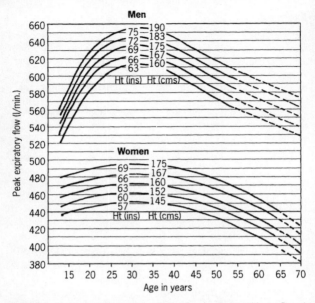

Fig. 25.1 Nomograms for peak expiratory flow in normal subjects. Based on data in Gregg IA, Nunn AJ (1973). *British Medical Journal* **3**:382.

physician and possibly a short (1 week) course of oral prednisolone 20–40 mg daily.

- Change to nebulized bronchodilators on admission.
- Viral infections are potent triggers of asthma so consider postponing elective surgery with a symptomatic URTI.
- Ensure anaesthetist is aware of asthma and discuss adding nebulized salbutamol 2.5 mg to premedication.
- Clearly document any allergies or drug sensitivities, especially aspirin/NSAIDs.
- Ensure patients are prescribed prn nebulized bronchodilators after surgery.

Postoperatively

Most well-controlled asthmatic patients have few problems with routine surgery, especially if they continue their routine medication.

- If there is increasing SOB and wheeze immediately following surgery consider:
  - underestimated severity of asthma preoperatively
  - drug reaction (antibiotics, anaesthetic agent, NSAIDS can all provoke bronchospasm)

- failure/inability to take usual medication (sedation, pain)
- inadequate bronchodilator therapy.

- Remember other conditions result in wheeze. LVF and PE are both potent triggers to bronchospasm. Also consider fluid overload and pneumothorax.

Acute severe asthma

See p. 283.

Chronic obstructive pulmonary disease (COPD)

COPD encompasses chronic bronchitis and emphysema. The majority of patients with COPD have been tobacco smokers for a significant period of their lives. Some elderly patients may have severe COPD despite stopping smoking many years previously. Other factors associated with COPD include occupational exposure to dusts and atmospheric pollution, poor socioeconomic status, repeated viral infections, α_1-antitrypsin deficiency, and regional variation within the UK (the incidence being highest in the north and west).

Symptoms of COPD usually start after the age of about 55 years. The most common symptom is breathlessness, often combined with cough, wheeze, and sputum production. Symptoms are frequently severe by the time any medical help is sought. Patients frequently give a history of repeated exacerbations of respiratory symptoms during the winter months. The morning is usually the worst time for patients with both asthma and COPD. Other features that may help to distinguish asthma from COPD are shown in Table 25.1.

Table 25.1 Clinical features of asthma and COPD

Asthma	COPD
Symptoms may have been present in childhood, resolve in early adult life, and return later	Symptoms start in middle age or later life
Often woken in early hours of morning by cough and SOB	Sleep generally not disturbed once patient gets off to sleep
History of hay fever or eczema	Often no history of atopy
May have never smoked	History of tobacco smoking
Periods with no respiratory symptoms	Decreasing symptom free periods as age increases

Pathophysiology

The principal problems in COPD are the development of airflow obstruction and mucus hypersecretion, exacerbated by repeated viral and bacterial infections. Many patients have an element of reversible airflow obstruction. If this can be demonstrated it is treated as asthma. Progressive airflow obstruction may lead to respiratory failure.

Patients with predominantly emphysema may be thin, tachypnoeic, breathless at rest and, although hypoxic, develop CO_2 retention only as a late or terminal event. Patients with predominantly chronic bronchitis are frequently overweight with marked peripheral oedema, poor respiratory effort, and CO_2 retention. These classical stereotyped pictures of 'pink puffer' or 'blue bloater' are relatively infrequently seen compared with the majority of patients who have a combination of features.

Preoperative assessment

- Establish exercise tolerance – ask specifically about hills and stairs.
- Ensure any element of reversible airflow obstruction (asthma) is optimally treated. A trial of oral prednisolone may be worth considering combined with a medical review.
- Optimize treatment of heart failure if present.
- Check spirometry (this is much more informative than PEF in COPD).
- Check blood gases if patient has difficulty climbing one flight of stairs, is cyanosed, has an O_2 saturation of $\leq 95\%$ on air, or has any peripheral oedema.
- If the patient has a very poor exercise tolerance (< one flight of stairs) and is undergoing a procedure that will make breathing painful or difficult postoperatively, discuss with the anaesthetist whether HDU/ICU care would be appropriate postoperatively.
- Change to nebulized bronchodilators prior to surgery and continue for 24–48 h afterwards.

Postoperatively

- Mobilize early whenever possible.
- Regular physiotherapy to prevent atelectasis and encourage sputum clearance.
- Give O_2 as appropriate – see Table 41.2, p. 295.
- If the patient becomes pyrexial with more copious or purulent sputum send a sample for culture and start an antibiotic. Oral amoxycillin, trimethoprim, or clarithromycin is usually sufficient for mild exacerbations of COPD. If the patient is seriously unwell treat as postoperative pneumonia (p. 284).
- Continue with nebulized salbutamol 2.5 mg qds and ipratropium 500 μg qds until fully mobile and change back to inhalers 24 h before discharge. Salbutamol may be given more frequently but there is no benefit from higher doses of ipratropium.
- If the patient is very slow to mobilize consider referral to pulmonary rehabilitation programme if available.

Bronchiectasis

Bronchiectasis may be caused by genetic factors (e.g. cystic fibrosis, CF) or acquired following damage to the lower respiratory tract, especially severe, early childhood infections. Most patients have a chronic productive cough, which may be present throughout the year. There is frequently a component of asthma associated with chronic inflammatory changes in the airways. Once established, bacterial infections can be difficult or impossible to eradicate. *Pseudomonas aeruginosa* is a common pathogen that may be present for many years and be associated with intermittent exacerbations of respiratory symptoms.

The mainstay of treatment for bronchiectasis is regular physiotherapy, frequent courses of appropriate antibiotics, and treatment of any asthmatic symptoms. In CF there is also malabsorption due to pancreatic insufficiency, so appropriate dietary advice and pancreatic supplements are essential.

Patients with bronchiectasis need to be as fit as possible before undergoing any major surgery which will inhibit their coughing or require a general anaesthetic. For elective surgery this may mean a planned admission for i/v antibiotics and physiotherapy prior to surgery.

Preoperatively

- Before elective surgery the aim is to ensure that the patient is as fit as they can be. Discuss maximizing therapy with the chest physician looking after the patient. A course of i/v antibiotics and vigorous physiotherapy for 3–10 days immediately prior to surgery may be necessary.
- Refer patient for respiratory physiotherapy before operation and ensure patient will receive physiotherapy immediately postoperatively if they have severe bronchiectasis. Contact on-call physiotherapist if necessary.
- Maximize bronchodilatation: convert to nebulized bronchodilators.
- Increase dose of prednisolone by 5–10 mg/day if on long term oral steroids.
- Send sputum sample for M,C&S before operation so that results will be available if patient needs antibiotics postoperatively.
- Inform anaesthetist.
- Prior to major surgery, consider starting i/v antibiotics on admission. Use current or most recent sputum culture to guide appropriate prescribing. If in doubt assume the patient has *P. aeruginosa* in their sputum and use a combination such as ceftazidime and gentamicin or imipenem and gentamicin.
- Consider checking spirometry and blood gases.
- If patient has more respiratory symptoms than usual, consider postponing elective surgery and refer to chest physician.

Postoperatively

- Ensure regular physiotherapy available: three times daily and at night if severely affected.
- Adequate oxygenation; check SpO_2.
- Continue appropriate i/v antibiotics for at least 3 days postoperatively or until discharged.
- Maintain adequate nutrition, especially if any malabsorption.
- Refer to chest physicians early if any deterioration in respiratory symptoms.

Cystic fibrosis (CF)

Almost all patients with CF have symptoms from their bronchiectasis and will require treatment as outlined above. Always inform the patient's CF physician of an admission to a surgical ward; 80% of CF patients have pancreatic malabsorption. Maintaining adequate nutrition after surgery is essential and the advice of an experienced CF dietician is essential.

Restrictive pulmonary disease

Restrictive pulmonary disease may be caused by intrinsic lung disease (such as pulmonary fibrosis) or by extrinsic conditions in which the lung parenchyma is normal but there is a failure of the respiratory mechanism to provide an adequate air supply to the lung. Extrinsic conditions include disease of the chest wall (kyphoscoliosis, severe obesity) or other abdominal problems producing significant splinting of the diaphragm. CXR changes will be according to the underlying condition.

Pulmonary fibrosis

Pulmonary fibrosis makes patients breathless because they have lungs that are hard to inflate and have impaired ability to take up O_2. Initially there is an inflammatory reaction centred on the alveoli, impairing gas exchange. Over a period of time, which can vary from days to years, collagen is formed in and around the alveoli causing more marked impairment of gas exchange and smaller, stiffer lungs.

Pulmonary fibrosis is the final response of the lung to a number of different stimuli. Causes include those associated with autoimmune disorders (e.g. rheumatoid arthritis, scleroderma), inhaled dusts (e.g. asbestos), or ingested substances, especially drugs (e.g. amiodarone, chemotherapy agents, paraquat poisoning). Allergic response to inhaled substances can cause fibrosis if exposure is prolonged (e.g. bird fancier's and farmer's lung). Pulmonary infections relatively rarely trigger a fibrotic response. Treatment is usually with oral steroids but other immunosuppressive therapy may be used and young patients may be considered for lung transplantation if very severely affected.

Preoperatively

- Many patients are stable and only slowly deteriorate over some years. These patients may tolerate surgery relatively well.
- Inform the anaesthetist
- Check preoperative blood gases. A reduced PaO_2 reflects significant disease.
- Obtain lung function tests including spirometry, lung volumes, and gas transfer if these have not been done within previous 6–8 weeks.
- For those on steroids, increase dose starting with premedication (100–200 mg of hydrocortisone) and continuing an extra 5–10 mg of prednisolone per day until the patient goes home.
- Discuss seriously ill patients with chest physician.

Postoperatively

- Ensure adequate additional O_2, maintain $SpO_2 > 92\%$.
- Mobilize early.
- Treat any respiratory infection vigorously.
- Ensure patient is continuing to receive steroids in appropriate form, e.g. convert to i/v hydrocortisone while nil-by-mouth.

Restrictive pulmonary disease due to chest wall conditions

Chest wall or thoracic spinal deformities result in an increase in the work of breathing and a reduction of all lung volumes. Respiration is characterized by rapid shallow breaths and is easier in the sitting position. Blood gases often remain normal until late. CO_2 retention is a late sign and implies severe disease. The severity of the condition may be assessed using spirometry.

Postoperatively, sputum retention may be a major problem and good physiotherapy and analgesia are vital. Spinal disease will preclude certain regional anaesthetic techniques, such as epidural analgesia. Patients may develop respiratory failure with relatively minor postoperative problems and must be assessed regularly. A laparotomy in a patient who depends on their diaphragm for adequate ventilation because of underlying chest wall disease may cause respiratory failure in the early post-operative period.

Perioperative plan

- Follow the principles described under pulmonary fibrosis.
- Ask the anaesthetist whether postoperative HDU/ICU admission should be planned.
- Measure spirometry and consider checking arterial blood gases.
- Vigorous physiotherapy pre- and postoperatively.

- Early involvement of the ICU team and respiratory physicians if deterioration occurs.

Sleep apnoea syndrome

These patients develop recurrent apnoea and hypoxaemia during sleep. Many are overweight, middle-aged men, who present with complaints of snoring with periods of apnoea, disturbed sleep, and excessive daytime drowsiness. The patient may develop systemic and pulmonary hypertension, congestive cardiac failure, and respiratory failure with CO_2 retention. Two types of sleep apnoea are recognized:

- obstructive sleep apnoea, OSA (obstruction of the upper airway)
- central apnoea (due to intermittent loss of respiratory drive).

Both conditions result in intermittent respiratory arrest, which resolves when the patient responds to the hypoxia that develops. Patients frequently have marked daytime hypersomnolence because of repeated nocturnal arousal from hypoxia. The condition is diagnosed in a sleep laboratory by monitoring O_2 saturation and nasal airflow; additional tests including measurement of respiratory and abdominal muscle activity, EEG, and EMG activity (polysomnography) may be required in some patients.

Treatment

- Weight reduction and management of associated conditions such as airflow obstruction, hypertension, and cardiac failure may be successful.
- Continuous positive airway pressure (CPAP) applied overnight by a nasal mask is often used with good effect.
- A few patients require surgery to the upper airway.

Operative risks

Patients with sleep apnoea syndrome are at risk of respiratory failure perioperatively as they are extremely sensitive to all sedative drugs, especially opioid analgesics. The risk of developing respiratory complications after major abdominal or thoracic surgery is high.

Perioperative plan

Suspected sleep apnoea

- Take a history from the patient and, if possible, their sleeping partner. Ask the patient about daytime hypersomnolence and how easily they would fall asleep during common tasks such as reading, talking to someone, or driving.
- Ask the partner about snoring and whether any apnoeic spells have been observed at night; the patient is usually unaware of these but spouses may be very worried.

- Obesity and collar size >17 inches are risk factors for OSA.
- Consider a medical opinion in patients with peripheral oedema, O_2 saturation ≤92%.

Previously diagnosed sleep apnoea
- Ensure patient is optimally treated for any associated medical conditions.
- If on inhalers, change to nebulized bronchodilators.
- Ensure patient will be able to continue taking usual medication by an appropriate route postoperatively.
- If the patient is receiving CPAP at night, ensure that ward staff are familiar with setting it up.
- Examine the patient; heart failure and peripheral oedema suggests severe OSA.
- Measure blood gases and pulse oximetry to determine the normal PaO_2 and whether the patient retains CO_2.
- Alert the anaesthetist concerned. Regional anaesthesia will often be preferred to minimize the use of sedative agents. Regional techniques may provide effective postoperative analgesia, avoiding the requirement for opioids. Consider the use of NSAIDs.
- Contact the chest physiotherapist.
- Do **not** write up for night sedation.

Postoperative care
- Patients are best managed in the HDU/ICU.
- After major surgery some patients may need ventilation for a few hours until they are stable enough to wean from the ventilator.
- Continuous pulse oximetry should be used on the ward.
- Nurse the patient sitting up whenever possible.
- There is debate about the optimum method of O_2 supplementation. Aim to maintain the O_2 saturation that the patient maintained preoperatively, titrating the O_2 to the minimum required. A few patients may develop CO_2 retention with O_2 therapy. This is detected by blood gas analysis in those patients at risk who become difficult to wake or develop signs of CO_2 retention.

Further reading
Boushra NN (1996). Anaesthetic management of patients with sleep apnoea syndrome. *Canadian Journal of Anaesthesia* 43:599–616.

Hirshman CA (1991). Perioperative management of the asthmatic patient. *Canadian Journal of Anaesthesia* 38:R26–32.

Nunn JF, Milledge JS, Chen D, Dore C (1988). Respiratory criteria of fitness for surgery and anaesthesia. *Anaesthesia* 43:543–51.

Nel MR, Morgan M (1996). Smoking and anaesthesia revisited (editorial). *Anaesthesia* 51:309–11.

Pederson T, Viby-Mogensen J, Ringsted C (1992). Anaesthetic practice and postoperative pulmonary complications. *Acta Anaesthesiologica Scandinavica* 36:812–8.

Perioperative Cardiopulmonary Evaluation and Management (1999). Supplement to *Chest* 115:43S–171S.

Schwilk B, Bothner U, Schraag S, Georgieff M (1997). Perioperative respiratory events in smokers and non-smokers undergoing general anaesthesia. *Acta Anaesthesiologica Scandinavica* 41:348–55.

Smetana GW (1999). Preoperative pulmonary evaluation. *New England Journal of Medicine* 340:937–44.

Wong DH, Weber EC, Schell MJ, Wong AB, Anderson CT, Barker SJ (1995). Factors associated with postoperative pulmonary complications in patients with severe chronic obstructive pulmonary disease. *Anesthesia Analgesia* 80:276–84.

Endocrine and metabolic disorders

Andrew Hattersley and John Saddler

Diabetes

Diabetes affects 2% of the population and 6% of patients over 60 years in the UK. Diabetes underlies 1 in 6 vascular surgical admissions, and presents many perioperative problems. It may also present on the surgical ward for the first time.

Liaise closely with the local diabetes team. Most hospitals will have a diabetes specialist nurse who can advise on appropriate insulin regimes and will have access to a diabetologist if needed. All diabetes nurses (and many diabetic patients) will have practical knowledge about treatment regimes so ask for advice!

The principal problems encountered are the control of blood glucose and dealing with the complications – retinopathy, nephropathy, ischaemic heart disease, peripheral vascular disease, cerebrovascular disease, neuropathy, and a reduced response to infection.

Autonomic neuropathy may result in abnormal responses to general and regional anaesthesia.

History

- Ask about previous episodes of uncontrolled hyperglycaemia and their trigger.

- Ask how patient assesses their own diabetic control and their insulin regime.
- Ask for symptoms of IHD.
- Ask for symptoms suggesting autonomic neuropathy: postural hypotension, gastric distension, diarrhoea, excessive sweating, urinary retention.

Examination

- Blood pressure is elevated in many type 2 diabetics. Aim for 160/90 or less before elective surgery. Postural hypotension may be a sign of autonomic neuropathy if the patient is normally hydrated.
- Foot examination: Assess the vascular and neurological supply of the feet – if either is compromised there is a high risk of developing ulceration.

Investigations

- *Blood glucose*: Aim for sugars in the range 6–10 mmol/l. See below.
- *Creatinine and electrolytes*: Renal impairment is present in up to 30% of diabetics at some point in their life.
- *Urine analysis for ketones and proteinuria*: If ketones are present check blood gases and/or HCO_3^- to exclude ketoacidosis. Proteinuric diabetic patients are at increased risk of postoperative renal failure.
- *ECG* (if over 30 years): Increased risk of ischaemic heart disease.

Maintaining euglycaemia

Tight control perioperatively is unnecessary. It is better to have a high blood sugar rather than a low one if a patient has reduced consciousness from anaesthesia. Glucose levels will fluctuate depending on food intake, intravenous fluids, insulin and physical and psychological stresses. Do not expect constant values, especially in IDDM (type 1).

For most patients combinations of diet, oral hypoglycaemic agents and/or subcutaneous insulin can usually control glucose. An insulin pump should be reserved for critical times (see perioperative regime) as it requires blood glucose to be measured 1–2 hourly, putting strain on the patient and nursing staff if continued for long periods.

Short-acting subcutaneous insulin allows rapid alterations of glucose levels. It has a peak action at 2–3 h with little effect after 6 h. When using a subcutaneous sliding scale blood glucose should only be measured before meals. Glucose control on a sliding scale is safe rather than optimal, so switch patients to their preoperative regime before discharge (with minor modification if needed).

Dealing with hyperglycaemia

- Hyperglycaemia up to 20–25 mmol/l without ketoacidosis is not a medical emergency. High glucose levels can result in thirst, dehydration, and impaired wound healing, and should be reduced in a controlled manner. If the patient is not immediately perioperative give an additional small dose (4–8 U) of subcutaneous soluble insulin.

- Ketoacidosis is the presence of acidosis (pH <7.2 or HCO_3^- <15 mmol/l) and ketosis (at least ++ ketones on urine testing) with elevation of blood glucose. Rarely, it may occur with only minor elevation of glucose. It is a medical emergency requiring physician review. Ask for the on-call medical specialist registrar.

Dealing with hypoglycaemia

Hypoglycaemia (blood glucose less than 3.5 mmol/l) can lead to convulsions, unconsciousness, and permanent cerebral dysfunction if not rapidly and effectively treated. In a conscious patient give a sweet drink followed by biscuits or sandwiches. If unable to eat, give 50 ml of 50% dextrose i/v. This can be irritant to veins and should be given slowly via a large-bore cannula. If venous access is not possible give glucagon 1 U i/m or rub glucose gel (e.g. Hypostop) on the gums.

Radiology and endoscopy in the diabetic patient

Investigations such as barium enemas and upper endoscopy should be considered as minor operations. Manage as described below.

There are certain points to remember:

- Metformin can cause GI disturbance, particularly diarrhoea. Before embarking on extensive GI investigations, reduce or discontinue the drug to see if GI symptoms settle. Radiological contrast can precipitate lactic acidosis in patients on metformin particularly if there is renal impairment. Metformin must be discontinued at the time of a contrast radiographic procedure and re-started 2 days later.
- Radiology involving contrast. I/v contrast agents in diabetic patients with nephropathy can precipitate acute renal failure. Non-contrast imaging may be safer, e.g. ultrasound, MR, etc.

Perioperative period

Insulin treated diabetes

The basic principles of glycaemic control during this period are:

- Avoid hypoglycaemia, as anaesthesia or sedation will mask the symptoms of impending coma.
- Avoid profound hyperglycaemia, because of the potential for acidosis, ketosis, and electrolyte disturbances. Hyperglycaemia also causes an osmotic diuresis leading to dehydration.
- Aim to maintain blood glucose between 6 and 10 mmol/l. Liaise with the anaesthetist to discuss the optimal regime.
- Use a variable infusion rate of insulin.
- Glucose infusion is also needed.

- K^+ should be added to the glucose unless the patient has renal impairment, since insulin facilitates intracellular K^+ uptake.
- Use separate cannulae for each of the infusions, to ensure each solution is delivered reliably. Whenever possible use a syringe driver for the insulin and an infusion pump for the dextrose.

A suggested prescription is outlined in Box 26.1. The current blood glucose level determines the infusion rate of insulin. There are two insulin infusion rates; the first is a lower initial rate, and the second is a higher rate which can be used if the blood glucose level is not maintained below 10 mmol/l. Patients who would normally require >0.75 U/kg of insulin per day should commence on the higher insulin infusion rate from the outset. A rough guide to anticipated hourly insulin requirements is to divide the total normal daily insulin requirement by 24.

A less sophisticated system, where insulin, glucose, and K^+ are added to the same infusion bag (the GKI regimen), has been widely used in the past. This delivers insulin and glucose in balanced proportions, so the infusion rate is not so critical. It may be acceptable in areas where frequent patient monitoring is unavailable, and is outlined in Box 26.2.

Ideally, insulin-treated diabetics should be scheduled first on the operating list. The infusions can be discontinued when the patient is eating and drinking normally. At this stage, the subcutaneous regime can be reinstated.

After major surgery it may be necessary to limit the amount of 5% dextrose received by the patient. In this situation change to 10% dextrose at 50 ml/h or dextrose saline 0.18% (with KCl) at 100 ml/h.

Box 26.1 Perioperative insulin prescription

- Infuse 1 l 5% dextrose with 20 mmol KCl at 100 ml/h.
- Add Actrapid insulin 50 U to 50 ml 0.9% (normal) NaCl and infuse by syringe pump according to the table below:

Blood glucose (mmol/l)	Initial infusion rate (ml/h = U/h)	Rate if blood glucose is not maintained <10 mmol/l (ml/h = U/h)
<5	0	0
6–10	1	2
11–15	2	4
16–25	4	8
>25	6	10

- Commence infusions early on the morning of surgery.
- Measure blood glucose 2 hourly before surgery, and hourly during surgery using glucose reagent sticks and an electronic meter.
- Postoperatively, check blood glucose 2 hourly initially, then 4 hourly once good control has been established.

Box 26.2 The GKI regime

- Add 15 U Actrapid insulin and 10 mmol KCl to 500 ml 10% dextrose and infuse at 100 ml/h.
- Measure blood glucose 1–2 hourly.
- If blood glucose measurements fall below 6 mmol/l, take down the bag and make up a new solution containing 10 U Actrapid insulin and 10 mmol KCl in 500 ml 10% dextrose. Infuse at 100 ml/h.
- If blood glucose measurements rise above 12 mmol/l, take down the bag and make up a new solution containing 20 U Actrapid insulin and 10 mmol KCl in 500 ml 10% dextrose. Infuse at 100 ml/h.

Diabetes not treated by insulin

- Patients with diet-controlled diabetes require no special preparation, if their glucose and electrolytes are normal. Insulin and dextrose infusions (as detailed above) can be instituted if blood glucose levels become consistently raised above 15 mmol/l in the perioperative period.
- Ideally, discontinue long-acting sulphonylureas (chlorpropramide, glibenclamide) 24–48 h prior to surgery. Replace with shorter-acting sulphonylureas (e.g. tolbutamide) if necessary. If long-acting agents are continued, watch for hypoglycaemia perioperatively. Metformin can be continued as it does not cause hypoglycaemia.
- Omit oral hypoglycaemic drugs on the day of surgery. If these patients are undergoing minor surgery, and will be eating and drinking soon after their procedure, no further special preparation is necessary.
- Monitor glucose levels every 2 h initially. Start insulin and dextrose infusions if glycaemic control is poor.
- If more major surgery is planned, or if diabetes is not well controlled on drugs, manage in the same way as insulin-treated diabetics, with insulin and dextrose infusions as outlined above.

Table 26.1 indicates when to use an insulin infusion in either non-insulin or insulin-treated patients depending on the type of surgery planned.

Table 26.1 When to use an insulin infusion in diabetics

	Non-insulin treated diabetes	Insulin-treated diabetes
Minor surgery	Rarely	Usually
Major surgery	Commonly	Always

Steroid therapy

Adrenal or pituitary disease resulting in over- or undersecretion of steroids is extremely rare. In contrast, a very large number of patients are steroid-dependent from medical therapy with high dose steroids.

Preoperative preparation for patients taking steroids

Glucocorticoid drugs are prescribed for two main reasons:

- Replacement therapy for adrenal or pituitary disease.
- Anti-inflammatory therapy or immunosuppression: This is the commonest use of these drugs, which are prescribed for a wide range of medical conditions. These include asthma, rheumatoid arthritis, polymyalgia, temporal arteritis, skin disorders, connective tissue diseases, and hypersensitivity states.

There are a number of unwanted effects that occur with larger doses and prolonged administration:

- Increased susceptibility to, and severity of, infections.
- Impaired wound healing.
- Increased peptic ulceration, especially if the patient also takes NSAIDs.
- Metabolic effects: Hyperglycaemia and water and electrolyte imbalance may occur. Preoperative serum electrolyte and glucose analysis is important.
- Muscle wasting and weakness: Care must be taken in moving and positioning these patients.
- Osteoporosis with susceptibility to fractures after relatively minor injury (e.g. moving patient while asleep).
- Skin and blood vessel fragility: Difficulty may be experienced with setting up i/v infusions. Pressure sores are more common.
- Adrenocortical suppression will result in a blunted response to any stress. Surgery, anaesthesia, an underlying illness, or sudden withdrawal of steroid medication after prolonged therapy can all precipitate acute adrenal insufficiency. All surgical procedures in these patients must be covered with increased steroid administration. A suggested regime is shown in Table 26.2.

Hypoadrenalism

Hypoadrenalism can present to surgeons with vomiting, diarrhoea, and weight loss. It should be considered in all patients who are hypotensive and dehydrated, particularly if serum K^+ is raised. Adrenal insufficiency may occur in patients on steroid treatment, particularly if they have been taking high dose steroids (greater than a replacement dose) for more than 3 months.

The equivalent physiological replacement doses of various steroids are given in Table 26.3.

Table 26.2 Perioperative steroid therapy

Steroid therapy	Operation	Perioperative steroid cover
Currently on steroids		
<10 mg prednisolone per day (or equivalent – see Table26.3)	Any	Assume normal HPA response Additional steroid cover not required (continue maintenance)
10 mg prednisolone per day (or equivalent)	Minor surgery	25 mg hydrocortisone at induction
	Moderate surgery	Usual preoperative steroids + 25 mg hydrocortisone at induction and 100 mg/day for 24 h
	Major surgery	Usual preoperative steroids + 25 mg hydrocortisone at induction and 100 mg/day for 48–72 h
Patient stopped steroid therapy		
< 3 months	See above	Treat as if on steroids
> 3 months	Any	No perioperative steroid therapy necessary
High dose immunosuppression		
	Any	Usual immunosuppressive doses during perioperative period

Source: Nicholson G, Burrin JM, Hall GM (1998). Perioperative steroid supplementation. *Anaesthesia* **53**:1091–104.

Table 26.3 Equivalent steroid doses

Prednisolone	5 mg
Prednisone	5 mg
Cortisone acetate	25 mg
Hydrocortisone	20 mg
Dexamethasone	750 μg
Methylprednisolone	4 mg
Betamethasone	750 μg
Deflazacort	6 mg
Budesonide (Enterocort CR)	No strict physiological dose equivalent, as the steroid is predominantly delivered to the intestine, with systemic availability around 10–20%. The drug is solely used for inflammatory bowel disease. Perioperative steroid therapy should be given as if the patient were on at least 10 mg prednisolone daily, irrespective of budesonide dose

Steroids vary in their mineralocorticoid effect, higher in hydro-cortisone and cortisone and very low in betamethasone and dexamethasone.

Diagnosis of hypoadrenalism

Do a Synacthen test. Measure cortisol level before and 30 min after a 250 μg injection of artificial ACTH (Synacthen). Cortisol levels should not be measured in patients on steroid replacement as they can be misleading due to varying degrees of cross-reaction with a cortisol assay. Patients who are have been taking steroids > 3 months should be assumed to be steroid dependent in the perioperative period. No further testing of these patients is required.

Thyroid disease

Perioperative management of known thyroid disease

Thyroid surgery is usually performed for:

- a generalized goitre, especially for cosmetic reasons
- symptoms of respiratory obstruction
- a discrete nodule to exclude malignancy
- the treatment of recurrent thyrotoxicosis.

There are a number of complications that can follow thyroid surgery. They include:

- Airway impairment: Haemorrhage into the wound may compress the trachea and can require urgent decompression if breathing becomes obstructed. Tracheomalacia may also contribute to post-operative dyspnoea. Laryngeal nerve injury, particularly if bilateral, may produce significant tracheal obstruction.
- Hypocalcaemia, due to parathyroid gland damage or removal.
- Thyroid crisis can rarely follow surgery if hyperthyroidism has been inadequately controlled (see below).

Hyperthyroidism

Defer elective surgery in hyperthyroid patients because of the increased cardiovascular risk. Treat first with carbimazole or propylthiouracil. If surgery cannot be postponed, hyperthyroid patients can be prepared with β-adrenergic blockade using propranolol (10–40 mg qds) or nadolol (80 mg bd) to reduce the resting heart rate below 90/min. KI may reduce gland vascularity but is little used.

Thyroid crisis may arise in undiagnosed or inadequately prepared hyperthyroid patients. This is rare but life-threatening. Features include hyperthermia, tachyarrhythmias, and hallucinations. Treatment (in ICU/HDU) comprises:

- oxygen

- active cooling
- steroids: hydrocortisone 100–300 mg i/v
- β-adrenergic blockade: propranolol 1 mg boluses to 10 mg i/v initially
- correction of dehydration and electrolyte abnormalities.

Hypothyroidism

- Correct hypothyroidism with thyroxine before elective surgery.
- Thyroxine can precipitate or considerably worsen IHD – seek the advice of a physician. Correction of hypothyroidism usually takes 3 months.
- Hypothyroidism after total thyroidectomy is treated with a replacement dose of 100–150 μg thyroxine directly. Do not use i/v triiodothyronine (T_3).
- Patients on thyroxine may discontinue therapy for a few days perioperatively if they are unable to take medication by mouth, as the drug has a long half-life.
- Hypothyroid patients are more sensitive to narcotics and anaesthetic agents, so these agents must be administered in reduced doses. Hypothermia will also aggravate circulatory and respiratory depression.
- Emergency patients who are found to be acutely hypothyroid should be considered for i/v T_3. Refer to a specialist physician.

Thyroid enlargement

A goitre or thyroid nodule in a patient presenting for surgery may be an incidental finding. Nodules and goitres are extremely common even in areas without iodine deficiency (30% from autopsy studies) but thyroid malignancy is rare (1 in 10–30 000). Urgent investigation of goitre is thus rarely required perioperatively. It is important to exclude a large retrosternal goitre causing thoracic outlet obstruction. This is normally only seen in thyroids detectable on physical examination or on routine PA CXR. It should be assessed radiologically by thoracic inlet views and by a flow-volume loop on respiratory function tests.

Interpreting thyroid function tests

TSH is the key indicator of thyroid disease. Thyrotoxicosis cannot be diagnosed unless the TSH is suppressed, nor primary hypothyroidism if the TSH is not elevated. Table 26.4 aids the interpretation of thyroid function tests using total thyroxine and TSH. Some labs measure free thyroxine which is unaffected by changes in protein binding.

Unsuspected thyroid disease

Thyroid disease is common, ten times more so in women. Approximately 2% of women will develop thyrotoxicosis, 4% hypothyroidism,

Table 26.4 Interpretation of thyroid function tests

		TSH		
		High	*Normal*	*Low*
Total thyroxine (T_4)	High	? TSH-secreting pituitary tumour	Euthyroid with high thyroid-binding globulin e.g. Pill Pregnancy	Free T_3 raised Thyrotoxicosis Thyroiditis
	Normal	Subclinical hypothyroidism (TSH 10–20 mu/l)	Normal	Free T_3 raised Thyrotoxicosis Thyroiditis Free T_3 normal Past Grave's Ophthalmic Grave's Thyroid nodules (at risk of future thyrotoxicosis)
	Low	Primary hypothyroidism or thyroiditis (TSH >20 mu/l)	Sick euthyroid Low thyroid binding globulin Secondary hypothyroidism	Secondary hypothyroidism

NB: In any patient with acute illness, thyroid function tests may be altered. This is called 'sick euthyroid'. Most commonly serum thyroxine is reduced, but TSH is normal. No treatment or further investigation is required.

and up to 30% have thyroid nodules or goitre. Thyroid disease can present for the first time on surgical wards. The presentation in surgical wards is likely to differ from those patients who present in endocrine outpatient clinics.

Hyperthyroidism
Hyperthyroidism should be exclude if the following occur: weight loss, diarrhoea, abnormal liver function tests, change in bowel habit, AF, anxiety and stress, heat intolerance, weight loss despite a normal or increased appetite, and difficulty getting to sleep. These features are common in surgical patients, and only one or two symptoms may be present in patients with thyrotoxicosis. Examination may reveal a goitre that may be generalized, or a single nodule. A bruit suggests thyrotoxicosis. Exophthalmos is rare but if present a diagnosis of Grave's disease can be made. Examine for tachycardia, AF, and LVF.

Hypothyroidism
Recent onset of constipation may suggest hypothyroidism. This is associated with weight gain rather than weight loss. Hypothyroidism can occur in the absence of goitre.

Obesity

Obese patients pose a number of problems to the anaesthetist and surgeon. They include:

- Cardiovascular dysfunction: There is an increase in blood volume and in cardiac work. Hypertension is common, as is coronary artery disease and atherosclerosis. Diabetes is also more common in obese subjects.

- Respiratory compromise: Vital capacity and functional residual capacity are reduced, and closing volume is increased. Pulmonary blood will be shunted past inadequately ventilated dependent lung regions, and hypoxaemia will result. These changes are accentuated in the supine and head-down positions and may last for several days postoperatively.

- Miscellaneous factors: Transport and positioning of patients may be difficult. Venous access may be a problem, and maintenance of an airway and tracheal intubation can be difficult. Hiatus hernia, which increases the risk of pulmonary aspiration, is more common. There is an increased incidence of wound infection and dehiscence. Regional anaesthetic techniques (e.g. epidural blocks) and surgery are technically more difficult.

Preoperative preparation

- Dieting is definitely an option for obese patients in whom elective surgery is planned.

- Evidence of cardiac disease should be sought. Hypertension and heart failure can be treated as necessary. An ECG should be performed and a CXR may be useful.

- Use the appropriate sized blood pressure cuff (2/3 arm circumference).

- Proton pump inhibitors may be prescribed if symptoms of gastric reflux are present (p. 197).

Postoperative care

- Respiratory factors: All obese patients should receive supplemental O_2 therapy postoperatively. A pulse oximeter is useful to determine the adequacy of oxygenation. Sitting the patient up will improve ventilation. Chest physiotherapy will be helpful, particularly if the patient has undergone abdominal surgery. Obese patients may occasionally require a period of postoperative ventilation, particularly after prolonged or more major surgery. It is important also to treat postoperative pain adequately.

- Infections are more common, particularly in the wound and in the chest, and should be checked for and treated with appropriate antibiotics.

- Thromboembolism is more likely. Prophylactic measures, such as subcutaneous heparin, compression stockings, and early mobilization will help to reduce the incidence of DVT.

Rare endocrine disorders

Phaeochromocytoma

Surgical removal of a phaeochromocytoma poses formidable anaesthetic challenges. The management must involve detailed liaison between anaesthetist and endocrinologist, and is outside the scope of this book.

Cushing's syndrome

Cushing's syndrome is treated surgically by hypohysectomy or bilateral adrenalectomy. Steroid replacement therapy will be needed immediately postoperatively, the exact dose schedule to be determined by the anaesthetist and endocrinologist.

Conn's syndrome

Conn's syndome may be due to adrenal hyperplasia or an aldosterone-secreting tumour. Patients with this syndrome may undergo curative surgery or have unrelated procedures. Medical therapy may only partially correct hypokalaemia, so this will need monitoring. If aldosterone antagonists cannot be given by mouth then i/v sodium carenoate can be substituted.

Further reading

Breivik H (1996). Perianaesthetic management of patients with endocrine disease. *Acta Anaesthesiologica Scandinavica* 40:1004–15.

Choban PS, Flancbaum L (1997). The impact of obesity on surgical outcomes: a review. *Journal of the American College of Surgeons* 185:593–603.

Gavin LA (1992). Perioperative management of the diabetic patient. *Endocrinology and Metabolism Clinics of North America* 21:457–75.

Milaskiewicz RM, Hall GM (1992). Diabetes and anaesthesia: the past decade. *British Journal of Anaesthesia* 68:198–206.

Oberg B, Poulsen TD (1996). Obesity: an anaesthetic challenge. *Acta Anaesthesiologica Scandinavica* 40:191–200.

Shenkman Z, Shir Y, Brodsky JB (1993). Perioperative management of the obese patient. *British Journal of Anaesthesia* 70:349–59.

Renal disorders

Anthony Nicholls

Renal impairment

The diagnosis of renal impairment is easily made when a high serum creatinine is found. Assessment of the significance of minor elevations of creatinine depends on the age and size of the patient. Renal impairment is very common in elderly patients undergoing surgery and is a significant risk for postoperative renal failure. Although it is impractical to measure renal function precisely in surgical patients, the serum creatinine should measured routinely according to the schedule on p. 23 and in anyone in whom there is concern about their renal status. Clearly, the greatest risk arises in those with the most severe renal impairment.

Causes

The common causes of renal failure may have relevance for surgical care.

- Ischaemic renal disease is the cause of renal impairment in 25% of affected patients over 65 years. Strongly associated with atheroma at other sites: carotid, cerebral, coronary, aorta, peripheral vessels. Patients undergoing aortic or peripheral arterial surgery with renal impairment almost invariably have atherosclerotic renovascular disease. Such patients should have a renal ultrasound scan preoperatively (look for asymmetric renal shrinkage).

- Obstructive uropathy accounts for a further 25% of affected males over 65 years, usually due to benign prostatic disease. Again, ultrasonography will be diagnostic.

- Diabetes is the cause of renal impairment in 20% of all patients. Diabetic nephropathy is strongly associated with accelerated atherosclerosis at all sites.

- Glomerulonephritis often leads to protein loss and hypoalbumin-aemia. Apart from the risk of renal failure postoperatively, there is an increased risk of poor wound healing and pressure sores.
- Hypertensive nephrosclerosis is common. Hypovolaemia or hypotension will increase the risk of worsening renal function, while accelerated hypertension will itself be hazardous.
- Other causes of renal failure include polycystic disease, reflux nephropathy and chronic tubulointerstitial disease. These disorders pose no particular risks beyond those of renal impairment itself.

Clinical implications

Renal impairment is commonly associated with fluid and electrolyte disturbances, particularly hyperkalemia, acidaemia, and fluid retention.

Severe renal impairment is complicated by anaemia. The decision to transfuse may need advice from a renal physician. Blood transfusions should be given through a white-cell filter. This avoids sensitizing the patient to foreign HLA antigens, which may induce cytotoxic anti-body formation and compromise future transplantation.

Impairment of renal function affects the metabolism and/or excretion of many drugs, and hence their dosage. The BNF gives comprehensive advice on prescribing in renal impairment.

History taking

- Check for reduced exercise tolerance: anaemia or other cardio-respiratory problems may be contributory.
- Ask about appetite and nausea: the patient may be malnourished.
- Ask for drug intolerance or allergy.

Examination

- Assess fluid balance.
- Signs of fluid overload include hypertension, oedema, and elevation of the JVP. It is more important to establish whether JVP is elevated than accurately measure the pressure. Oedema over the shins or sacrum is easy to detect, but in those who have lost weight, it is often only evident in the wasted tissues of the calves.
- Dehydration: Check for postural hypotension (> 20 mmHg fall in systolic BP moving from supine to on standing) and reduced skin turgor. Oedema is highly unusual in dehydration, but not imposs-ible in the presence of a very low serum albumin (see nephrotic syndrome below). Skin turgor is best assessed by gently pinching a skin fold on the forearm. The turgor of the skin overlying the clav-icles is an unreliable sign in the elderly, but useful in younger patients.
- A raised respiratory rate may be due to acidosis ('air hunger') or pulmonary oedema.

Investigations

- Serum creatinine is the key measure of renal function. Kidney function is not the sole determinant of serum creatinine: it also depends upon muscle bulk, body weight, age, and sex.
- The glomerular filtration rate (GFR) can be estimated by the Cockroft and Gault formula, where the age is in years, weight in kg, and creatinine in μmol/l. Multiply by 0.85 for women.
- $$\text{GFR} = \frac{(140 - \text{age}) \times \text{weight} \times 1.24}{\text{creatinine}} \text{ ml/min}$$
- Serum urea is of little help in assessing renal function. Urea rises in dehydration, GI bleeding, sepsis, and catabolism. Urea falls in malnutrition and starvation. A disproportionate rise or fall in urea relative to creatinine may unravel these problems.
- Electrolytes: Na^+ usually normal. Hypokalaemia may occur with high-dose diuretics. Hyperkalaemia less common except in advanced renal failure unless due to combination of renal impairment and drug therapy: ACE inhibitors, aldosterone antagonists, K^+ supplements, NSAIDs.
- Serum HCO_3^- (or pH and standard HCO_3^-): Acidosis is common in renal failure. It aggravates hyperkalaemia and may cause tachypnoea.
- Hb low in advanced renal failure due to erythropoietin deficiency. Patients tolerate modest anaemia (Hb 9–12 g/dl) well unless elderly or with cardiorespiratory disease.
- Ca^{2+} may be low in renal failure.
- Albumin often low due to poor nutrition even if no urinary loss of protein.

Preoperative preparation

- BP should be 110–170 systolic and 70–95 diastolic.
- Fluid balance should be near normal. A slightly 'wet' patient is safer than a dehydrated one. A central line will help in cases where assessment is difficult. Rehydrate patients preoperatively with 0.9% NaCl. Significant dehydration may result in reduction in renal blood flow and a further deterioration in renal function. Avoid this at all times.
- Start i/v 0.9% saline infusion at a rate of 1 l/12 h while the patient is nil-by-mouth.
- Consider transfusion if Hb <9 g/dl and major surgery is planned. Transfuse at a higher level if there is co-existing cardiorespiratory disease in an elderly patient. Beware of inducing fluid overload.
- *Hyperkalaemia*: Defer surgery if K^+ >6.0 mmol/l. K^+ 5.5–6.0 mmol/l is usually safe if suxamethonium can be avoided. Correction of

acidosis with 1.26% $NaHCO_3$ will lower K^+ (check Ca^{2+} to avoid tetany). Resonium 30 g rectally will lower K^+ within 2– 3 h. If drugs contributing to hyperkalaemia (ACE inhibitors, aldosterone antagonists, K^+ supplements, NSAIDs) have been prescribed it may take 24–48 h off medication to correct hyperkalaemia. In emergencies, K^+ can be lowered by an infusion of insulin and dextrose or by administration of a nebulized β-agonist (e.g. salbutamol 2.5 mg). Cardiac toxicity is reversed by i/v Ca^{2+} (e.g. 10% $CaCl_2$ 10 ml i/v). The section on electrolyte disorders details the treatment of hyperkalaemia (p. 309).

- *Biliary surgery and jaundice*: The risk of postoperative renal failure is very high when there is a combination of renal impairment and hepatobiliary disease. See p. 201 for fuller details.

- *Emergency surgery*: The finding of renal impairment as a new biochemical abnormality raises the possibility of acute renal failure complicating the underlying surgical emergency. Alternative explanations include obstructive uropathy (commonly due to prostatic disease), or previously undetected chronic renal disease. Insert a bladder catheter and measure residual urine volume. Consider CVP monitoring. Measure hourly urine output postoperatively. As soon as is practical get a renal tract ultrasound examination to evaluate the cause of renal impairment.

- Patients *undergoing aortic surgery, emergency abdominal surgery*, or any surgery in the presence of sepsis are at particular risk of developing renal decompensation.

Postoperative care

- Avoid NSAIDs at any stage. They increase the risk of acute-on-chronic renal failure.

- Care with i/v doses of opioids. Metabolites of morphine that are both sedative and depress respiration may accumulate in renal failure. PCA morphine or regional analgesia are often the best regimes following major surgery (see pain control p. 54).

- Give appropriate i/v fluids postoperatively. Replace losses carefully and give normal maintenance requirements – based around the normal daily urine output of the patient. Do not allow the patient to become dehydrated as a permanent deterioration in existing renal function may occur.

- Bladder catheter and hourly urine output monitoring. A urine output of <30–40 ml/h should be investigated. A CVP line will assist with correct fluid status. If oliguria supervenes refer to Chapter 43 (p. 299).

- Daily creatinine, electrolytes, Ca^{2+}, until stable.

- Check Mg^{2+} postoperatively.

Table 27.1 Perioperative prescribing in renal failure

	Diuretics	Phosphate binders (CaCO$_3$, Al(OH)$_3$)	Vitamin D analogues	β-blockers	ACE inhibitors	Vasodilators	Morphine/ pethidine	Anti-biotics	Immuno-suppressives
Continue therapy i/v until able to absorb from gut	✓								
Give normal preoperative dose and resume when stable postoperatively			✓	✓		✓			✓
Omit preoperative dose and resume when stable postoperatively					✓[a]				
Drugs that may need dose adjustment in renal failure		✓		✓			✓	✓	

[a] Discuss with anaesthetist.

Dialysis patients

The underlying cause and complications of renal failure may have relevance for surgical care (see p. 173). This section focuses on specific issues in dialysis patients.

Vein care

- *Haemodialysis patients* depend on good vascular access for their survival. Peritoneal dialysis (PD) patients may need haemodialysis in the future. Preserve large forearm veins during surgery and anaesthesia. Cannulation of these veins may result in their loss and prejudice long-term renal care for the patient. Small cannulae in veins on the back of the hand are preferred. Veins on the ulnar aspect of the forearm are also suitable as these are rarely used for dialysis. Avoid the cephalic or brachial veins.

- *During surgery* an arm with a fistula in it should be lightly wrapped in soft gauze or cotton wool and placed to ensure blood flow will not be compromised. Take the blood pressure in the opposite arm. Arterial cannulae should be placed in the radial rather than the brachial artery, and only used when strictly necessary.

Scheduling dialysis

- Haemodialysis. Dialyse the patient a few hours before a surgical procedure. This ensures that the serum K^+ is in the normal range at the time of anaesthesia. Dialysis patients commonly have marginal elevation of serum K^+ in the range 5.5–6.5 mmol/l before dialysis. Use of suxamethonium during anaesthesia will cause the K^+ to rise by about 1 mmol/l, which would be hazardous in the face of marginal hyperkalaemia. Delay haemodialysis for 24–48 h after surgery in order to prevent heparin-induced bleeding postoperatively. Monitor K^+ daily to ensure this delay is safe.

- PD leads to steady-state biochemistry: the serum K^+ on any particular day will be similar to the following day provided dietary intake is constant. Continue PD to right up to surgery, but drain the peritoneal cavity preoperatively for optimal respiratory function. There is no urgency to re-commence PD immediately postoperatively: 24 h free of dialysis is of no significance. PD is usually delayed for some weeks after abdominal surgery to allow adequate healing.

- If a period of temporary haemodialysis is planned postoperatively, request that the anaesthetist place a temporary central venous dialysis catheter under anaesthesia. This is convenient and comfortable for the patient.

Postoperative considerations

- *Bleeding*: Platelet function in renal failure may be impaired. Coagulation is usually normal. Check the history for bleeding, e.g.

after needling or previous operations. If in doubt, check both co-agulation tests and the bleeding time (normally <10 min) using an automated device (contact your haematology department). Correct coagulation with FFP as necessary. Improve platelet dysfunction with i/v DDAVP (desmopressin) 0.3 μg/kg in 50 ml 0.9% saline given i/v over 30 min.

• *Perioperative fluids*: Ensure adequate replacement fluids are given. Maintenance fluids are around 500–750 ml/day. Some patients on dialysis pass some urine; allow extra intake to compensate for this. Make allowance for sweating, diarrhoea, etc. as described on p. 70. Do not overload with potassium.

• *Third space losses*: After major surgery, especially abdominal surgery, third space losses (wound oedema, paralytic ileus) need to be replaced with i/v NaCl intra- and postoperatively to maintain circulating volume. With normal renal function a diuresis removes these sequestered fluids over subsequent days as soon as they are reabsorbed from third spaces. In a dialysis patient resorption of third space losses may lead to intravascular fluid overload unless anticipated by fluid removal on dialysis in parallel with the reduction in sequestration. If this fluid is not removed, pulmonary oedema may develop. Accurate charting of administered fluids helps prevent this problem.

Nephrotic syndrome

Nephrotic syndrome means heavy proteinuria sufficient to deplete serum albumin and cause oedema. It is commonly due to primary glomerular disease, but occasionally as part of a systemic disorder (SLE, amyloid, diabetes). Some patients will be on, or have recently received steroid therapy. The physiological disturbances relevant to surgery include:

• malnutrition and muscle wasting secondary to protein loss
• intravascular volume depletion due to diuretic therapy and hypo-albuminaemia
• blood hypercoagulability due to increased platelet stickiness, loss of antithrombin-III in the urine and volume depletion
• skin fragility due to malnutrition, oedema, ±steroid therapy
• increased risk of infection due to loss of immunoglobulins in the urine, malnutrition, ±steroid therapy
• poor wound healing (factors as above).

Surgery in patients with nephrotic syndrome should be avoided if possible. For many patients nephrotic syndrome will be a temporary stage in the evolution of their underlying kidney disease. Remission, with or without the use of immunosuppressive therapy, is fairly common, and provides a more favourable state for surgery. Other patients will progress to renal failure, but without heavy protein loss and oedema. Surgery is then less hazardous as serum albumin levels are usually normal, volume status normal or increased and blood coagulability normal or reduced.

Examination

- *Fluid balance assessment* is tricky. Oedema is not relevant as a sign of intravascular volume overload but assessment of the JVP is critical. If this cannot be seen assume the patient to be intravascularly depleted. The only reliable sign of fluid overload is elevation of the JVP (or CVP if a line is present) as hypertension can occur in the face of intravascular volume depletion.
- *Dehydration*: Check for postural hypotension (>20 mmHg fall in supine systolic BP on standing) and reduced skin turgor over the clavicles. The classic sign of intravascular volume depletion in nephrotic syndrome is the combination of an apparently dry upper part of the body with soggy legs – reduced turgor over the clavicles together with massive leg oedema.

Investigations

- Serum creatinine to assess renal function.
- Electrolytes: Na^+ often low in nephrotic syndrome, especially if over-diuresed. Hypokalaemia may occur with high dose diuretics.
- Total calcium may be low, but most labs correct for the albumin concentration.
- Albumin: Patients with levels of >25 g/l are not at major risk, but extreme protein loss will result in serum albumin levels <20 g/l. At this level complications as outlined above are likely.

Preoperative preparation

- BP should be 110–170 systolic and 70–95 diastolic.
- Intravascular fluid balance should be near normal. A slightly 'wet' patient is safer than a dehydrated one. Place a central line preoperatively and normalize CVP unless the JVP is clearly seen. Consider the use of 4.5% human albumin solution if the serum albumin is <20 g/l.
- DVT prophylaxis is mandatory (see p. 48).
- Pressure sore prevention should start preoperatively.
- Drug kinetics: Many drugs are bound to serum albumin, so free levels of some drugs will be increased. This is most important for benzodiazepines, which have a greater effect in nephrotic patients. Other agents, particularly aminoglycosides, have an increased volume of distribution with lower blood levels for any given dose.

Postoperative care

· Perioperative fluid replacement should be with colloid.
· Abdominal surgery: Nephrotic syndrome predisposes to many complications of abdominal surgery as outlined above.
· Avoid malnutrition: parenteral nutrition may be needed.
· Sutures may need leaving in place longer than usual.
· Monitor urine output and renal function closely. The risk of post-operative renal failure is high.

Further reading

Cranshaw J, Holland D (1996). Anaesthesia for patients with renal impairment. *Hospital Medicine* 55:171–5.

Neurological disorders

Richard Hardie and Chris Day

General principles

Death in neurologically disabled patients is most commonly a consequence of immobility. Typical postoperative complications include chest infection, UTIs, pressure sores, DVT, and PE. Except in the terminal stages of disease, these are preventable by good nursing, careful handling, and other appropriate prophylactic measures.

Ask about personal activities of daily living and level of independence. Patients will usually have established a personalized programme of care and maintenance. Medical and nursing staff on surgical wards should recognize this and both seek and accept advice from patients and their carers. Preventable complications arising perioperatively may not simply extend the length of hospital stay, but might also destroy the confidence of the patient and carers in the hospital for the future.

Depending upon the anatomical site of the underlying neurological lesion, specific clinical features are important and may be exacerbated or precipitated by anaesthesia and/or surgical intervention. Good practice should anticipate these. Table 28.1 relates specific neurological disorders to surgical risks.

Table 28.1 Important neurological conditions and postoperative risks

Site	Examples	Increased risks
Cerebrum	stroke head injury	impaired consciousness confusion seizures dysphasia
Lower brainstem	(pseudo-) bulbar palsy from stroke multiple sclerosis motor neurone disease myasthenia	dysphagia dysphagia dysphagia aspiration
Spinal cord	trauma multiple sclerosis transverse myelitis	hypoventilation (high cervical) neuropathic bladder and bowel saddle anaesthesia and sacral sores
Anterior horn cell	motor neurone disease old polio	pure motor weakness
Peripheral nerve/root	Guillain–Barré syndrome hereditary neuropathy (Charcot–Marie–Tooth syndrome)	mainly distal weakness possibly hypoventilation glove and stocking sensory loss
Neuromuscular junction	myasthenia gravis respiratory muscle involvement	fatiguable weakness, particularly of facial, bulbar, axial, and proximal limb muscles
Muscle	muscular dystrophies polymyositis	non-fatiguable pure motor weakness

Perioperative prescribing

- Pre-existing cerebral damage causes increased susceptibility to all centrally acting drugs, especially hypnotics and other sedatives including opioids. **Reduce the dosage of these agents accordingly.**
- Drugs that lower seizure threshold (e.g. tricyclics, major tranquillizers) should be used cautiously.

Ventilation

- *Clinical assessment* Exercise tolerance may be unavailable as a guide to fitness as immobile patients may not be capable of enough exercise to become short of breath. Weakness may affect the respiratory muscles insidiously, especially the diaphragm. This is most significant when sleeping supine, because of reduced respiratory drive and mechanical disadvantage.
- *Lung function tests* before surgery may demonstrate unexpectedly restricted vital capacity, particularly if done both lying and standing.

- *Oxygenation*: Special attention should be paid to adequate oxygenation, chest physiotherapy and early mobilization. If respiratory function is impaired, supplemental O_2 should be given postoperatively. Pulse oximetry is essential. However, significant hypoventilation may coexist with a normal saturation so arterial blood gas analysis may be necessary to determine adequacy of ventilation.

Swallowing

- Patients with bulbar weakness may already be both poorly nourished and at high risk of aspiration postoperatively. It may be advisable to keep them nil-by-mouth if in doubt after surgery.
- A malnourished patient will tolerate the catabolic stress of surgery badly and should not be starved postoperatively.
- If normal feeding will be delayed, enteral feeding can be given (n/g, jejunostomy, or PEG) or TPN considered. Involve the speech therapist and dietician at an early stage.

Pressure areas

Immobile, undernourished patients are at high risk of pressure sores, for example with motor neurone disease, but even more so if spinal cord injury or multiple sclerosis impairs cutaneous sensation. Scrupulous attention must be paid not just to careful handling, but also to seating, skin traction, plaster casting, and positioning on the operating table. Low pressure beds, mattresses, and cushions are expensive and often in short supply. 'Consultant clout' may be necessary to ensure ward nurses obtain essential equipment.

Bowel management

Be vigilant for the development of subacute intestinal obstruction secondary to constipation. Patients should be well hydrated and receive early prophylactic suppositories or laxatives if necessary.

Bladder management

Neuropathic bladders require careful management. Patients may have significant chronic retention and, if long-standing, reflux nephropathy or stones, increasing the risks of infection. Intermittent self-catheterization (ISC) is increasingly recognized as preferable to a long-term in-dwelling catheter. ISC should be continued in hospital wherever possible, if necessary with the assistance of nursing staff. The temptation to insert a catheter just for convenience must be resisted.

Deep venous thrombosis (DVT)

Any patient with a paralysed lower limb is at high risk of DVT (40–80%) and PE (1–10%). They should always have graduated antiembolism stockings, intraoperative pneumatic compression and, unless there is a clear contraindication, subcutaneous heparin. Other neurological patients should be considered at least in the moderate risk category. (See p. 48 for more details.)

Early mobilization and rehabilitation

All patients should get out of bed and exercise as soon as possible after surgery. This is equally important for postoperative cases with chronic disabilities. These patients should be referred for assessment to physiotherapists and occupational therapists. Advice from colleagues in neurology or rehabilitation medicine may also be helpful.

Cerebrovascular disease

Cerebrovascular disease is almost as common as IHD, but may be clinically silent. Normally cerebral perfusion is maintained during hypotension by autoregulation. If this fails cerebral perfusion may be is compromised.

The majority of strokes (about 80%) are ischaemic and survival is more likely than after intracerebral haemorrhage, but the distinction can only be made by early cranial imaging. Those who have had a definite previous stroke may not have been thoroughly investigated at the time.

History

- Enquire about all relevant vascular risk factors. Record details of previous cerebral events, asking carefully about lateralization and duration of symptoms. The definition of transient ischaemic attack (TIA) is restricted to symptoms lasting less than 24 h. A longer-lasting episode with full recovery is more correctly regarded as a minor completed stroke, implying that permanent damage was sustained.

- More than one event in the same arterial territory suggests significant large-vessel stenosis (aorta or carotid artery) with distal embolism. Otherwise, embolic stroke is uncommon without overt cardiac disease, of which the most important type is AF.

- In those with permanent neurological disability after a stroke, ask about personal activities of daily living and level of independence.

- IHD is the commonest cause of death in those with cerebrovascular disease. Ask specifically for cardiac symptoms.

Examination

- Briefly test higher mental function as a baseline on admission.
- Check visual fields for a gross hemianopia; speech for intelligibility and dysphasia; look for evidence of residual facial and/or hemiparesis; observe stance and gait.
- Listen for carotid bruits, although their value is unclear.
- Ensure BP is controlled at < 170/90.

Investigations

- FBC, looking at Hb and platelet count.
- ECG to document AF and look for ischaemic changes.
- INR in those on warfarin.
- Carotid ultrasound estimates the degree of stenosis. Patients presenting for major surgery with a history of TIA or stroke, who have not been previously investigated by carotid ultrasound, should have this preoperatively. Neurological consultation will be necessary if high-grade stenosis is demonstrated. Severe stenosis (>70%) in asymptomatic patients may justify elective endarterectomy because of the high risk of stroke after major surgery, but, in general, endarterectomy is reserved for symptomatic patients.

Perioperative prescribing

- *Aspirin*: It may be safe to omit aspirin for a day or two, but 300 mg suppositories are available.
- *Warfarin.* See p. 145.

Postoperative care

- Cerebrovascular and cardiovascular disease commonly co-exist. Supplemental O_2 may decrease morbidity. It may need to be continued for several days after major surgery.
- Treat hypovolaemia, anaemia, and hypotension promptly.
- Nurse high-risk patients in a high-dependency area.

Epilepsy

- *Risks*: Well-controlled epilepsy does not confer increased perioperative risk, as most anaesthetic agents are anticonvulsant. Patients commonly suffer from either generalized tonic–clonic or complex partial seizures. Complex partial seizures are transient, and associated with fleetingly abnormal behaviour.
- *Causes*: Most chronic seizure disorders are idiopathic (without structural abnormality on cranial imaging), but known causes include head injury, cerebrovascular disease, neurosurgery, intracranial tumour, and alcohol abuse.
- *Pharmacology*: Almost all anti-epileptic drugs (AEDs) induce liver enzymes and hence their own metabolism. Phenytoin and phenobarbitone may cause elevation of alkaline phosphatase and γ-GT and may interact with other drugs metabolized by the liver such as warfarin. Sodium valproate is an inhibitor of liver enzymes.
- *Monotherapy* is favoured in most patients, so patients receiving two AEDs are likely to be more difficult to control.

History

- *Nature of fits*: Review seizure type(s), current frequency, and adequacy of control.
- *Drugs*: Establish exact drug regime, including any controlled-release formulations. Verify patient compliance, particularly if doses seem high: toxicity may develop if they have not actually been taking what has been prescribed.
- *Shunts?* Check for previous neurosurgical shunt insertion. Prophylactic antibiotic cover will be needed for procedures that may induce bacteraemia (as for subacute bacterial endocarditis prophylaxis, p. 76).

Investigations

Check levels of phenytoin or carbamazepine if seizure control is poor. This may guide management if seizures occur postoperatively. Other agents are not worth measuring.

Perioperative prescribing

- Continue usual AED dosage if possible. Phenytoin need only be given once daily (half-life > 24 h).
- Patients nil-by-mouth preoperatively can safely be given their morning doses of AEDs unless there are specific instructions from the anaesthetist.
- Carbamazepine is available as a rectal preparation, but other drugs can be given via a n/g tube if necessary.
- i/v preparations are available for most AEDs: consult the BNF.

Postoperative care

- Maintain i/v access until fully recovered from anaesthesia.
- Avoid hyponatraemia, hyperventilation. or inadvertent AED withdrawal which may lower seizure threshold.

Dementia

Senile dementia is a hidden disability because of its insidious onset and a deceptive preservation of social skills until relatively late. It is characterized by persistent global disturbance of higher mental functions in a patient with normal alertness, and may affect about 10% of those over 65.

History and examination

- All elderly patients should be screened for dementia by a brief mental state examination and corroborating history from relatives.
- Adequate documentation on admission is crucial if a patient becomes confused subsequently.

- Review medication and try to minimize it. Some drugs may cause confusion and should be stopped.

Investigations

Na$^+$, Ca^{2+}, creatinine, glucose, thyroid function to exclude a treatable cause of cognitive impairment.

Perioperative prescribing

- Cerebral damage may increase susceptibility to centrally acting drugs.
- A sedative drug may be required for disruptive behaviour, but this may depress respiration, causing hypoxia and worsening confusion. Haloperidol (2.5–10 mg) and chlorpromazine (25–100 mg) both have a wide therapeutic index and are relatively safe. Alternatively, benzodiazepines can be used. These can be reversed with flumazenil if necessary.

Postoperative care

- Ensure adequate nursing levels and a safe ward environment.
- Support fluid intake and nutrition.
- Anticipate increased confusion at night; consider using a well-lit side room.
- Return the patient to a more familiar environment as soon as possible. Although demented patients might initially be thought inappropriate for day case surgery, this may minimize disruption. Plan this in advance with the anaesthetist. The carers may need extra support at home.
- The use of cot sides is controversial. Confused patients may injure themselves more when falling over cot sides than from a normal bed. Cot sides are no substitute for nursing care.

Parkinson's disease

Parkinson's disease (PD) is the second commonest cause of neurological disability after stroke. Its onset is insidious so it may go undiagnosed until admission for surgery. Then it tends to be diagnosed by the nurses and therapists rather than the medical staff! In such cases, get an assessment preoperatively from a neurologist or geriatrician with an interest in PD, but surgery need not usually be delayed. Treatment should normally wait till after surgery as there is no urgency. Advanced PD is associated with dementia and reduced ventilation.

Perioperative prescribing

- Continue established anti-PD therapy, possibly via a n/g tube. This will avoid postoperative akinesia. Dispersible Madopar can be substituted for any other L-dopa preparation. Selegiline syrup is available.

- Avoid metoclopramide and prochlorperazine. These are centrally acting dopamine receptor antagonists that may worsen PD. Domperidone does not cross the blood–brain barrier and is safe, as is ondansetron.

Myasthenia gravis (MG)

- *Pathology*: An autoimmune condition affecting post-junctional (neuromuscular) acetylcholine receptors (ACh-R). ACh-R antibodies reduce the number of receptors and duration of response. Associated with thymoma or other autoimmune illnesses.
- *Clinical features*: Characterized by muscular fatiguability resulting in ptosis, diplopia, facial weakness, and bulbar problems. Often progresses to involve upper limb and respiratory function.
- *Treatment* is with regular anticholinesterases (pyridostigmine, neostigmine). These may be combined with anticholinergics (atropine, propantheline) to reduce muscarinic side-effects such as bradycardia and abdominal cramps.
- *Immunosuppression* is commonly used (prednisolone and/or aza-thioprine). A thymoma may require surgery. In crises, plasma exchange may result in an improvement in muscular function.
- *Crises*: Acute exacerbations of MG occur if inadequate doses of anticholinesterases are prescribed, or absorption affected (myasthenic crisis). Excessive dosage of anticholinergics impairs neuro-muscular transmission, precipitating a cholinergic crisis from depolarizing block. These can sometimes, but not always, be distinguished by an edrophonium test, but a neurologist may be needed to clarify the problem.
- Patients with stable MG may present for any type of surgical procedure.

Perioperative problems

The majority of well-controlled myasthenics undergoing minor or moderate surgery do well. However, recovery from major surgery may be complicated.

- Some myasthenics with compromised respiratory function will require postoperative ventilation – see further reading.
- Bulbar palsy may result in ineffective cough and aspiration.
- Muscular weakness may result in respiratory complications including sputum retention, infection, and ventilatory failure.
- Steroid cover may require supplementation.
- Hypokalaemia and aminoglycoside antibiotics may worsen weakness.

- Cardiomyopathy is a rare complication.
- Absorption of anticholinesterases may be unpredictable post-operatively.

Perioperative plan

- Discuss with anaesthetist as early as possible and consider whether admission to ICU is advisable postoperatively.
- Work out the planned perioperative anticholinesterase regime with the anaesthetist. A n/g tube may be necessary for administration.
- Patients on pyridostigmine orally preoperative will need i/v neostigmine while unable to absorb from the gut. Pyridostigmine 60 mg po is approximately equivalent to 1–1.5 mg neostigmine s/c or i/m. Parenteral neostigmine needs to be given in divided doses 4 hourly or more often. For example, a patient stable on pyridostigmine 120 mg qds will need a total daily dose of neostigmine of 4–6 mg, so prescribe 1 mg 4 hourly i/m. Parenteral neostigmine may need to be combined with atropine or preferably glycopyrrolate. The anaesthetist or neurologist will advise.
- Alert the physiotherapy team – with major surgery intensive chest physiotherapy will be required pre- and postoperatively.
- Increase steroid cover if indicated (p. 167).
- If significant difficulties develop postoperatively, ask for assistance from the ICU team. Myasthenic patients may develop respiratory failure with minimal signs. Measuring the vital capacity and assessing the strength of the cough are good guides. Check the SaO_2, blood gases, and a CXR in patients giving rise to concern.

Myasthenic syndrome (Eaton–Lambert syndrome)

Perioperatively myasthenic syndrome presents similar problems to myasthenia gravis. It can be associated with underlying malignancy, usually an oat cell carcinoma of the lung. There is a pre-junctional reduction in release of acetylcholine. The condition does not respond to anticholinesterases.

Further reading:

Naguib M, El Dawlatly AA, Ashour M, Bamgboye EA (1996). Multivariate determinants of the need for postoperative ventilation in myasthenia gravis. *Canadian Journal of Anaesthesia* 43:1006–13.

Bone and joint disorders

Paul Marshall

General principles

The rheumatic diseases affect the bones, joints, and connective tissue. Skeletal abnormalities may themselves complicate the management of anaesthesia in particular with relation to the airway. Deformities may make the use of regional anaesthesia including spinals and epidurals difficult or impossible. Some disorders are associated with relevant systemic features including anaemia. Use of NSAIDs and steroids is common and side effects are potentially serious.

Some causes of bone and joint disorders have particular relevance for surgical care.

- *Rheumatoid arthritis*: Symmetrical deforming arthropathy with systemic features. See below.

- *Other connective tissue disorders*: These include systemic lupus erythematosus (SLE), progressive systemic sclerosis (PSS), and other rare conditions. Autoimmune multisystem disorders with a chronic course are commonly treated with steroids.

- *Spondyloarthropathies*: These mainly affect the spine and insertions of tendons and ligaments. Systemic features are commonly present, e.g. ankylosing spondylitis. This condition may cause fixed flexion neck deformity making tracheal intubation impossible. Reduced chest expansion and associated restrictive ventilatory defect are common. Aortic regurgitation may also occur.

- *Scoliosis*: In this condition, there is progressive lateral curvature of the spine associated with progressive ankylosis and an associated restrictive ventilatory defect. Congenital scoliosis may be associated with hypoplasia of the odontoid process resulting in atlantoaxial

instability. This may make tracheal intubation hazardous. (Asymptomatic atlantoaxial instability can also occur in Down's syndrome.)
- *Osteoarthritis*: There are no systemic features, but this is a disease of the elderly and intercurrent disease is common.

All these conditions may be associated with reduced mobility and consequent poor aerobic fitness. Functional assessment of cardio-respiratory status is often difficult. Decreased mobility may predispose to thromboembolic disease and DVT prophylaxis is important. Keep the period of immobility associated with surgery to a minimum.

Rheumatoid arthritis

Although not as common as osteoarthritis this condition affects 3% of the population and is associated with specific anaesthetic problems in relation to the airway as well as relevant systemic features.

Preoperative assessment

The following are important aspects of the history and examination.

Articular disease

Although many joints may be affected, and deformities may make i/v access and other procedures difficult, it is the effects of the disease on the airway which are most important.
- *The cervical spine*: Ask about headaches, neck pain, and possible neurological symptoms. Carefully assess the neck. Note any deformity and range of movement. Assess the angle between maximum flexion and extension achieved. Radiological changes occur in up to 86% patients with rheumatoid arthritis but may be asymptomatic particularly when the patient is on steroids. Atlantoaxial subluxation may make tracheal intubation and patient transfer hazardous as the cervical cord may be compromised with extremes of flexion or extension. Subaxial subluxation can also occur and may be exacerbated by flexion or extension. Fixed flexion deformities occur later in disease again making tracheal intubation difficult.
- *Temporomandibular joints*: Assess mouth opening as arthritis of these joints may limit mouth opening and make intubation difficult.
- *Cricoarytenoid joints*: Laryngeal involvement is common. Rarely stridor and upper airway obstruction may occur.

Systemic disease
- *Cardiovascular system*: An asymptomatic pericarditis may occur with an effusion. Progression to constrictive pericarditis is rare. Myocardial or valve involvement is uncommon.
- *Respiratory system*: There are CXR changes in up to 12.5% of patients with rheumatoid arthritis. Pulmonary fibrosis and pleural effusions may occur. Nodules in the lung are rare.

- *Haemopoietic system*: Normochromic normocytic anaemia is associated with active disease. Drugs may cause marrow suppression. Bleeding may contribute, particularly with NSAIDs.
- *Renal system*: Interstitial nephritis and amyloid may occur. The toxic effects of treatment (especially NSAIDs) are potentially serious.
- *Nervous system*: Peripheral neuropathy can occur. Both symptoms and signs in arms and or legs may be secondary to cervical spine compression.

Table 29.1 gives an investigation schedule for patients with RA.

The automatic ordering of flexion and extension views of the cervical spine preoperatively is controversial, particularly if it does not alter anaesthetic technique.

Table 29.1 Preoperative investigations in RA

All patients	To exclude
Full blood count	GI loss, drug effects
Creatinine and electrolytes	Renal involvement, drug toxicity
ECG	Ventricular hypertrophy. Low voltages might suggest pericardial effusion
CXR	Pulmonary fibrosis, pleural effusion, pericardial effusion
Selected patients	**Indications**
Cervical spine radiograph	Anaesthetist requests
Pulmonary function tests	Unexplained dyspnoea
Indirect laryngoscopy	Hoarseness, stridor
Echocardiography	Pericardial/valvular involvement

Drug review and possible side effects

- *NSAIDs*: gastric erosions, renal impairment including acute renal failure.
- *Disease-modifying drugs (e.g. gold, penicillamine)*: proteinuria, marrow suppression
- *Immunosuppressive agents (azathioprine, methotrexate)*: marrow suppression
- *Steroids*: hypokalaemia, hypertension, impaired glucose tolerance.

Perioperative prescribing

- *Continue disease-modifying drugs* (except azathioprine) up to the time of surgery. Azathioprine has been associated with major wound complications and should be discontinued 3 weeks before surgery.

- NSAID use has been associated with an increased risk of bleeding complications after major joint surgery. Aspirin has irreversible effects on platelet function and some surgeons prefer to stop it 10 days before major joint surgery. This decision will also depend on why the patient is taking aspirin. It may be appropriate to continue NSAIDs up until surgery using agents with a short half-life, e.g. diclofenac.
- Stop NSAIDs immediately if the patient is volume depleted or if there is significant deterioration of renal function.
- Institute DVT prophylaxis. (See p. 48.)
- Plan postoperative pain control and counsel patient in conjunction with relevant staff. PCA may be difficult if the hands are affected.
- Increased steroid cover will be necessary for anything more than minor surgery. (See p. 166.)
- Preoperative blood transfusion is not usually necessary unless there is associated blood loss.
- A protective neck collar at induction of anaesthesia is advisable if there is cervical instability.

Postoperative care

- Maintain adequate fluid intake and monitor renal function.
- Continue NSAIDs unless contraindicated using rectal or i/v routes if oral route unavailable.
- Maintenance of mobility associated with good pain control is important. If the patient is immobilized chest physiotherapy and passive exercises may be required.
- Continue steroid cover and reduce to maintenance level.
- Consider prophylaxis (e.g. ranitidine 150 mg bd) against gastric erosion/peptic ulceration in patients at risk.
- Resume rheumatoid medication as soon as practicable.
- Continue some form of DVT prophylaxis until patient is fully mobile.

Further reading

Campbell RSD, Wou P, Watt I (1995). A continuing role for preoperative cervical spine radiography in rheumatoid arthritis? *Clinical Radiology* 50:157–9.

Keystone EC, Musing ELS, Mak VCW (1996). Preoperative management of medications in the rheumatoid patient. *Current Opinion in Orthopaedics* 7:6–9.

MacArthur A, Kleiman S (1993). Rheumatoid cervical joint disease – a challenge to the anaesthetist. *Canadian Journal of Anaesthesia* 40:154–9.

Skues MA, Welchew EA (1993). Anaesthesia and rheumatoid arthritis. *Anaesthesia* **48**:989–97.

MacKenzie CR, Sharrock NE (1998). Perioperative medical considerations in patients with rheumatoid arthritis. *Rheumatic Diseases Clinics of North America* **24**:1–17.

Matti MV, Sharrock NE (1998). Anesthesia on the rheumatoid patient. *Rheumatic Diseases Clinics of North America* **24**:19–34.

Gastroenterological disorders

Tawfique Daneshmend and Alasdair Dow

Acid-peptic ulceration including oesophagitis

A history of acid-peptic ulceration of the upper digestive tract affecting the duodenum, stomach, or oesophagus will often be obtained in patients presenting for elective or emergency surgery unrelated to the upper GI tract.

Surgery for acid-peptic disease itself (elective surgery for peptic ulcer, gastro-oesophageal reflux disease; emergency surgery for perforated peptic ulcer or oesophagus; or surgery for acute GI bleeding) is not the purpose of this chapter. The management of these patients is addressed in standard surgical texts.

Chronic peptic ulceration should now be rare. Since over 90% of (previously idiopathic) gastric and duodenal ulceration is associated causally with *Helicobacter pylori*, in ideal circumstances previous eradication of this bacterium should have eliminated the need for continuing medical therapy. Most patients currently on acid-suppressing therapy usually require this for control of acid reflux, not ulcers.

Risks

- Acid aspiration during anaesthesia.
- Acute ulceration ± bleeding after major surgery.

Preoperative care

Major gastro-oesophageal reflux disease
- Advise anaesthetist.
- Preoperative therapy to reduce risks of regurgitation during anaesthesia (prophylaxis of acid aspiration). Omeprazole 20 mg bd for 3 days preoperative results in maximal acid suppression. Omeprazole 40 mg on the preceding evening then 40 mg 2–6 h before surgery (as recommended in the BNF) is almost as effective. Some anaesthetists use ranitidine preoperatively and sodium citrate 30 ml just before induction.

Give specific drugs as follows:
- Antacids: Continue current formulation or change to oral sodium citrate 30 ml qds.
- H_2 receptor antagonists: Change to ranitidine 50 mg i/v tds until able to take H_2 receptor antagonist orally.
- Proton pump inhibitors: Continue on oral therapy if possible (open and dissolve capsule contents in water and give via naso-gastric tube). Pantoprazole 40 mg can be given by slow i/v injection over >2 min.

Table 30.1 Perioperative drug therapy for patients with acid-peptic disease

NSAIDs and aspirin	Stop
Steroids	Switch to i/v, see Chapter 23
Antacids	Change to oral sodium citrate 30 ml qds
Proton pump inhibitors	Continue on oral therapy if possible (open and dissolve capsule contents in water and give via n/g tube). Consider i/v pantoprazole (see above)
H_2 receptor antagonists	Change to ranitidine 50 mg i/v tds until able to take it po

Hepatic disease

Patients with hepatic disease may need surgery for problems directly related to their liver disease – particularly for control of GI bleeding. Other patients present for unrelated surgery with stable compensated chronic liver disease. Those with alcoholic liver disease may develop delirium secondary to alcohol withdrawal (see p. 231).

Acute hepatocellular disease is usually due to injury by either viruses or toxins (usually drugs). In contrast acute jaundice, especially post-operatively, may be caused by additional mechanisms such as haemo-lysis (infection, cold agglutinins, transfusion reaction), biliary tract obstruction (by stone or ligature), and congestive cardiac failure (causing hepatic venous congestion).

Chronic liver damage results in cell necrosis, fibrosis and cell regeneration. In the early stages the liver is enlarged, later becoming small and shrunken as cirrhosis progresses. The fibrosis results in portal hypertension, and the cell necrosis eventually causes liver failure.

Causes

- In children: congenital, biliary atresia, metabolic diseases, viral hepatitis.
- In adults: hepatitis B or C virus infection, alcohol, primary biliary cirrhosis, chronic active hepatitis, haemochromatosis, idiopathic.
- Hepatocellular disease may be acute or chronic. Patients can be categorized according to hepatic or non-hepatic surgery.

Risks

- Decompenastion of chronic liver disease (i.e. development of hepatic failure) precipitated by sepsis, hypotension, bleeding, and catabolism.
- Bleeding.
- Acute renal failure.

History

- May help identify the type and cause of liver disease.
- Ask for previous symptoms of upper GI bleeding, ulcers, or past intervention, e.g. ulcer surgery, variceal sclerotherapy or resection, surgical shunt, or TIPSS.

Examination

- Look for signs of chronic liver disease and for decompensation, e.g. oedema, ascites, liver flap, jaundice.
- Assess conscious level.
- Assess nutritional state.
- Score the patient according to the Child–Pugh classification (Table 30.2). This is the most useful guide to grading surgical risk.

Investigations

- Serology for hepatitis viruses A, B, and C.
- FBC, creatinine, urea, electrolytes, LFTs.
- Clotting studies.

Preoperative therapy

Remember universal precautions against BBVs.

Control of GI bleeding

- Upper GI blood loss is treated as for any shocked patient (p. 253). Consider HDU/ICU admission.

Table 30.2 Child–Pugh prognostic scoring of chronic liver disease

Marker	Score		
	0	**1**	**2**
Renal function (creatinine level)	Normal	<177 μmol/l	>177 μmol/l
Glasgow coma scale	15	10–14	<10
Respiration	Normal	Ventilated or PaO_2< 8 kPa	
Age	≤60	>60	
INR	≤1.3	>1.3	

Child–Pugh score	Risk	Mortality at 1 month
<2	Low	12%
2–3	Medium	40%
>3	High	74%

- Variceal bleeding may be controlled by endoscopic injection sclerotherapy, endoscopic variceal band ligation. Tamponade using a four-lumen Sengstaken–Blakemore tube is much less effective.
- These procedures may be combined with drugs such as vasopressin, glypressin, or octreotide to reduce splanchnic blood flow (and thereby portal hypertension).
- Seek the help of an experienced endoscopist or gastroenterologist.
- The safe insertion, management and removal of a Sengstaken–Blakemore tube requires much experience.
- Patients with GI bleeding not responding to medical therapy should be considered for urgent surgery before further deterioration occurs.
- Correct clotting abnormalities with FFP.
- Vitamin K is usually of little benefit in the presence of intrinsic liver disease.

Management of ascites
- Massive ascites may need abdominal paracentesis.
- Up to 10 l may be removed in a day.
- Give albumin 20% solution 100 ml i/v with every third litre of ascites drained to maintain intravascular volume.
- Gelatin solution 500 ml may be substituted for albumin.
- The safest method is to use a peritoneal dialysis catheter (e.g. Bonano) and insert it about 5–10 cm below the umbilicus in the midline.
- Beware spontaneous bacterial peritonitis.

Fluid and electrolyte imbalance

- Hyponatraemia is common in liver failure/decompensation, partly because of diuretics.
- Consider fluid balance and possible fluid/water overload.
- Avoid infusion of saline, normal, or otherwise.
- Hyperkalemia may occur because of potassium sparing diuretics (spironolactone, amiloride).
- Consider switching to loop diuretics if K^+ >5.0 mmol/l, but this may contribute to hyponatraemia.
- Renal impairment is a serious complication of hepatic disease, and requires specialist help. Contact renal physician or ICU team.
- Establish an i/v line for patients unable to take oral fluids: use glucose saline 2000 ml/day, and add K^+ if serum K^+ <4.0 mmol/l. Beware of fluid overload and worsening hyponatraemia.
- In severe hepatic disease hypoglycaemia is common: substitute with glucose 10–20% at 50–100 ml/h, and monitor blood glucose frequently.
- Cross-match blood and FFP as appropriate to procedure.

Precautions

- Remember that portal hypertension will dramatically increase blood loss during all abdominal procedures.
- Warn the operating theatre staff if the patient has positive hepatitis viral serology.
- ICU care will be needed for Child's category B and C patients, and for patients undergoing portosystemic shunting procedures.

Postoperative care

- Morphine i/v for analgesia, usually by intermittent boluses, but beware of longer half-life in liver disease and chance of increasing encephalopathy.
- Avoid any high protein enteral feeds: low-protein, high-carbohydrate is best.
- Close monitoring of renal function with hourly urine output.
- Hypotension or hypoxia may result in severe hepatic decompensation unless treated urgently. Patients with chronic liver impairment may develop a vasodilated pattern of hypotension requiring inotropic therapy on ICU.
- Changes in conscious level may represent hepatic encephalopathy, without classical signs such as flapping tremor. Seek expert advice from a gastroenterologist.
- Following major surgery a daily coagulation screen should be performed. A raised INR is one of the most sensitive indicators of liver synthetic function. Regular (6–12 hourly) bedside estimations of

blood glucose estimations (e.g. BM stick) should be carried out until stable.

- Changes in liver function should be expected whenever a patient with underlying liver disease has a major GI bleed. Many will progress to multi-organ failure with mortality over 50%.

Obstructive jaundice

Jaundice in the context of liver disease is discussed in the preceding section. Jaundice arises more often from biliary obstruction, without significant liver disease being present.

Causes of obstructive jaundice include:

- gallstones
- pancreatic cancer
- sclerosing cholangitis
- cholangiocarcinoma
- surgical damage to the biliary tree.

Normal current practice is to decompress a potentially infected biliary tree by ERCP before any definitive surgery. This reduces perioperative morbidity and mortality, but they remain high.

Perioperative risks

- *Acute renal failure:* Bilirubin itself may have toxic effects on the kidney. Sepsis is common, and bacteraemia is triggered by operation on an infected biliary tree.
- *Septic shock and multiorgan failure.*
- *Bleeding:* Platelet count may be low from septicaemia. Fat-soluble clotting factor deficiency may prolong the INR.
- *High mortality:* If cholangitis is present, then the presence of three or more of the following factors predicts a mortality as high as 50%:
  - major cardiorespiratory disease
  - pH<7.4
  - bilirubin >90 mmol/l
  - platelet count <150 × 10⁹/l
  - albumin <30 g/l.
- If possible, decompress an *infected biliary tree* by ERCP rather than by open surgery.

Preoperative preparation of the jaundiced patient

- Avoid morphine as it constricts the biliary sphincter. Use pethidine.
- Avoid dehydration. Give 1000 ml 0.9% saline i/v over 6–12 h preoperatively before the induction of anaesthesia (unless CCF present).

- Monitor urine output via a bladder catheter.
- Give 500 ml 10% mannitol over 20–30 min either an hour before, or following induction of anaesthesia.
- Correct coagulation defects.
- Prophylactic antibiotics as in Chapter 17.

During surgery

- Hourly urine output monitoring.
- Give further mannitol (100 ml 10%) if urine output <60 ml/h.

Postoperative care

- Monitor urine hourly.
- Give 100 ml mannitol 10% over 15 min if urine output <50 ml/h for 2 consecutive hours.
- Keep careful fluid balance, using a CVP if necessary.
- Check electrolytes and creatinine daily.

Table 30.3 Perioperative prescribing in liver disease

Diuretics	Usually switch to i/v aldosterone antagonists such as sodium carenoate
NSAIDs	Stop
Isoniazid/methyldopa	Stop
Alcohol	Stop
Anticoagulants	Discontinue if INR or APTR >2.0

Malnutrition

Malnutrition is common in surgical practice, typically in the following situations:

- Gastrointestinal surgery for chronic GI disease (e.g. Crohn's disease).
- In elderly patients with chronic heart, pulmonary, or renal disease.
- Postoperatively in patients with prolonged ileus or with major complications.

History should determine cause and duration of malnutrition.

Examination should look for signs of causative illness (e.g. ulcerative colitis, anorexia nervosa) and include assessment of nutritional status (weight, skin fold thickness, upper arm girth)

Investigations

- Height and weight: compare these to previously documented values and calculate BMI.
- CXR: for signs of opportunistic infection.

- Hb, red cell indices. If abnormal check B_{12}, folate, and ferritin.
- Electrolytes, Ca^{2+}, Mg^{2+}.
- LFTs: hepatic disease may be causative or consequent.
- CK MM fraction may be elevated due to muscle breakdown in severe malnutrition.

Therapy

- Consider transfusion of packed cells if Hb < 9 g/dl.
- Contact hospital nutrition team or ICU team for advice on subsequent nutrition. **Do not begin TPN without senior advice.** See section on nutrition (p. 87).
- Contact anaesthetist as operative risk may be high.
- Arrange pressure area assessment through senior nurse on ward.
- Contact tissue viability nurse for existing skin damage.

Postoperative care

The section on nutrition (Chapter 18, p. 87) gives specific guidance on postoperative nutritional support.

Table 30.4 Perioperative prescribing for malnourished patients

Multivitamin preparations	Switch to i/v preparation
Insulin	May require sliding scale i/v: see Chapter 26
H2 blockers	Switch to ranitidine 50 mg i/v tds
Anticoagulants	Stop if central feeding line to be inserted Otherwise continue

Inflammatory bowel disease

Patients with inflammatory bowel disease (IBD) may require surgery for their disease itself, or need other forms of surgery by chance.

The main risks of surgery in these patients results from the following factors:

- Immunosuppressive therapy: Poor wound healing, increased infection rate, pressure sores.
- Chronic malnutrition: As above.
- Fluid and electrolyte depletion: Risk of renal failure, cardiac arrhythmias.

It follows that surgery has least risk when the patient is on minimal immunosuppressive therapy together with minimal disease activity. Elective surgery should be deferred until the patient is in the best possible condition. Urgent surgery, either for IBD, or in those with incidental IBD, may mean a less than ideally prepared patient.

Bowel perforation or toxic bowel dilatation necessitates emergency surgery, and the risks are always high.

History and examination

- Assess disease activity: recent weight gain/loss, blood loss in stools, general condition.
- Identify of complications, e.g. fistulae, abscesses.
- Assess nutritional state (see section on malnutrition above).

Investigations

- Hb, ESR.
- Electrolytes, creatinine, urea, LFTs, serum albumin. **Do not take blood from a dedicated TPN line.**
- Erect chest and abdomen plain films may be necessary for surgical evaluation.
- Stools for culture and microscopy.

Therapy

- Hypokalemia < 4.0 mmol/l should be treated with i/v infusions containing K^+ preferably added by the manufacturer or by pharmacy (see hypokalaemia, p. 308). In severe diarrhoea 120–240 mmol K^+/day may be required
- Anaemia Hb < 9 g/dl indicates blood transfusion.
- ESR > 30 mm/h and active rectal bleeding usually indicates active disease: liaise with senior surgical and medical staff
- Hypoalbuminaemia < 30 g/l will require intensive nutritional supplementation.
- Severe acute colitis may present with all the signs of haemorrhagic shock and resuscitation should be immediate. Urgent surgery may be required.
- Pain may require i/v opioids: pethidine is often preferred to morphine because the former causes less smooth muscle spasm. i/v PCA probably provides the best pain control.
- If patient is likely to require a stoma during surgery, contact stoma care team for preoperative counselling.

Postoperative care

As for major bowel surgery.

- In patients on steroids, postoperative anastamotic breakdown may occur with few specific signs. Pulmonary infections and other septic complications may also present late.
- Enteral nutrition may be delayed for some days: consider TPN via a dedicated feeding line. Contact nutrition team or ICU team.
- Check Hb, electrolytes, and creatinine daily.

Table 30.5 Perioperative prescribing in IBD

Rectal steroids	Replace with i/v hydrocortisone prior to surgery, and afterwards if colostomy is performed
Oral steroids	Replace with i/v hydrocortisone while patient is nil-by-mouth. See Chapter 26, p. 167
Sulphasalazine	Continue up to day of operation
NSAIDs	**Avoid**, because of GI bleed risk

Further reading

Lai EC, Tam PC, Paterson IA, Ng MM, Fan ST, Choi TK, Wong J (1990). Emergency surgery for severe acute cholangitis. The high risk patients. *Annals of Surgery* 211:55–9.

Lai EC, Chu KM, Lo CY *et al.* (1992). Surgery for malignant obstructive jaundice: analysis of mortality. *Surgery* 112:891–6.

Lehnert T, Herfarth C (1993). Peptic ulcer surgery in patients with liver cirrhosis. *Annals of Surgery* 217:338–46.

Haematological disorders

Richard Lee and John Purday

Anaemia

Defined as a haemoglobin concentration below the normal for the age and sex, anaemia is common in patients undergoing surgery. It usually results from blood loss (acute or chronic) but also from failure of production or haemolysis and is conventionally diagnosed when the haemoglobin (Hb) concentration is < 13 g/dl in an adult male and < 12 g/dl in an adult female. However, most anaesthetists would be happy with a Hb > 10 g/dl depending on the patient's physiological reserves and the expected blood losses. If in doubt, the anaesthetist must be contacted.

The common causes of anaemia in the surgical patient are:

- *Blood loss* which is either acute, as in trauma when the body will often also show signs of hypovolaemia, or may be chronic when compensatory mechanisms have increased plasma volume thereby preserving circulating volume.

- *Bone marrow failure* due to infiltration by tumour or suppression by drugs, e.g. cytotoxic drugs, indomethacin, and chloramphenicol. These patients often present with symptoms and signs related to the failure of platelet or white cell production such as bleeding or infection.

- *Megaloblastic anaemias* due to either folate or vitamin B_{12} deficiency. Folate stores can commonly become depleted in pregnancy, malnutrition, malabsorption and haemolysis. B_{12} deficiency is usually due to parietal cell and intrinsic factor antibodies (pernicious anaemia) but can rarely be due to gastrectomy, intestinal blind loops or Crohn's disease.

- *Complex anaemias* due to problems with production and breakdown of Hb, e.g. renal failure, rheumatoid arthritis, and hypothyroidism.

- *Haemolytic anaemias* are either inherited (e.g. the thalassaemias, sickle cell, and spherocytosis); acquired, e.g. auto-immune (often drugs or infections); or physical (mechanical heart valves, disseminated intravascular coagulation – DIC, and jogging).

History

- Often difficult to diagnose clinically.
- Associated with non-specific symptoms of fatigue, dyspnoea, palpitations, headaches, and angina; the severity often reflects the speed of onset more than the degree of anaemia because there is less time for adaptation in the cardiovascular system and in the O_2-dissociation curve of Hb.
- Symptoms from the commonest causes should be elicited including relevant family history; always enquire about aspirin, NSAIDs, and alcohol.
- Important areas for enquiry include the respiratory and cardiovascular history which may be worsened by the anaemia or make its impact greater. For example, angina may be worsened by a decrease in the O_2-carrying capacity of the blood.

Examination

- Look for signs of hypotension in acute blood loss and signs of cardiac failure in chronic anaemia.
- Also, look for signs from the common causes (as previously listed).

Investigations

Blood counts should be performed routinely prior to surgery according to the schedule on p. 24, but also in anyone:

- at risk of anaemia
- undergoing major surgery
- with other significant medical problems, especially heart or lung disease.

Much can be deduced from the Hb and MCV alone, but in many instances, a blood film gives additional useful information. Confirmatory tests such as ferritin, B_{12}, and folate levels, reticulocyte count, direct Coombs test, ESR, liver and renal function, and bone marrow should be requested as appropriate. Further investigations (what and when) of any abnormalities will be dictated by the clinical situation.

Preoperative preparation

Ideally, patients scheduled for elective surgery should have their FBC checked in the weeks approaching the operation so that abnormalities such as anaemia can then be investigated and corrected in time. If delaying surgery is possible, it is more appropriate and far safer to treat the underlying cause and to raise the Hb slowly with simple, effective measures, e.g. oral iron or B_{12} injections. Transfusing a patient with chronic anaemia may precipitate heart failure.

Perioperative considerations

Blood transfusion

When should a red cell transfusion be given? A better appreciation of the potential risks of allogeneic blood has led to a more conservative approach to transfusion support. Although in general blood transfusion is safe, the associated risks are important because they may have permanent implications for the patient. Patients who need transfusion may be anxious about the risks of blood and require reassurance.

Unfortunately, there are no evidence-based guidelines that set clear target levels for transfusion. In addition as Hb decreases cardiac output increases, owing to a decrease in blood viscosity, and O_2 delivery may be maintained.

- Maintenance of circulating volume is crucial perioperatively. Carefully consider the fluids administered to prevent significant haemodilution, which is commonly seen in patients actively bleeding.

- Most healthy patients without evidence of cardio-respiratory compromise can function with a Hb of 8–10 g/dl. However, although unsupported by clinical evidence, a Hb of 10 g/dl (haematocrit of 30%) is often quoted as the lowest acceptable level.

- Each case must be assessed with a view to coexistent disease, expected intra-operative blood loss, and whether acute or chronic. Decide the acceptable Hb for the patient and aim to maintain this level with a combination of i/v blood and clear fluids.

- Patients with significant ischaemic heart or respiratory disease will need a Hb of at least 10 g/dl to avoid problems such as angina.

- Patients requiring urgent surgery may need preoperative blood transfusion if found to be unacceptably anaemic preoperatively. The advantages of preoperative transfusion include, better Hb function (release of O_2 peripherally), and a more stable blood volume before surgery. Whenever possible transfuse these patients the day before operation.

- Jehovah's Witnesses have a special consent form to refuse blood products; once this is signed, any doctor who gives blood can be charged with assault. The use of cell saver and isovolaemic haemodilution techniques (see later) is often allowed and should be discussed with the patient.

· If in doubt it is usually best to contact the anaesthetist.

Complications of blood transfusion

· *Mismatch*: Most commonly due to giving the wrong blood to the patient. The transfusion must be immediately stopped, the unit returned to the blood bank and FBC, clotting, and serum samples sent. Signs and symptoms of a transfusion reaction are present and a haematologist should be contacted.

· *Transfusion reactions*: Aute allergic reactions with fever, sweating, tachycardia and urticaria are not uncommon (2%). Antipyretics and antihistamines (paracetamol 1 g and chlorpheniramine 10 mg i/v) may be given and the transfusion continued slowly (over 4 h). The blood should be stopped if a haemolytic reaction is suspected (hypotension, back and chest pains, oliguria, and haemoglobinuria). Manage this as a mismatched transfusion. i/v hydrocortisone 100 mg may be necessary for severe reactions.

· *Metabolic*: With large volume, rapid infusions acidosis and hypocalcaemia (from the citrate anticoagulant) and hyperkalaemia.

· *Hypothermia*: Particularly in large volume transfusion unless the blood is adequately warmed.

· *Circulatory overload*: Particularly in patients with cardiac failure.

· Dilutional coagulopathy – clotting factors and platelets only survive a few days. In patients with normal underlying coagulation check for this complication after the equivalent of a 60% circulating volume transfusion.

· *Cross-infection*: The BBVs, e.g. HIV, hepatitis B and C (although screened, donors may donate prior to seroconversion) and also bacteria and malaria.

· *Massive transfusion* exacerbates all these problems but can also lead to acute lung injury after several days.

Group & save or cross-match?

· Once grouped and saved, blood can usually be cross-matched within half an hour if the antibody screen is negative. Many patients need only be grouped and saved prior to surgery.

· Patients who should be cross-matched include those patients who have a decreased preoperative Hb and those operations with a high chance of intra-operative blood loss (see p. 24).

Suggested procedure for transfusion
Always follow your hospital's policy.

· Check unit of blood against blood form and patient's arm band.

· Only use a blood giving set, and if multiple units are planned an approved blood warmer should be considered.

- Give a unit over 2–3 h unless there is active bleeding where the rate should be determined by clinical circumstances.
- Look for signs of an allergic reaction (as above) which are likely to present early. (This is difficult in rapid transfusion.)
- In cases of severe haemorrhage, type specific blood may be obtained usually within 10 min – provided the sample has reached the laboratory!

Blood conservation techniques

With increasing awareness of the complications of blood transfusion, these techniques are becoming more widespread.

- Many larger centres have facilities for patients to pre-donate their own blood (with or without the use of erythropoietin) in the weeks leading up to the surgery. This is only of use in elective surgery.
- Haemodilution techniques allow for the removal of 1–2 units of blood at the start of an operation, which are immediately replaced by saline. During the surgery, the blood lost by the patient has a lower Hb and the whole blood is re-infused at the end of the procedure. The blood should not be out of the patient for longer than 4 h.
- Blood salvage techniques include the use of cell savers and re-infusion of drains and can be used for:
  - Procedures with expected blood loss greater than 1 l, e.g. aortic aneurysm repair, hip revisions, trauma, major spinal and urological surgery, etc.
  - Jehovah's Witnesses where blood loss > 1 l is expected.
  - Contraindications to the re-infusion of salvaged blood include tumour and bacterial contamination.

Postoperative care

Considerable fluid redistribution occurs following major blood loss in the first 24–48 h. The Hb should be checked regularly if blood continues to be lost. A portable meter such as the Haemocue is the most convenient method. In most patients, the Hb should be measured the day after any surgery where significant blood loss has occurred.

Indications for postoperative blood transfusion are similar to those for perioperative transfusion. Patients with proven iron deficiency, in whom the cause has been removed, should continue with oral iron for at least 3 months after the Hb has been normalized in order for iron stores to be replenished.

Coagulation disorders

Abnormalities of coagulation are common in patients on surgical wards, often in association with bleeding.

- Trauma or surgery may reveal congenital disorders in adult life.

- Acquired disorders are due to lack of coagulation factor synthesis, increased loss due to consumption or massive blood loss, or the production of substances that interfere with their function.

- A family history may be elicited (haemophilia A and B are sex linked recessives, von Willebrand's disease is autosomal dominant with variable penetrance) but cannot be relied on. A family history is absent in 30% of haemophiliacs!

- Response to previous haemostatic challenges (tonsillectomy, dental extractions) may indicate the severity of the coagulopathy, e.g. in severe haemophilia A (factor VIII <2%) bleeding occurs spontaneously; in mild haemophilia (factor VIII 5–30%) bleeding occurs only after trauma.

- Concurrent and past medical problems such as liver disease, malabsorption (vitamin K deficiency), infection, malignancy (DIC), autoimmune disease (SLE, RA) as well as medications (anticoagulants, aspirin, and NSAIDs) may be relevant.

Laboratory investigations

The usual screening tests of bleeding (Table 31.1) include a platelet count, prothrombin time or international normalized ratio (PT/INR),

Table 31.1 Laboratory investigation results in common bleeding disorders

Disorder	Platelet count	INR	APTT	TT	Fibrinogen	Other
Haemophilia A	N	N	↑	N	N	↓ VIII
Haemophilia B	N	N	↑	N	N	↓ IX
vWD	N (usually)	N	↑	N	N	↓ VIII, vWF ↑ bleeding time
Liver disease	N or ↓	↑	↑	N	N or ↓	↓ V
Vitamin K deficiency	N	↑	↑	N	N	↓ II, VII, IX, X
DIC	N or ↓	↑	↑	↑↑	N or ↓	↑ FDPs, d-dimers ↓ II, V, VIII
Massive transfusion	↓	↑	↑	N or ↑	N or ↓	N FDPs
Heparin (unfractionated)	N (rarely ↓)	N or ↑	↑↑	↑↑	N	^ anti-Xa
Heparin (LMW)	N (rarely ↓)	N	N	N	N	^ anti-Xa
Warfarin	N	↑↑	↑	N	N	↓ II, VII, IX, X
Lupus anticoagulant	N	N or ↑	↑↑	N	N	DRVVT +ve, cardiolipin antibody

activated partial thromboplastin time (APTT), thrombin time (TT), fibrinogen. Specific factor assays are dictated by the pattern of abnormalities in the initial screen and usually follow discussion with a haematologist. Circulating anticoagulants, e.g. antibodies to factor VIII or von Willebrand factor, are often secondary to SLE, RA, or malignancy. Management is difficult and surgery should be avoided if possible. Lupus anticoagulants are not uncommon, are often not associated with SLE, and are considered a risk for thrombosis rather than bleeding; however, they may be of no clinical significance if transient (e.g. following viral infections).

Preoperative preparation

- An unexpected abnormality in the coagulation screen should be investigated before surgery by seeking advice from a haematologist.

- Anticoagulation guidelines in the UK recommend that for minor surgical procedures the warfarin dose is stopped or adjusted to achieve an INR of approximately 2.0 on the day of surgery; for major surgery, warfarin should be stopped at least 3 days before, and depending on the thrombotic risk of the condition for which the patient is anticoagulated, the INR can be monitored and if necessary heparin instituted once the INR is below the lower limit of the therapeutic range. It typically takes 4 days for the INR to reach 1.5 after warfarin is stopped if the INR is normally 2–3 (the elderly may take longer).

- Anticoagulation in patients with prosthetic heart valves can be temporarily discontinued for 4 days before surgery and restarted as soon as possible after surgery as the short-term risk of thromboembolism in these patients is small. When it is not possible to restart warfarin immediately post surgery, and in patients deemed at especially high risk of thromboembolism, the use of heparin for an interim period may be considered. In emergency surgery, FFP may need to be given. See p. 145 for further details.

   All these patients are best discussed with the anaesthetist, haematologist and cardiologist.

- Previously untreated mild haemophilia requires strenuous efforts at avoiding blood products. If factor concentrates are necessary, the treatment of choice is now recombinant factors in accordance with established guidelines. Always involve a haemophilia specialist. DDAVP or tranexamic acid may be used in addition, if appropriate.

- Abnormalities due to liver disease or vitamin K deficiency should be given vitamin K (phytomenadione) 10 mg slowly i/v. FFP (15 ml/kg) may be needed in addition if the presenting symptom is bleeding.

Perioperative and postoperative management

DIC is probably the commonest cause of a significant coagulation abnormality in the surgical setting, particularly in the peri- and postoperative phase. It is associated with infections (especially gram −ve bacteraemia), placental abruption, amniotic fluid embolism, major trauma, burns, hypoxia, hypovolaemia, and severe liver disease. Haemorrhage, thrombosis, or both may occur. Chronic DIC is associated with aneurysms, haemangiomas, and carcinomatosis.

The laboratory abnormalities are variable, depending on the severity of the DIC, and reflect both consumption of platelets and coagulation factors as well as hyperplasminaemia and fibrinolysis.

- Treatment should be aimed primarily at removal or control of the underlying cause whilst support is given to maintain tissue perfusion and oxygenation.

- Abnormal coagulation parameters in the presence of bleeding or need for an invasive procedure are indications for haemostatic support. Transfusion of platelets (for advice see under thrombocytopenia) and FFP (15 ml/kg initially or 4 U in an average adult) should help restore platelets, coagulation factors and the natural anticoagulants, antithrombin, and protein C. Cryoprecipitate (10 U initially) may also be necessary if the fibrinogen level cannot be raised above 1 g/l by FFP alone.

- The indications for heparin and concentrates of antithrombin and protein C are not established. Anti-fibrinolytics such as tranexamic acid are generally contraindicated in DIC. Intramuscular injections, aspirin, and NSAIDs should be avoided in any patient at risk of bleeding; the i/v and subcutaneous routes are acceptable.

Massive transfusion of stored blood perioperatively may cause significant dilutional coagulation disorders owing to the lack of factors V, VIII, and XI. DIC, which can be precipitated by shock, is often also present. In addition, thrombocytopenia is a frequent occurrence. Therapy consists of replacement FFP and platelets as guided by coagulation tests.

Guidelines for fresh frozen plasma administration

- The usual starting dose is 12–15 ml/kg which raises the coagulation levels 12–15%.

- FFP takes 20 min to thaw and the infusion should be commenced within 2 h of thawing and be complete within 4 h of thawing.

- Definite indications for use are life-threatening haemorrhage with overdose of coumarin anticoagulants or vitamin K deficiency and acute DIC.

- Conditional indications include massive blood transfusion (bleeding is usually secondary to thrombocytopenia) and liver disease.

- Regular checks of coagulation should be made to assess the underlying trend and the efficacy of treatment.

Thrombocytopenia

Thrombocytopenia may be due to:

- failure of platelet production, either selectively (hereditary, drugs, alcohol, viral infection) or as part of general marrow failure (aplasia, cytotoxics, radiotherapy, infiltration, fibrosis, myelodysplasia, megaloblastic anaemia)
- increased platelet consumption, with an immune basis (ITP, drugs, viral infections, SLE, lymphoproliferative disorders) or without an immune basis (DIC, TTP, cardiopulmonary bypass)
- dilution, following massive transfusion of stored blood to bleeding patients (usually after transfusion of more than one blood volume).
- splenic pooling (hypersplenism)

Note: renal failure and aspirin can impair platelet function.

Laboratory features

Unexpected thrombocytopenia should always be confirmed with another sample and a blood film.

- The blood film will exclude pseudo-thrombocytopenia due to platelet clumping (caused by EDTA anticoagulant with a prevalence of 0.1%) and may provide diagnostic clues such as leukaemic cells, leuco-erythroblastic picture, giant platelets (e.g. May–Hegglin anomaly), large platelets (e.g. ITP), small platelets (e.g. Wiskott–Aldrich syndrome), red cell fragmentation (DIC, TTP).
- Abnormal coagulation associated with thrombocytopenia suggests the possibility of DIC or liver disease or rarely von Willebrand's disease type IIB.
- The bone marrow will distinguish marrow failure from other causes of thrombocytopenia.
- Platelet antibody tests have not been shown to be important for routine diagnosis and management, but may be useful in special circumstances, e.g. anti-HPA-1A in neonatal alloimmune thrombocytopenia.

Clinical features

Spontaneous bleeding is rare above a platelet count of $50 \times 10^9/l$. Minor bleeding (purpura, epistaxis) may occur below this level. Serious spontaneous haemorrhage (GI bleeding, haematuria, cerebral haemorrhage) is unlikely above a count of $10 \times 10^9/l$ unless there is concurrent coagulopathy or infection. For a given degree of thrombocytopenia, the risk of bleeding is lower in ITP than in marrow failure – probably because young platelets in ITP are larger.

Preoperative preparation

- Unexplained thrombocytopenia should be investigated before elective surgery as the appropriate precautions will be determined by the underlying cause.

- Minor procedures such as bone marrow biopsy may be performed without platelet support provided adequate pressure to the wound is applied.

- For procedures such as insertion of central lines, transbronchial biopsy, liver biopsy or laparotomy, the platelet count should be raised to at least $50 \times 10^9/l$. For epidural or spinal anaesthesia the platelet count should be $100 \times 10^9/l$.

- For operations in critical sites such as the brain or eyes, the platelet count should be raised to $100 \times 10^9/l$.

- In ITP platelet transfusions should be reserved for major haemorrhage. Preparation for surgery entails the use of steroids or high dose immunoglobulins initially.

Platelet transfusions

A standard adult therapeutic pack has the platelets from 6 blood units and contains $>240 \times 10^9$ platelets. Transfusion will on average raise the platelet count by $20–40 \times 10^9/l$ in an adult, providing there are no complicating risk factors such as sepsis or splenomegaly.

Platelets must be given either through a fresh blood-giving set or through a special platelet giving set.

Perioperative management

- Efforts directed at minimizing trauma and achieving surgical haemostasis pay dividends.

- Monitor platelet count and give platelets as necessary to maintain a safe level till wound healing is well advanced.

- If microvascular bleeding continues despite a platelet count of $>50 \times 10^9/l$ suspect DIC; if confirmed by coagulation tests give FFP and cryoprecipitate as appropriate.

- Intramuscular injections and analgesics containing aspirin or NSAIDs should be avoided.

- Remember with renal failure and aspirin abnormal platelet function may cause bleeding with normal platelet counts. DDAVP (desmopressin) 0.3 μg/kg in 50 ml 0.9% saline over 30 min may improve platelet function in renal failure.

Sickle cell disease

The term sickle cell disease (SCD) refers to the group of clinically significant haemoglobinopathies which have in common the inheritance of sickle Hb, either in the homozygous state (HbSS, sickle cell anaemia) or in combination with another Hb β-chain abnormality such as Hb C (HbSC disease), Hb D (HbSD disease) or β-thalassaemia (HbS/β-thal).

It is estimated that there are now over 10 000 patients with SCD in Britain. SCD is endemic in parts of Africa, the Mediterranean, Middle East, and India. The highest incidence is from equatorial Africa; therefore, **all black patients should have a sickle test preoperatively.**

Susceptibility to sickling is proportional to the concentration of HbS. In the heterozygous state (sickle cell trait), sickling is uncommon, as the HbS concentration is <50%. HbC and HbD in association with HbS enhances the sickling process whereas HBF impedes it. Apart from hypoxia, hypothermia, pyrexia, acidosis, and dehydration (often associated with infection) are known to precipitate sickle crises. The pathology of SCD is primarily a result of vaso-occlusion by sickled red cells leading to haemolysis and tissue infarction.

Clinical features

- The manifestations of SCD do not become apparent before 3–4 months of age when the main switch from fetal to adult Hb occurs.

- There is great variability, not only between patients, but also within individual patients at different periods of life; many remain well most of the time.

- Vaso-occlusive crises are the most common cause of morbidity and mortality. The presentation may be dramatic with acute abdomen, 'acute chest syndrome', stroke, priapism, and painful dactylitis. By the time patients reach adulthood most will have small fibrotic spleens. A less acute complication is proliferative retinopathy due to retinal vessel occlusion and neovascularization (more common in HbSC disease).

- Aplastic crises are characterized by temporary shutdown of the marrow manifested by a precipitous fall in the Hb and absence of reticulocytes. Infection with parvovirus B19 and/or folate deficiency are often responsible.

- Sequestration crises occur mainly in children. Sudden massive pooling of red cells in the spleen can cause hypotension and severe exacerbation of anaemia with fatal consequences unless transfusion is given in time.

- Haemolytic crises, manifest by a fall in Hb and rise in reticulocytes and bilirubin, usually accompany vaso-occlusive crises. Chronic haemolysis leads to gallstones in virtually all patients with SCD though many remain asymptomatic.

Laboratory features

- The Hb is usually 6–9 g/dl, much lower than symptoms suggest. Reticulocytes are usually increased and the film shows sickled cells and target cells. Howell–Jolly bodies are present if the spleen is atrophic. Leucocytosis and thrombocytosis are common reactive features. In sickle cell trait the Hb and film are normal.

- Screening tests for sickling which rely on deoxygenation of HbS are positive in both HbSS and HbAS.
- Hb electrophoresis distinguishes SS, AS, and other haemoglobinopathies. Quantitation of the HbS level is important in certain clinical situations where a level <30% is aimed for to prevent repeated sickling. It is not necessary to wait for the results of electrophoresis before embarking on emergency surgery; a positive sickle test and the blood picture usually allow distinction between SCD and sickle cell trait. A mixed race patient always has trait.

Management

- As no effective routine treatment exists for SCD care is directed toward prophylaxis, support and treatment of complications. Folic acid supplements, pneumococcal and H. Influenzae type B (HIB) vaccinations and penicillin prophylaxis are recommended from an early age, preferably within a comprehensive care programme.
- For crises: Rest; rehydration with oral/i/v fluids; antibiotics if infection is suspected; maintain PaO_2; keep warm; prompt and effective analgesia including opioids.
- Blood transfusions may be life-saving, but the indications are limited. Exchange transfusions have a limited role in some vaso-occlusive crises (acute chest syndrome, stroke). Always discuss with a haematologist.

Preoperative preparation

Always seek expert advice from an anaesthetist and haematologist well before surgery. A sample for group and antibody screen should be sent well in advance as previously transfused sickle cell patients often have red cell antibodies.

Perioperative and postoperative care

Special attention must be given to the potential problems of hypoxia; dehydration, infection, and pain associated with anaesthesia and surgery in both SCD and sickle cell trait patients.

- Dehydration must be avoided by allowing oral fluids as late as possible, giving pre- and post-operative i/v fluids.
- Hypoxia must be prevented. Measure pulse oximetry and give O_2 where indicated.
- Regional anaesthesia is not contraindicated and tourniquets can be used if limbs are meticulously exsanguinated prior to inflation.

Haemoglobin SC disease

- Results from double heterozygosity for HbS and HbC.
- Affects 0.1% of American blacks.

- Intermediate in severity between sickle cell disease and trait.
- Patients develop anaemia, splenomegaly, jaundice, aseptic necrosis of the femoral head, hepatic disease, retinal disease, and bone marrow and splenic infarcts.
- Myocardial necrosis has been described after general anaesthesia.
- Management principles are as for sickle cell disease.

Rare blood disorders

Hereditary spherocytosis

- Autosomal dominant condition in which red cells have a smaller surface to volume ratio and are abnormally permeable to Na^+.
- The inflexible red cells are phagocytosed in the spleen resulting in microspherocytic anaemia with marked reticulocytosis. The cells' increased osmotic fragility is diagnostic.
- Splenomegaly is common. Splenectomy leads to a 50–70 % increase in red cell survival.
- Splenectomy should not be performed in children under 10 years of age, and should be preceded by pneumococcal, meningococcal and HIB vaccine and then lifelong oral penicillin, to help avoid infection.
- There are no particular anaesthetic considerations.

Glucose-6-phosphate dehydrogenase (G6PD) deficiency

- X-linked trait with variable penetrance in people from the Mediterranean and American blacks.
- The disease may afford some protection against malaria and is therefore prevalent in endemic areas.
- The G6PD enzyme is responsible for the production of NADPH which is involved in the cell's defence against oxidative stresses such as infections (usually viral, but also septicaemia, malaria, and pneumonia) or oxidative drugs (aspirin, quinolones, chloramphenicol, isoniazid, probenecid, primaquine, quinine, sulphonamides, naphthalene, and vitamin K).
- Additionally, drugs producing methaemoglobinaemia, such as sodium nitroprusside and prilocaine, are contraindicated, as patients are unable to reduce methaemoglobin, thereby diminishing O_2-carrying capacity.
- Classically, ingestion of broad (fava) beans results in haemolysis (favism).
- Usually the haemolysis of red cells occurs 2–5 days after exposure causing anaemia, haemoglobinaemia, abdominal pain, haemoglobinuria, and jaundice.

- Diagnosis is made by demonstration of Heinz bodies and red cell G6PD assay.
- Treatment includes discontinuation of the offending agent and transfusion may be required.

Thalassaemias

Thalassaemias are due to absent or deficient synthesis of α- or β-globin chains of Hb. The severity of these disorders is related to the degree of impaired globin synthesis.

- The hallmark of the disease is anaemia of variable degree.
- Diagnosis is confirmed by Hb electrophoresis and/or globin chain analysis.
- The disease is prevalent in peoples of Mediterranean (mainly β), African (α and β) and Asian (mainly α) extraction.
- Patients with α-thalassaemia have mild or moderate anaemia.
- Those with severe β-thalassaemia, also called thalassaemia major, are transfusion dependent.
- Since there is no iron excreting mechanism, the iron from the transfused blood builds up in the reticuloendothelial system, until it is saturated, when iron is deposited in parenchymal tissues, principally the liver, pancreas, and heart.
- Preoperative preparation should include assessment of the degree of major organ impairment (heart, liver, pancreas) secondary to iron overload.
- High-output congestive cardiac failure with intravascular volume overload is common in severe anaemia and should be treated pre-operatively by transfusion.
- Previous transfusion exposure may cause antibody production and therefore cross-matching may be prolonged.
- The exceedingly hyperplastic bone marrow of the major thalas-saemias may cause overgrowth and deformity of the facial bones leading to airway problems and make intubation difficult.

Further reading

Davies SC, Roberts-Harewood M (1997). Blood transfusion in sickle cell disease. *Blood Review* 11:57–71.

Dewhirst WE, Glass DD (1990). Hematological diseases. In Katz, Benumof, Kadis, eds. *Anaesthesia and uncommon diseases.* Philadelphia: WB Saunders, 378–436.

Guidelines for the use of fresh frozen plasma (1992). *Transfusion Medicine* 2:57–63.

Guidelines on platelet transfusions (1992). *Transfusion Medicine* 2:311–18.

Guidelines on therapeutic products to treat haemophilia and other hereditary coagulation disorders (1997). *Haemophilia* 3:63–77.

Guidelines on oral anticoagulation, 3rd edn (1998). *British Journal of Haematology* 101:374–87.

McClelland DBL ed. (1996). *Handbook of Transfusion Medicine*, 2nd edn. London: HMSO.

Stehling L (1996). Anaemia, haemoglobinopathies – anaesthetic considerations. In Prys-Roberts, Brown, eds. *International practice of anaesthesia*. Oxford: Butterworth-Heinemann, 1/42/1–1/42/10.

Vichinsky EP, Habernkern CM, Neumayr L *et al*. (1995). A comparison of conservative and aggressive transfusion regimens in the perioperative management of sickle cell disease. *New England Journal of Medicine* 333:206–13.

Vipond AJ, Caldicott LD (1998). Major vascular surgery in a patient with sickle cell disease. *Anaesthesia* 53:1204–6.

White RH, McKittrick T, Hutchinson R, Twitchell J (1995). Temporary discontinuation of warfarin therapy: changes in the international normalized ratio. *Annals of Internal Medicine* 122:40–2.

The geriatric patient

Anthony Nicholls

Surgical epidemiology in the elderly

Surgical mortality increases with age. Chronic medical disorders, delays in seeking surgical opinion and diagnostic delays increase morbidity and mortality. Medical causes of postoperative mortality outnumber surgical causes by 3 to 1. Cardiorespiratory disease is the commonest cause of postoperative death but infectious complications of abdominal surgery are also important.

- Autopsy studies of postoperative deaths in the elderly show pneumonia to be the commonest cause of death as well being the most commonly missed diagnosis. Other infections (including peritonitis), cardiac failure and PE also often undiagnosed before death. Cardiac deaths are common even in those without clinical evidence of heart disease.

- The commonest surgical procedures in the elderly are biliary procedures, hernia repair, colonic surgery for cancer, vascular procedures, prostatic resection, cataract removal, joint replacement, and repair of hip fracture. The combination of age and overt cardiovascular disease results in mortality as high as 15% in patients over 70 with heart disease undergoing all forms of surgery.

- Surgery for hip fracture poses a major challenge. Mortality after hip fracture is 7% at 1 month, 13% at 3 months and 24% at 12 months. Only 40% of 1 year survivors are independent for the full range of activities of daily living.

It is in the elderly that the most difficult decisions about whether or not surgery should be undertaken will be encountered. The risk of death will usually be significant and should not be underplayed in the consent process. The natural history of medical problems in the elderly may render surgical intervention futile.

Clinical problems in the elderly

Elderly patients with chronic heart, lung, renal, neurological, or other organ-specific disease need perioperative care along the lines suggested elsewhere in this book. Apparently fit elderly patients should always be evaluated carefully for cardiorespiratory disease, but successful outcomes of surgery in the elderly will also need an approach beyond that of organ-specific medicine.

The core skills of geriatric care are the search for hidden problems, the anticipation of unusual presentation of disease and the management of multiple pathology. Elderly care, and in particular rehabilitation after surgery, focuses more on functional disability rather than single-organ pathology. The key factors leading to ill-health in the elderly usually relate to one of the following areas:

- limited homeostatic reserve: temperature regulation, nutrition, immune response, renal function, pulmonary reserve, cardiac output
- falls and poor balance
- impaired mobility
- sensory impairment: visual and hearing loss
- urinary or faecal incontinence
- cognitive impairment: dementia, confusion and delirium
- iatrogenic disease, usually from medication.

The physiology of ageing

The physiological process of ageing is separate from clinical disease and functional impairment of any organ system may be exposed by the stress of surgery.

Respiratory system

- Total lung capacity decreases by 25% during ageing.
- Residual volume increases and inspiratory capacity decreases.
- Muscular strength and lung elasticity are reduced.
- Ageing impairs gas exchange, with lower PaO_2 in the elderly.

- Kyphosis also reduces lung capacity.

Heart

- Ejection fraction decreases with age.
- The physiological response to stress is blunted.
- The risk of silent coronary disease increases.
- Arterial wall stiffness increases and autoregulation of blood flow to brain and kidney is impaired.

Kidney

- Glomerular filtration rate decreases with age.
- Muscle bulk is reduced so creatinine production is lower. Modest elevation of the serum creatinine may conceal significant renal impairment.
- Ageing also impairs tubular function with reductions in both renal concentrating ability and free water clearance.
- Responses to both fluid loading and dehydration are diminished.

Nervous system

- Postural reflexes are impaired.
- Hearing, sight, and cognition diminish.

GI tract, nutrition, and metabolism

- Metabolic rate decreases with age.
- Muscle mass is reduced and chronic malnutrition is common.
- Gut transit time is increased but food absorption decreased.
- The reduced turgor and elasticity of skin makes it a less reliable indicator of hydration or nutrition.
- Bone density and mass are reduced.

Immune response

- Specific and non-specific immune responses are blunted.
- The white cell response to infection is reduced.
- Central temperature regulation may be compromised: infection may be present without significant fever.

Medical evaluation and stabilization before surgery

- Risk assessment is necessary for proper informed consent.
- Minimizing risk depends on the timing of surgery and perioperative precautions.

- Functional assessment of cardiac and lung function may be needed before elective surgery: treadmill testing and lung function tests will reliably identify those at highest risk.
- Urgent or emergency surgery may need to be delayed until full medical evaluation and optimal care of medical problems.

Prevention and management of postoperative complications

Infection

Trials in the elderly show that antibiotic prophylaxis with cephalo-sporins reduces wound infection rates by up to 45% in abdominal and orthopaedic surgery. Give first dose up to 2 h before surgery and continue for 24 h (see p. 78).

Venous thrombosis

PE is a common cause of death in the elderly. Venous thrombosis pro-phylaxis should be routine for most surgery in the elderly. Prophylaxis should be started on admission to the surgical ward in most elderly patients whether or not surgery is ultimately undertaken. See Chapter 13, p. 76.

Nutrition

- Malnutrition is associated with increased surgical morbidity and mortality in the elderly.
- Trials of nutritional supplementation show reduced length of hos-pital stay and reduced minor postoperative complications without reduced mortality.
- Oral protein supplementation is safe and beneficial, with nocturnal n/g feeding reserved for those with evidence of significant malnu-trition on admission.
- Parenteral nutrition has similar indications in the elderly as in other age groups. See section on nutrition (Chapter 18, p. 87).

Urinary tract management

- Urinary retention, incontinence, and infection are common post-operative complications in the elderly.
- Short-term catheterization is indicated for urine output monitor-ing in many elderly patients, particularly those with cardiac and renal disease. It is also helpful in immobile patients after orthopaedic and abdominal surgery.
- Urinary retention in elderly men can be minimized by catheter removal within 24 h if practical. The catheter should normally be removed last thing at night with the opportunity for normal voiding the following morning.

- Intermittent catheterization may be preferable to placement of an indwelling catheter.

Delirium

- Up to two thirds of elderly patients develop delirium postoperatively. These patients suffer increased length of stay, more complications, increased mortality, and increased risk of subsequent institutional care.
- Advanced age, history of cognitive impairment, severe illness, and history of heavy alcohol intake predispose to postoperative confusion. Precipitating factors include metabolic disturbance, dehydration, infection, hypoxia, alcohol withdrawal, urinary retention, change in environment, and various medications especially opioids.
- Aggressive management of infection, hypoxia, and hypotension in the elderly will reduce the frequency of delirium, but despite optimal care many elderly patients will suffer a period of confusion. The inevitability of this complication may need careful explanation to relatives.
- Detailed management and assessment of confusion is in Chapter 47, p. 326.

Rehabilitation

- Postoperative rehabilitation of the elderly will include:
  - physiotherapy directed at mobilization
  - occupational therapy to restore independence in activities of daily living
  - geriatrician advice on optimal medical therapy
  - social assessment
  - psychological support of patient and family
  - specialist nursing care.
- Transfer to an elderly care bed once immediate surgical support is no longer necessary has been shown to shorten hospital stay for many conditions, especially hip fracture.
- The section on team work on the surgical ward gives more guidance (Chapter 23, p. 115).

Medical follow up

- Elderly patients who develop significant medical problems during their surgical admission, or whose surgical admission was precipitated by a medical problem, should normally have medical or geriatric follow-up on discharge to reduce hospital readmission.
- Typical scenarios include falls leading to hip fracture, cardiac disease with systemic embolism, postoperative cardiac failure or infarction, drug toxicity.

Further reading

Committee of Management (1998). Symposium: Care of elderly people. *Prescribers Journal* **38**:197–255.

Morrison RS, Chassin MR, Siu AL (1998). The medical consultant's role in caring for patients with hip fracture. *Annals of Internal Medicine* **128**:1010–20.

Alcohol intoxication and chronic alcoholism

Colin Berry

Introduction

Alcoholism is drinking which results in impairment of physical and social health. Alcohol consumption contributes to 15–30% of male and 8–15% of female hospital admissions in the UK. Equivalent figures in the USA are slightly higher.

The causes of hospital admission are physical complications of excessive drinking, alcohol-related trauma, or neuropsychiatric illness related to alcohol consumption. Additionally, alcohol withdrawal symptoms commonly arise in patients admitted for unrelated medical or surgical problems.

Physical complications

- Many of the physical complications of alcohol abuse have implications for surgical and anaesthetic care, particularly after trauma.

Acute intoxication and coma

- Usually treated conservatively. Prevent airway obstruction and aspiration of vomit. May require ICU admission.

- Blood alcohol concentration >400 mg/100 ml puts patients at risk of respiratory arrest. Other causes for coma must also be sought in these patients (e.g. head injury, other drugs, methanol, metabolic causes, infection).
- Alcoholic coma has a mortality of up to 5%.

Alcoholic liver disease
Three phases are described:

- Fatty liver is reversible with abstinence and rarely causes illness.
- Alcoholic hepatitis is usually a progression from fatty liver. Characterized by abdominal pain, weight loss, jaundice and fever. Histological changes can be reversed by abstinence. Survival may be improved by corticosteroids in the early stages. Usually progresses to cirrhosis in women.
- Alcoholic cirrhosis is characterized by jaundice, ascites, portal hypertension, and hepatic failure. Cirrhosis is irreversible but abstinence may result in stabilization and increased life expectancy.

Pancreatitis
Both chronic and acute pancreatitis can be caused by alcohol misuse. The mortality rate in acute pancreatitis is 10–40%

Upper GI bleeding
- Gastritis, erosive gastric ulcers and Mallory–Weiss oesophageal tears.
- Oesophageal varices in those with severe liver disease and portal hypertension.

Cardiovascular disease
- *Cardiac arrhythmias*: Atrial fibrillation complicates both binge drinking and chronic alcohol misuse. Ventricular arrhythmias are also reported.
- 7–11% of *hypertension* in men (1% in women) can be attributed to alcohol ingestion in excess of 40 g per day. Intracerebral and sub-arachnoid haemorrhage are more common irrespective of the severity of hypertension.
- *IHD*: Modest alcohol intake may offer cardio-protection, but the incidence of IHD increases if alcohol intake exceeds 30 g/day (e.g. $1\frac{1}{2}$ pints of beer).
- *Alcoholic cardiomyopathy* is caused by a direct toxic effect of alcohol (not by thiamine deficiency). Commonest in men aged 30–60, it is characterized by a dilated hypokinetic LV with a decreased ejection fraction. Patients may present with congestive cardiac failure and oedema, which may be exacerbated by low serum albumin.

Metabolic effects

- Hypoglycaemia may complicate acute alcohol intoxication, alcoholic liver disease, and pancreatic disease. It is more common in children and adolescents. Malnutrition can be another cause.
- Ketoacidosis may present after binge drinking in association with vomiting and fasting. Blood alcohol concentrations may not be elevated at the time.
- Metabolic alkalosis may be seen after prolonged vomiting.

Convulsions

- Alcoholic convulsions are most commonly seen 7–48 h after cessation of drinking.
- They are typically tonic–clonic with loss of consciousness. Several fits over a period of a few days are common.
- Hypokalaemia and hypomagnesaemia predispose to convulsions.
- Convulsions are normally self-limiting but can be fatal if associated with trauma or sustained unconsciousness.
- Other causes for convulsions must be ruled out (e.g. hypoglycaemia, intracranial bleeds, tumours, abscesses).

Malnutrition

Many features of chronic alcohol misuse can be attributed to the ingestion of 'empty calories' (i.e. calories with no nutritional value) and loss of appetite. Common complications include:

- *Anaemia*: macrocytosis: direct toxic alcohol effect, megaloblastic change, folate deficiency, iron deficiency, poor diet, upper GI blood loss.
- *Marrow toxicity*: neutropenia: marrow toxicity, folate deficiency; thrombocytopenia can complicate clotting deficiencies.
- *Cerebellar degeneration* due to toxicity and thiamine deficiency.
- *Amblyopia* (blurring, red green blindness): thiamine and B_{12} deficiency.
- *Wernicke's encephalopathy* and *Korsakoff's psychosis*: thiamine deficiency.
- *Peripheral neuropathy*: B vitamin deficiency.
- *Immunodeficiency* with increased prevalence of respiratory infections (including TB). Neutropenia and the poor housing and sanitation conditions encountered by chronic alcoholics exacerbate this.
- *Skin diseases*: psoriasis, eczema, rosacea, fungal infections, and acne are commoner in heavy drinkers.

Trauma

- Alcohol slows reaction time, decreases co-ordination and balance, and impairs judgement. This leads to accidental injury and major trauma.
- The risk of road traffic accident increases as blood alcohol rises. Injuries are more serious in motor vehicle accidents where alcohol is involved.
- 30% of pedestrians killed in motor vehicle accidents by day have a measurable blood alcohol concentration. This figure increases to 70% at night.
- 26–54% of home and leisure injuries are related to alcohol. It is particularly associated with family violence and child abuse.

Preoperative assessment of alcohol abusers

History

- Quantify excessive drinking.
- Ask about weight loss and history of GI bleeding.
- Enquire about recurrent accidents, infections.
- Loss of social status may be important.

Examination

This may yield little in all but advanced cases, but look for:
- fetor
- spider naevi, ascites, jaundice, bruising
- malnutrition, neglect
- tremor, peripheral neuropathy, psychosis, encephalopathy, convulsions (withdrawal)
- hypertension, cardiac failure, arrhythmias.

Investigations

- Haematology: increased MCV, iron deficiency, marrow depression, coagulation defects.
- Blood alcohol concentration may be important. 80 mg/dl is the legal driving limit in the UK: 200 mg/dl causes severe intoxication; and >500 mg/dl is frequently fatal.
- Glucose.
- Electrolytes: hypokalaemia is common.
- Triglycerides are often raised.
- Liver enzymes: raised γ-GT and aminotransferases.
- Albumin: marker for malnutrition.

- Coagulation may be abnormal due to clotting factor deficiency.
- ECG: conduction defects, bifid T-wave, ST changes (similar to digoxin changes), arrhythmias (commonly AF).
- Echocardiogram if suspicion of alcoholic cardiomyopathy: dilated LV, decreased ejection fraction, reduced LV function.
- CXR may show aspiration pneumonia, TB, or lung cancer.

Perioperative management

- Avoid non-emergency surgery in the presence of acute alcohol toxicity.
- If emergency surgical intervention is unavoidable, ensure adequate rehydration with careful attention to electrolyte imbalance (special attention to hypokalaemia and hypoglycaemia).
- Correct clotting abnormalities with FFP and/or platelets as appropriate.
- Treat anaemia (e.g. iron deficiency, upper GI bleeding) with appropriate transfusion.
- Assume the patient has a full stomach and take routine pre-anaesthetic precautions.
- Give intravenous vitamins (high potency B and C).
- Patients with liver failure require intensive care if surgical intervention is required.
- Patients with GI bleeding and cirrhosis are in danger of developing hepatic failure. Insert a gastric tube (with care in the presence of varices) to stop digestion of blood.
- Anticipate alcohol withdrawal symptoms. Treat with chlordiazepoxide (10–50 mg 4 times daily) if patient can take oral medication or chlormethiazole if intravenous therapy is required.
- An infusion of chlormethiazole 0.8% (8 mg/ml) is initially given at 3–7.5 ml (24–60 mg)/min until the patient is lightly sleeping, and then reduced to 0.5–1 ml (4–8 mg)/min to maintain sedation. **Overdosage with chlormethiazole can cause profound respiratory depression.**
- An infusion of ethanol 5% (add 50 g ethanol to 1 l 0.9% saline or any other crystalloid) can be used to prevent alcohol withdrawal in the immediate perioperative period. This may be preferable to attempting withdrawal at this vulnerable time. Alternatively, oral or n/g administration of alcoholic drinks may be appropriate (within limits)!
- Look for and treat unusual infection in potentially immunocompromised patients.

Further reading

Chick J (1993). Alcohol problems in the general hospital. *British Medical Bulletin* 50:200–10.

Cherpitel C (1993). Alcohol and injuries: a review of international emergency room studies. *Addiction* 88:923–37.

Edwards G, Anderson P, Babor TF *et al.* (1994). *Alcohol policy and the public good.* Oxford: Oxford University Press.

Imrie CW (1996). Diseases of the pancreas: acute pancreatitis. In Weatherall D *et al.*, ed. *Oxford textbook of medicine*, 3rd edn, vol 2. Oxford: Oxford University Press, 2027–33.

Tønnesen H, Rosenberg J, Nielsen HJ, Rasmussen V, Hange C, Pedersen IK, Kehlet H (1999). Effect of perioperative abstinence on poor postoperative outcome in alcohol misusers: randomised controlled trial. *British Medical Journal* 318:1311–6.

Tønnesen H, Kehlet H (1999). Preoperative alcoholism and postoperative mortality. *British Journal of Surgery* 86:869–74.

Misuse of drugs

Colin Berry

Epidemiology

One in four of the UK population aged over 16 has taken an illegal drug at some stage in their life. Substance abuse is commonest in the lowest income groups in urban areas. High rates of regular illicit drug usage occur in many societies, and contribute to violent and accidental injury.

In the USA around a half of patients admitted with violent assault-related trauma, and a quarter of those with road traffic trauma, test positive for cocaine metabolites on urine or blood screening. Doctors working in both emergency and elective settings must suspect drug related-illness in many patients.

History

- Chronic abusers may give explicit details of their recent drug-taking activity.
- Other patients conceal their activities for fear of legal recrimination.
- In those with reduced consciousness, get a history from those present at preceding events or from paramedics attending the scene prior to arrival in hospital.

Street drugs in common use fall into four groups (Table 34.1). Healthcare workers should be aware that it is common to take combinations of drugs. The effects of alcohol must also be considered.

Table 34.1 Street drugs in common use and principal effects

Agent	Pharmacological effects
Cannabis	Tachycardia, abnormal affect e.g. euphoria, anxiety, panic, psychosis, poor memory, fatigue (chronic use)
Stimulants (cocaine, amphetamines, Ecstasy)	Tachycardia, labile blood pressure, excitement, delirium, hallucinations, hyper-reflexia, tremors, convulsions, mydriasis, sweating, hyperpyrexia, exhaustion, coma
Hallucinogens (LSD, phencyclidine, ketamine)	Tachycardia, hypertension, weak analgesic, altered judgement and perceptions, toxic psychosis, dissociative anaesthesia
Opioids (morphine, heroin, opium)	Euphoria, respiratory depression, hypotension, bradycardia, constipation, pinpoint pupils, coma

Opioids

Opioid misuse (mostly heroin in the UK) is either by intravenous injection or inhalation. One per cent of the British population has taken heroin at least once in their lives.

Physical signs of opioid use

- coma
- small pupils
- needle marks (limbs/groins – sometimes hidden by tattoos)
- difficult venous access
- associated illness (infections/SBE).

The most lethal side effect of opioids is respiratory depression and subsequent coma. Treatment of coma is well documented for all accident and emergency departments. The use of the specific opioid antagonist naloxone (200 μg every 2 min to a total of 1 mg) may be used as both a diagnostic and therapeutic adjunct when treating opioid-induced coma but the basic principles of resuscitation must take priority.

Medical complications of opioid addiction

- Opioid addicts commonly develop venous conditions such as emboli and abscesses, which may need surgery.
- Addicts also present with injuries from assault and trauma.
- A serious complication of intravenous drug use is bacterial endocarditis. This affects 2 out of every 1000 drug injectors per year. Right-sided endocarditis is commonest in this group and can be associated with pulmonary abscesses and embolic phenomena from vegetations. Left-sided endocarditis is also common.

Infection risks for patient and staff

- Intravenous drug abusers commonly share needles.
- The incidence of blood borne infections is increased, particularly HIV and hepatitis viruses. In 1990, 6% of male injectors and 6.5% of female injectors were found to be infected with HIV in London. Of the 50–80% of injectors who have been infected with hepatitis B, 1–10% will become carriers. As many as 60% of injectors in the UK may be infected with hepatitis C (see p. 97).
- Social exclusion and economic deprivation lead to poor housing and sanitation. These in turn lead to an increased rate of all types of infection especially pneumonia, tuberculosis and infestations.

Analgesia for the opioid misusing patient

- Patients who are misusing opioids have the same rights to adequate analgesia following trauma or surgery as any other patient.
- There are common perceptions among medical staff that addicts may overemphasize their analgesia needs in order to satisfy their drug dependence. This may be true in a minority of cases but should not be an obstacle to providing good analgesia.
- In many cases, analgesia can be provided without using opioids. Combinations of regional nerve blocks, epidurals and NSAIDs will avoid the need for prescribed opioids where contra-indications to these do not exist.

Opioid analgesia for the opioid addict

- Opioids should be administered in the same way as for normal patients with doses titrated to effect.
- PCA removes the burden of administration from medical and nursing staff and allows the patient a sense of control over their well being. The in-built safety mechanism of drowsiness stops the patient from overdosing when this technique is used but the usual observations and precautions must be observed.
- PCA machines may need to be programmed to allow for the tolerance demonstrated by chronic opioid users. Larger doses may need to be prescribed to achieve the same analgesic effect as in a non opioid addict.
- The use of analogue pain scores can be useful to make an accurate assessment of the efficacy of pain control.
- Patients in need of longer-term analgesia following surgery will benefit from the support of a psychiatric team specializing in drug misuse.
- A small group of 'ex-addicts' will have great fears about being prescribed opioids if they have been 'cured' of their addiction for fear of becoming addicted again. This is a tiny risk and should not be a

cause of inadequately treated postoperative pain. Discussion with the patient of the techniques involved, with the help of the psychiatric team, can overcome most of these difficulties.

Cocaine and crack cocaine

Cocaine can be taken orally, nasally, intravenously, or smoked. Crack is a manufactured free base of cocaine, which is smoked in a highly concentrated form.

Perioperative hazards

- *Pharmacology*: Cocaine toxicity is a serious problem in the perioperative period. Most effects are mediated by central and peripheral adrenergic stimulation owing to inhibition of dopamine re-uptake, increased dopamine release, and increased levels of adenyl cyclase.
- *Cardiovascular effects*: 40% of presenting symptoms are cardiovascular and include tachycardia, hypertension, aortic dissection, arrhythmias, accelerated coronary artery disease, coronary spasm, infarction, and sudden death. Intracerebral vasospasm can lead to stroke, rigidity, hyper-reflexia, and hyperthermia.
- *Lung injury*: Inhalation of cocaine can cause alveolar haemorrhage or pulmonary oedema.
- *Renal failure* has been reported following renal infarction and secondary to rhabdomyolysis.
- *ACTH secretion* is increased after acute ingestion of cocaine, probably due to the secretion of corticotrophin releasing factor.
- *Psychiatric symptoms* range from a feeling of elation and enhanced physical strength to full toxic paranoid psychosis.
- *Chronic effects*: weight loss, digestive problems, psychological dependence.

Perioperative care

- Patients *intoxicated with cocaine* may need managing in intensive care until they are stabilized.
- *Monitoring*: ECG, BP, and pulse oximetry are minimal requirements.
- *Reversing drug effects*: Most of the life-threatening side-effects of cocaine result from vasospasm. They can be reversed with combinations of vasodilators, anti-arrhythmics, α-blockers and β-blockers (Table 34.2). The use of these agents in patients after major surgery should only be undertaken with arterial, CVP, and pulmonary artery pressure monitoring.
- **Combinations of local anaesthetic and vasoconstrictors (or any vasopressor) should be avoided. Tachycardia or a hypertensive crisis could result.**

Table 34.2 Drug therapy for cocaine intoxication

Signs	Treatment
Hypertension, tachycardia	Labetolol, esmolol
Arrhythmias	Lidocaine (lignocaine)
Myocardial ischaemia	GTN, calcium antagonists
Tremors or convulsions	Benzodiazepines

- *Toxic intra-arterial injections of cocaine* have led to critical limb and organ ischaemia. Successful treatment has included regional plexus blockade with local anaesthetic in association with intravenous heparin. Other treatments have included stellate ganglion block, intra-arterial vasodilators, urokinase, and early fasciotomy.

Ecstasy (3,4-methylenedioxymethamphetamine – MDMA)

Epidemiology

Classed as a hallucinogenic stimulant, Ecstasy is taken in tablet form at a dose of 75–100 mg. Several similar drugs are sold as Ecstasy but all have a similar effect. Ecstasy use is reported in 9% of those aged between 16–19 years.

Drug effects

Effects are experienced about half an hour after ingestion and can last up to 6 h. Users experience a mild rush followed by a feeling of serenity. Anxiety, paranoia, hallucinations, and psychosis have been reported.

Risks

It is estimated that 20 people die from Ecstasy every year in the UK.

Many cases present with hyperthermia (body temperatures in excess of 39°C) and DIC. Other postmortem findings associated with ecstasy related deaths include liver necrosis, myocardial fibrosis, perivascular haemorrhage, and neuronal degeneration. Hyperthermia is associated with dehydration during physical exercise in night clubs, and adequate water intake has been a key to education in this area.

Some deaths result from dilutional hyponatremia and cerebral oedema. Ecstasy may stimulate antidiuretic hormone (ADH) release and the use of isotonic drinks is now recommended.

Surgical and anaesthetic risks

Although no specific acute surgical problems arise from the use of Ecstasy, suspect Ecstasy use in all young patients admitted for whatever cause. This is especially true at night and at weekends. Where suspicion exists, measurement of body temperature, serum electrolytes, and a clotting screen will help to exclude drug-related morbidity in the perioperative period.

Further reading

Brookhoff D, Campbell E A, Shaw LM (1993). The underreporting of cocaine related trauma: drug abuse warning network vs hospital toxicology tests. *American Journal of Public Health* 83:369–71.

Cheng DCH (1994). The perioperative care of cocaine abusing patients. *Canadian Journal of Anaesthesia* 41:883–7.

Farrell M (1991). Physical complications of drug abuse. In Glass IB, ed. *The international handbook of addiction behaviour*. London: Routledge, 120–5.

McKenzie D, Williams B (1996). Licit and illicit drugs, CCSA/ARF 1995 Canadian Profile. *Addiction Research Foundation*, 118–204.

Parliamentary Office of Science and Technology (1996). *Common illegal drugs and their effects – cannabis, ecstasy, amphetamines and LSD*. London: POST.

Ramsay M, Percy A (1996). *Drug misuse declared: results of the 1994 British crime survey*. London: Home Office.

Medical emergencies in surgical patients

This section provides a trouble-shooting guide to medical emergencies and other medical problems arising on the surgical ward.

Diagnostic approaches reflect the probabilities of diagnoses in a surgical (rather than acute medical) setting.

Presenting problems rather than diagnoses form the titles of the various chapters, and cross-references are given for overlapping symptoms.

Recognizing and managing seriously ill surgical patients

Iain Wilson and Anthony Nicholls

If seriously ill patients are recognized and treated early in the course of their condition, they have an improved chance of survival, less chance of requiring intensive care, and a reduced risk of cardiac arrest. Serious illness may be caused by any process that results in severe physiological derangement. If untreated, progression to organ system failure and death is common.

Patients who are severely ill may complain (but are often too ill to do so), may display abnormal signs, or have deranged physiological values and laboratory data. By responding to these at an early phase, deterioration may be stopped.

The principles of management of this group of patients includes:

- recognition of the patient
- initial treatment
- liaison with senior colleagues and other specialities including intensive care
- overall management plan.

Recognition of the patient

During patient assessment the following suggest impending or established critical illness.

Circulation

- hypotension (<100 mmhg systolic)
- tachycardia (130/min)
- bradycardia (<45/min)
- new arrhythmia
- post cardiac arrest
- excess surgical bleeding.

Respiration

- airway problems
- post respiratory arrest
- respiratory rate >30/min
- SpO_2 <95% on O_2.

Neurological status

- deteriorating conscious level or unexplained confusion
- seizures.

Renal

- oliguria (<30 ml/h)
- polyuria (>200 ml/h).

General

- fever >39.5°C
- patient causing concern to nursing, physiotherapy, or medical staff.

Laboratory

- metabolic acidosis (base excess <−5 mmol/l); pH <7.25
- K^+ >6 mmol/l.

Initial treatment

The priority is to ensure adequate oxygenation and cardiac output:

- airway, breathing and circulation
- obtain help (see below)
- assess conscious level

- consider underlying problem: the priorities are surgical bleeding, major heart or lung disease, and sepsis.

Different sections of this book deal with different problems:

- severe dyspnoea p. 281
- severe hypotension p. 249
- coma and confusion p. 326.

Many patients respond to first line treatment with a sustained improvement. Those who do not are a high risk group, even if they do not continue to deteriorate.

Liaison with senior colleagues and other specialities

Seriously ill patients need experienced doctors, as early expert intervention may be necessary. Senior surgical advice should be obtained, and if indicated, early intensive care or medical assessment requested. Relevant investigations should be requested.

Some patients will be able to continue on the ward with a revised management plan and regular assessment; others will require care on the HDU/ICU.

- The ICU offers closer observation and a higher staff to patient ratio to provide nursing and medical care. Invasive physiological monitoring is routine and inotropic support, ventilation, and renal replacement therapy may be instituted.

- The HDU allows a level of care between ICU and the ward. Ventilation and renal replacement therapy are not generally performed, but invasive monitoring and inotropic support are.

Overall management plan

A longer-term clinical management plan should be made for the patient and treatment goals established. Regular review of the patient is vital along with a flexible response to change therapy if indicated.

Further reading

Lee A, Bishop G, Hillman KM, Daffurn K (1995). The Medical Emergency Team. *Anaesthesia and Intensive Care* 23:183–6.

McQuillan P, Pilkington S, Allan A *et al.* (1998). Confidential inquiry into quality of care before admission to intensive care. *British Medical Journal* 316:1853–8.

Cardiorespiratory arrest

Iain Wilson and Anthony Nicholls

Impending cardiac arrest *244*
Cardiopulmonary resuscitation (CPR) *245*

Cardiac arrest occurs when a patient suddenly loses consciousness with no cardiac output. Immediate access to defibrillation and basic life support give the patient the best chance of survival. Cardiac arrest may occur with VF, pulseless VT, asystole, or electromechanical dissociation (also known as pulseless electrical activity – PEA). A variety of clinical conditions may lead to cardiac arrest. Some of these should be detected before cardiac arrest occurs.

Impending cardiac arrest

Cardiac arrest may occur unexpectedly in AMI, major PE, or with severe underlying heart disease. Otherwise cardiac arrest on a surgical ward will often be preceded by warning signs such as hypotension, tachycardia, chest pain, dyspnoea, fever, restlessness, or confusion. Hypoxaemia, hypovolaemia, and sepsis may progress to cardiac arrest unless rapidly diagnosed and corrected. Do not hesitate to ask the cardiac arrest team or the ICU team to help with a sick patient before they actually arrest. CPR for patients who are septic or hypovolaemic usually fails.

When a patient is identified as being severely ill and at risk of a cardiac arrest the following should be rapidly assessed:

- *Oxygenation*: Is the airway clear, and is the patient breathing adequately? Give high flow O_2 and manually support ventilation if necessary. Monitor using a pulse oximeter and measure blood gases. See the section on acute dyspnoea and respiratory failure (p. 281).
- *Is the patient conscious?* Is the patient narcotized or oversedated?

- *Is the patient hypovolaemic?* Most hypotensive patients should be given fluids as part of the initial management. Only if the patient has cardiac failure are i/v fluids ineffective (and may worsen pulmonary oedema), but this anxiety should not prevent fluids being given routinely to the vast majority of hypotensive patients. See the section on hypotension (p. 249).

- *Confusion or reduced conscious level* should be taken as a sign of significant clinical deterioration and a cause urgently sought. See p. 326.

- *Exclude sepsis.* Tachypnoea or confusion may be the first signs of septicaemia in a surgical patient. Check the temperature. Take blood for culture. Consider intra-abdominal problems: bile leak, bowel anastamosis leak. Give antibiotics if in doubt (p. 341).

- Check for *electrolyte disturbance* including metabolic acidosis.

- Consider *moving the patient to ICU.*

- *Treat pain.* Pain causes adrenaline (epinephrine) release and increases the risk of cardiac arrhythmia.

Cardiopulmonary resuscitation (CPR)

Whenever cardiac arrest occurs, the cardiac arrest team should always be summoned unless the patient is 'not for CPR'. Early defibrillation and basic life support are of the utmost importance.

The management of cardiac arrest is detailed in other texts, but protocols for basic and advanced life support are given in Figs 36.1 and 36.2 at the end of the chapter.

CPR in surgical patients

- CPR maintains a low cardiac output to the essential organs when performed properly. Occasionally open chest cardiac compression is used for patients with PEA following penetrating trauma, following recent sternotomy, or during abdominal or thoracic surgery.

- In VF or pulseless ventricular tachycardia, the first two shocks should be at 200J and thereafter 360J. As the duration of cardiac arrest increases, successful defibrillation becomes less likely.

- The outcome of cardiac arrest is best in patients with a witnessed cardiac arrest, with early CPR by someone trained in the technique, when ventricular fibrillation is present, and with early defibrillation. A poor outcome is likely with asystole, delayed treatment, and in patients with multisystem disease.

- PEA also has a poor prognosis, unless a cause is immediately identified and treated. If the underlying mechanism is hypovolaemia, which is aggressively managed, and immediate surgery performed, some of these patients will survive. Other causes of PEA include PE, major MI, tension pneumothorax, cardiac tamponade, and electrolyte problems.

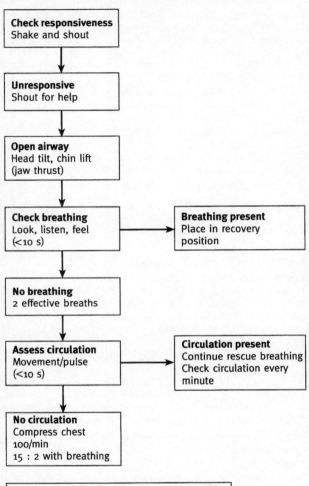

Fig. 36.1 Basic life support.

- Adrenaline (epinephrine) (1 mg i/v) is given regularly throughout CPR to preserve some vascular tone in an attempt to maintain cerebral circulation during resuscitation. Large doses are required due to hypoxia and acidosis. Use 1 : 10 000 solutions (1 mg/10 ml) intravenously, although a double dose may be given down an endotracheal tube if venous access is not available.

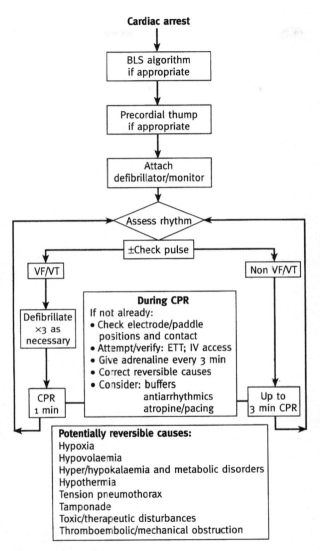

Fig. 36.2 The ALS algorithm for the management of cardiac arrest in adults. Note that each successive step is based on the assumption that the one before has been unsuccessful. Reproduced by kind permission of the Resuscitation Council (UK).

- $NaHCO_3$ is best administered with blood gas guidance, but is usually needed after 15 min of cardiac arrest in a dose of 50 ml of 8.4% given i/v. HCO_3^- should be given earlier if the arrest is due to a metabolic acidosis.

- As soon as practical, check the background details of the patient in an attempt to diagnose the underlying problem and to help decide whether prolonged resuscitation attempts are valid.

- Discontinue resuscitation if the patient does not respond to advanced life support measures. Although every patient is different, in practical terms resuscitation from VF is unlikely after 15–20 min of CPR, or from asystole or PEA after 10–15 min of CPR. However, in the case of hypothermia, or an accidental overdose of local anaesthetic drugs, expert advice from the cardiac arrest team or the ICU team should be obtained as prolonged resuscitation is occasionally indicated.

'Not for resuscitation' statements

Many of the patients on the wards are unsuitable for resuscitation owing to a poor overall prognosis or because of patient request. When this occurs it should be discussed with the patient, and/or his or her relatives, and be written clearly in the notes so that inappropriate resuscitation measures are not instituted in the event of a cardiac arrest. These orders should only be made by a senior doctor, be agreed with the junior medical and nursing staff and be signed and dated and reviewed on a regular basis in case the situation changes.

This is discussed in more detail in Chapter 10 (p. 37).

Further reading

Doyal L, Wilsher D (1993). Withholding cardiopulmonary resuscitation: proposals for formal guidelines. *British Medical Journal* 306:1593–6.

McQuillan P, Pilkington S, Allan A *et al.* (1998). Confidential inquiry into quality of care before admission to intensive care. *British Medical Journal* 316:1853–8.

O'Keefe S, Ebell MH (1994). Prediction of failure to survive following in-hospital cardiopulmonary resuscitation: comparison of two predictive instruments. *Resuscitation* 28:21–5.

Resuscitation Council (UK) (1998). *Advanced life support course provider manual*, 3rd edn.

Smith A, Wood J (1999). Can some in-hospital cardiopulmonary arrests be prevented? *Resuscitation* in press.

Stewart K (1995). Discussing cardiopulmonary resuscitation with patients and relatives. *Postgraduate Medical Journal* 71:585–9.

Wall JA, Palmer RN (1994). Resuscitation and patients' views. *British Medical Journal* 309:1442–3.

Hypotension

Iain Wilson and Anthony Nicholls

Basic principles

- Hypotension is defined as a systolic pressure < 100 mmHg and after surgery is most commonly due to hypovolaemia.
- Blood pressure is the product of cardiac output and peripheral resistance. Cardiac output is dependent on efficient cardiac filling and contractility. Changes in any of these parameters may result in hypotension.
- The earliest practical distinction to make in the management of a shocked patient is to decide whether the patient is hypovolaemic, has cardiac problems or has a vasodilated state (such as sepsis). This is best based on history and examination.
- Underlying cardiovascular conditions, and their drug treatment, may modify physiological responses to hypotension and confuse the clinical picture.
- Hypotension reduces coronary perfusion. In patients with coronary artery disease hypotension depresses cardiac contractility and may cause myocardial infarction. In such patients hypotension may persist after restoration of circulating volume.

Table 37.1 Common causes of hypotension in the surgical patient

Hypovolaemia	Actual blood loss or other fluid deficits: GI losses, third space losses, etc.
	Relative hypovolaemia associated with a vasodilated state (see below)
Defective cardiac pump	Cardiac failure
	Myocardial infarction
	Bradycardia or other arrhythmia
	Valvular heart disease
	Pulmonary embolism
	Tension pneumothorax
	Cardiac tamponade
	Drugs: β-blockers, some anti-arrhythmic agents
Vasodilated state	Sepsis
	High spinal or epidural anaesthesia
	Spinal shock
	Anaphylaxis
	Adrenal failure (also leads to volume depletion)
	Drugs: antihypertensive agents, anti-anginal agents, phenothiazines

- Untreated hypotension may progress to cardiac arrest and death. React to hypotension immediately. If the blood pressure cannot be measured, call for assistance even if the patient is still conscious.

Assessment of the hypotensive patient

- Assess ABC. Commence high flow O_2 therapy.
- Obtain a history and determine the time-scale of the hypotension, the underlying surgical diagnosis and any complicating medical factors. The timing of the hypotensive episode is important, as bleeding is much more likely soon after surgery, whereas thrombo-embolic complications occur later. Septic shock may occur at any time and is associated with fluid extravasation and hypovolaemia.
- Examine the patient. Absent or weak peripheral pulses with an altered conscious level indicate severe hypotension. Recent onset hypotension with associated dyspnoea is suggestive of tension pneumothorax or pulmonary embolism. The presence of bulging neck veins suggests a pump problem (cardiac failure or impeded filling from tension pneumothorax or pericardial tamponade). Empty neck veins in the supine position suggest hypovolaemia. Peripheral vasoconstriction with poor capillary refill (>2 s) occurs in both hypovolaemia or pump failure. Warm peripheries with an easily palpable pulse suggest a vasodilated state.
- Measure the pulse rate, BP, and O_2 saturation (pulse oximeter).

- Compare the BP readings to previous 'normal' BPs. Remember that hypertensive patients may be shocked with BPs that might normally be considered acceptable.
- Check recent urine output.

Immediate treatment plan for the hypotensive patient

- Call for assistance – surgical or medical according to the suspected underlying problem. Consider contacting the ICU team if the patient does not respond to simple management.
- Unless there is clear evidence to suggest a cardiac problem, start rapid i/v fluid replacement. Run in 1000 ml of crystalloid (or 500 ml colloid) as quickly as possible while you assess the underlying problem. The choice of fluids for continuing replacement is dealt with in Table 37.2. Although colloids may restore the circulation more quickly, (smaller volumes are required), either crystalloids or colloids are suitable for volume expansion.
- Young fit adults may lose a lot of fluid before becoming hypotensive, but much smaller degrees of volume depletion cause shock in the elderly or those with cardiac disease. Hypotensive drugs and

Table 37.2 Fluids for restoration of circulating volume in hypotensive patients

Fluid	Proprietary brands	Indications and hazards
Crystalloid		
0.9% NaCl		Resuscitation in hypovolaemia, sodium
Hartmann's solution		and water depletion: fistulae, vomiting, diarrhoea, ascites
Colloids		
Gelatin	Gelofusine	Short-term restoration of circulating blood volume
	Haemaccel	Half life 3–6 h
Etherified starch	Hespan	Short-term restoration of circulating blood volume
	eloHAES	Half-life > 6 h
	HAES-steril	
	Pentaspan	
Human albumin	HAS 4.5%	Not indicated for hypovolaemia
Blood		
Plasma reduced red cells		Blood loss >1500 ml or Hb <10 g/dl (hypovolaemia class III or IV – see Table 37.3)

anti-anginal medication may modify the response to hypovolaemia and exaggerate hypotension.

- A CVP line will prove useful in patients in whom the circulation is difficult to assess and in those not responding to simple measures. In expert hands this is quick and safe. In inexperienced hands it may be time-consuming, painful, unsuccessful, unreliable, and dangerous.

- Ensure that a nurse stays with the patient continuously. Record fluids given and clinical observations.

- Monitor the urine output via a urethral catheter.

- Assess the patient's response to first line measures. Estimate whether the patient is deteriorating or is reasonably stable. In a deteriorating patient consider whether the presumed diagnosis could be wrong and who should be contacted to obtain urgent advice. Ask for assistance before the situation worsens.

- Review the patient frequently.

Investigations in the hypotensive patient

Consider whether the following investigations may help determine the cause of the hypotension:

- *12-lead ECG*: acute MI, major PE, cardiac arrhythmia.
- *CXR*: pneumonia, pneumothorax, oligaemic areas in PE, pulmonary oedema, cardiac enlargement.
- *FBC*: haemorrhage.
- *Electrolytes*: Hyponatraemia with acute hypotension is typical of salt and water depletion.
- *Creatinine and urea*: Is the patient developing renal failure?
- *Arterial blood gases*: Hypoxia with a clear CXR and absence of airflow obstruction suggests PE. Circulatory failure leads to tissue hypoxia and metabolic (lactic) acidosis that depresses myocardial contractility.
- *Serum cortisol* should be checked and a bolus of hydrocortisone 100 mg i/v given if adrenal insufficiency is possible (previous steroid therapy). The stress of hypotension should cause a high cortisol level, and more sophisticated tests are not necessary in this setting.
- Cardiac tamponade is highly unlikely unless there has been thoracic surgery or trauma. Echocardiography is then the most useful investigation.

Further management plan for the hypotensive patient

Treatment of the underlying problem takes priority but remember the following:

- *Surgery*: Severe hypovolaemia due to haemorrhage may need surgical control. If this is likely, contact the surgeon, anaesthetist, and theatre as soon as possible. Ensure that there are adequate supplies of blood for transfusion.
- *ICU*: Patients who do not require surgery but remain shocked despite 1500 ml of rapid fluid replacement should be referred to the ICU team for possible admission. Patients with cardiac problems should be considered for CCU.
- *Documentation*: Remember to document your actions when time allows.
- *Communication*: Talk to the patient and the family.
- *Specific problems*: Plan specific management of common problems as detailed below.

Specific problems causing hypotension

Major haemorrhage

- *Access*: Insert two large (14 or 16 gauge) cannulae. The antecubital fossa is often the easiest site, although the external jugular, long saphenous, or femoral vein (long cannula required from theatre or A&E) can be used. A venous cut-down may occasionally be required.
- *Cross-match*: Blood should be taken at the time of cannulation for cross-match and other investigations. Order at least 8 units of blood for shocked patients with active bleeding.
- *Assess volume loss*: The degree of hypovolaemia is related to the patient's physical status (Table 37.3) although there is marked individual variation. The elderly, for example, do not always develop an

Table 37.3 Classification of hypovolaemia in a previously healthy patient

	Class I	Class II	Class III	Class IV
Blood loss: % circulating volume	<15	15–30	30–40	>40
Blood loss: ml (in adults)	<750	750–1500	1500–2000	>2000
Pulse	Normal	100–120/min	120/min Weak	>120/min Very weak
Systolic BP	Normal	Normal	Low	Very low
Diastolic BP	Normal	High	Low	Very low
Capillary refill	Normal	Slow	Slow	Absent
Mental state	Alert	Anxious	Confused	Lethargic
Respiratory rate	Normal	Normal	Tachypnoeic	Tachypnoeic
Urine output	>30 ml/h	20–30ml/h	5–20 ml/h	< 5 ml/h

appropriate tachycardia. Young patients may still have a normal systolic BP despite the loss of 1500 ml of blood. Restoration of a normal systolic BP does not indicate full resuscitation. In severe hypovolaemia (class III) blood is usually needed before a full cross match is possible. either use an emergency cross-match or obtain group-compatible blood quickly. In patients not responding to volume replacement and those with class IV hypovolaemia, administer uncross-matched group O Rhesus –ve blood (Table 37.4).

- *Surgery:* It is often impossible to replace brisk surgical bleeding with i/v infusions – these patients often need urgent surgery. Always reconsider this option, along with the likely operation required.

- *Contact the blood bank:* Speak to the blood bank technician personally to find out how long cross-matching will take and to confirm the samples have arrived. Ensure a porter is dispatched to bring the blood to you.

- *Warm blood:* When administering large volumes of i/v fluids a blood warmer should be used. Organize this via theatre.

- *Target haemoglobin:* Aim for a haemoglobin concentration of 8–10 g/dl by giving a balanced transfusion of blood and crystalloid or colloid. Measure the Hb or Hct regularly using a Haemocue or similar portable device during resuscitation if possible. Each 2 units of plasma reduced blood will require approximately 500 ml plasma expander (e.g. gelatin solution) or 1000 ml saline to achieve this. Checking the FBC via the lab may not keep pace with the situation.

- *Correct coagulation:* When bleeding is rapid and it is not practical to obtain regular coagulation results 2 units of FFP should be given after 6 units of transfused blood and then repeated after each 4 units of red cells. Platelet transfusions should be given if the count falls below 50 000/mm³. This does not usually occur until at least 10 units of blood have been given. Pre-existing coagulation abnormalities will need specific treatment (p. 210). FFP requires 20 min to thaw before being issued and platelets may need to be ordered from a regional centre. Repeat coagulation tests every few hours.

- *CVP line:* Central venous access is not indicated for initial fluid replacement, but is useful to guide fluid therapy once resuscitation is well underway. Catheterize the patient and monitor hourly urine output.

Table 37.4 Average times to obtain different types of blood

Type of blood	Time required for preparation
Full cross-match	30–40 min (less if antibody screen negative)
ABO compatible	10 min
Uncross-matched O Rhesus –ve	Available immediately in A&E or theatre

Septic shock

Sepsis may present in a variety of ways, sometimes as septic shock. **Consider septic shock as the diagnosis when any degree of fever accompanies acute hypotension.** Typically the hypotension is out of proportion from any estimated fluid and blood losses and does not respond to fluid replacement alone. Although some patients present with the classic warm vasodilated circulation of gram −ve endotoxic shock, many others present with diverse signs of different organ system dysfunction.

The goal of early identification and treatment of septic shock is to avoid progression to the syndrome of refractory hypotension and multi-organ failure. The mortality of late septic shock is high.

Diagnosis of septic shock

- *History:* Sepsis may often be suggested from the history − bowel perforation, postoperative pneumonia, infected urethral catheter, potentially infected central venous lines, etc. Physical examination may confirm this.

- *Signs:* These include hypotension, depressed conscious level, confusion, fever or hypothermia, renal failure and dyspnoea resulting from lung infection or acute respiratory distress syndrome (ARDS). The peripheral circulation may suggest a hypovolaemic picture.

- *Immediate investigations:* FBC, U&E, blood cultures, CRP, coagulation screen, urinary cultures, and CXR. A raised WBC and CRP are common, but when these are normal the diagnosis cannot be totally discarded.

- *Subsequent investigations:* Some patients particularly those with suspected intra-abdominal sepsis may require ultrasound, CT scanning, or laparotomy.

Treatment principles

- *Oxygenation:* Urgent control of any airway or respiratory problems.

- *Normalize circulation:* Fluid replacement with either crystalloids or colloids or blood products if indicated. Inotropes are often needed to restore the circulation. These can only be given on an HDU/ICU.

- *Surgery:* Urgent surgery may be required to treat the underlying problem (e.g. anastamotic leak). Inform the anaesthetist as early as possible to allow optimal resuscitation of the patient.

- *Antibiotics:* Broad-spectrum antibiotic cover should be commenced as soon as samples for culture and sensitivity have been taken. Suitable regimes are described in Table 37.5. In patients who have deteriorated while on antibiotics seek expert microbiological advice.

Table 37.5 Antibiotic treatment of the septicaemic patient

Clinical features	Organisms	Antibiotics	Comments
Skin generally red ± confluent or peeling rash ± diarrhoea ± confused	*Staph. aureus* Group A streptococcus	flucloxacillin 1–2 g qds i/v or clindamycin 450–900 mg qds i/v	
Catheter *in situ* or recently catheterized	Coliforms + *Pseudomonas* sp.	gentamicin 3–5 mg/kg i/v + cefotaxime 2 g tds i/v	
Severe cellulitis, blistering and dusky purple patches (necrotizing fasciitis)	Group A streptococcus	benzyl penicillin 2.4 g qds i/v + clindamycin 450 mg–1.2 g qds i/v. imipenem 500 mg qds i/v + clindamycin 450 mg–1.2 g qds i/v	Urgent plastic surgery opinion
Black blisters, foul smelling 'gas gangrene'	*Clostridium perfringens*	imipenem 500 mg qds i/v + clindamycin 1.2 g qds i/v + metronidazole 500 mg tds i/v	Urgent surgery. Consider hyperbaric O_2 therapy to stop toxin production
TPN/CVP line infection	Staphylococci including coagulase If TPN line consider fungal infection	vancomycin 1 g bd i/v add fluconazole 400 mg i/v od if fungus likely or proven	Discuss with microbiologist re Gram −ve cover
Postoperative pneumonia	Gram −ves	gentamicin 3–5 mg/kg i/v + cefotaxime 2 g tds i/v or imipenem 500 mg qds i/v or ceftazidime 1–2 g tds i/v	
No obvious focus, but treatment required on clinical grounds	Many possibilities	gentamicin 3–5 mg/kg stat i/v + cefotaxime 2 g tds i/v + metronidazole 500 mg tds i/v	Discuss with microbiologist

Tension pneumothorax

Consider this diagnosis if the history suggests it (recent CVP line, trauma, fractured ribs) (see also Chapter 41, p. 286).

- Look for specific signs and request immediate portable CXR. Affected side should have reduced air entry. May also have resonant percussion note and deviated trachea.

- If the patient's condition is life-threatening (BP < 90 mmHg, hypoxic on O_2 or unconscious) and will not permit the wait for CXR the tension must be urgently released. Insert a 21G (green) needle into the second intercostal space in the mid-clavicular line on the suspected affected side. Confirm the presence of pleural air by aspirating with a syringe and then use a 16 gauge cannula with a syringe attached. Insert until air is aspirated and then remove the needle and allow the air to escape. Insert a formal underwater seal drain.

- If a pneumothorax is confirmed on a CXR insert a formal underwater seal drain. Simple aspiration of a pneumothorax is never appropriate if it has caused hypotension.

- Seek further advice from the anaesthetic, or thoracic medical or surgical team on further management of the chest drain.

Hypotension of cardiac origin

Cardiac failure may result in hypotension (although sometimes LVF is associated with tachycardia and hypertension). A cardiac cause of hypotension is more likely if there is a relevant history of underlying heart disease or chest pain. Infarction may be silent in the postoperative phase, or it may have occurred during anaesthesia. Changes on a 12-lead ECG may be delayed for 24 h, but a rise in the CK-MB fraction occurs sooner. Total CK levels are commonly elevated after surgery and are of no diagnostic significance. Troponin-T levels are more specific in the diagnosis of acute MI, and rise sooner than the CK level.

See p. 267 for management details.

Underlying valvular heart disease will severely alter the patient's ability to respond to fluid depletion or sepsis. Invasive monitoring on ICU is usually required.

Anaphylaxis

Drug allergy can cause anaphylactic shock. The reaction is typically immediately after an i/v injection and presents with any of the following signs: hypotension, bronchospasm, cyanosis, coma, upper airway swelling (especially lips and face), and an urticarial skin rash. A widespread capillary leak occurs with resultant hypovolaemia. Adrenaline is the only effective drug that will treat both the respiratory and cardiovascular effects of anaphylaxis.

Management of a severe reaction

- Secure the airway and administer high flow O_2.

- Lie the patient supine.
- Stop any drug/fluid being administered that may be responsible for the reaction.
- Administer i/v **adrenaline (epinephrine) 1 in 10 000 in a dose of 1 ml (100 μg)** at intervals of 20–30 s until a response is seen. Monitor the ECG via the ward defibrillator.
- If i/v access is a problem, **give im adrenaline (epinephrine) 1 in 1000 in a dose of 0.5–1 ml (0.5–1 mg)** and repeat in 10 min if necessary.
- Call for help – anaesthetist or ICU team. With cardiovascular collapse, call the cardiac arrest team.
- Commence rapid infusion of crystalloid/colloid.
- Administer hydrocortisone 200 mg i/v and repeat after 6 h if still unstable.
- Consider the use of an antihistamine (e.g. chlorpheniramine 10–20 mg i/v).
- Consider i/v aminophylline 5 mg/kg over 15 min for resistant bronchospasm.
- Document the reaction afterwards and ensure that the patient is informed of the offending drug.

Mild reactions (systolic BP > 80 mmHg, minor bronchospasm)
- Secure the airway and administer high flow O_2.
- Obtain i/v access and commence rapid infusion of crystalloid/colloid.
- For bronchospasm give 5 mg salbutamol nebulized, if necessary combined with aminophylline as above.
- Administer hydrocortisone 200 mg i/v.
- Consider the use of an antihistamine (e.g. chlorpheniramine 10 mg i/v).

Further advice in anaphylaxis

- Do not confuse the i/m strength of adrenaline (1 : 1000) with i/v adrenaline (1 : 10 000).
- The action of adrenaline (epinephrine) is short (2–3 min) and many patients with a severe anaphylactic reaction will need repeated doses at regular intervals, or better, an infusion of 1 : 10 000 adrenaline starting at 5–20 ml/h on ICU. This may need to be continued for some hours.
- A diagnosis of anaphylaxis may be confirmed by taking a blood sample 1–5 h following the reaction and measuring mast cell tryptase. Contact the biochemistry laboratory for detailed instructions.

Hypotension associated with epidural or spinal (subarachnoid) anaesthesia

Spinal anaesthesia

Local anaesthetic (usually bupivacaine) is injected into the CSF at a lumbar level in this technique. It is most frequently used for surgery below the umbilicus. A sympathetic block is produced which may result in vasodilatation and hypotension, particularly when anaesthesia extends above the umbilicus. A few patients develop a bradycardia due to interference with the sympathetic nerve supply to the heart. Hypotension is controlled with i/v fluids and vasopressors such as ephedrine or methoxamine. Normally blocks wear off before a patient is discharged to the ward. However, since spinal anaesthesia may last 4–8 h, some patients may return to the ward with a significant degree of sympathetic blockade. They are less able to compensate for hypovolaemia or postural changes and may become severely hypotensive following postoperative haemorrhage or when sitting up when the block is still active.

Treatment:

- Lie the patient flat and elevate the legs on some pillows. **Do not put the patient head down as the block may become higher.** Give the patient O_2.
- Increase the rate of the i/v fluid.
- Check the height of the block by looking for altered sensation (gently pinch a skin fold). A block above the umbilicus suggests the spinal anaesthesia may well be contributing to the problem. If the block is below this then check for other factors known to cause hypotension and contact the anaesthetist responsible.
- If the systolic BP is <80 mmHg give 5–6 mg of ephedrine i/v and contact an anaesthetist.

Epidural anaesthesia

This is used in a similar way to spinal anaesthesia but the local anaesthetic solution is usually delivered via a small catheter into the epidural space. The catheter may be used postoperatively for a continuous infusion of local anaesthetic and/or opioid to provide postoperative pain relief (see p. 61). The sympathetic block produced by these techniques is usually less but may still occur. Hypotension can arise as a result of an epidural infusion, but other causes are more likely.

Treatment:

- Check what is in the infusion. If only opioid is being used then the epidural will not cause hypotension unless the patient has recently received local anaesthetic in theatre.
- If the patient is receiving a local anaesthetic infusion then treat the patient as described for spinal anaesthesia above.
- Most hypotension in this group of patients will be due to other causes.

Acute pulmonary embolism

See p. 268.

Acute gastric dilatation

A rare cause of hypotension. Treat urgently with a nasogastric tube.

Central venous pressure (CVP) monitoring

Physiological principles

- Blood volume cannot be directly measured at the bedside. Changes in blood volume produce changes in cardiac output, arterial pressure, and venous pressure. There is marked physiological variation in responses to changes in blood volume, so no single clinical sign can be used for monitoring volume.

- The CVP can be useful when there is difficulty estimating blood volume. In most normal patients the venous pressure reflects blood volume, although the relationship is non-linear.

- The CVP is the pressure of blood in the superior vena cava. It is the same as right atrial pressure. It represents the pressure of blood filling the right ventricle. Both venous return and cardiac function influence CVP.

- Normal CVP is 5–10 cmH$_2$O (4–8 mmHg).

- Isolated CVP readings are difficult to interpret (e.g. the same absolute reading could be obtained in an athlete participating in a marathon or in a hypovolaemic patient). Care is required in interpreting CVP readings and they rarely need to be measured immediately. The trend of CVP and its response to therapy provides an invaluable guide to treating the circulation.

- Under normal circumstances right and left atrial pressures are similar so the CVP will reflect physiology in both right and left ventricles.

Table 37.6 Interpreting CVP reading in hypotensive patients breathing spontaneously

CVP reading	Implication	Suggested action
Low (< 5 cmH$_2$O)	Low blood volume	Continue to volume load the patient
Normal range (5–10 cm H$_2$O)	Does not exclude continuing hypovolaemia	Fluid challenge (see below)
High (>10 cmH$_2$O)	Low circulating volume unlikely to be the sole cause of hypotension	Check for pump failure, over-transfusion, tension pneumothorax, cardiac tamponade, pulmonary embolism, cor pulmonale

• The CVP is not a reliable guide to left atrial pressure in many cardiorespiratory diseases (LVH, valvular heart disease, left or right ventricular failure, cardiomyopathy, serious respiratory disease or thromboembolic disease). A pulmonary artery catheter can provide more accurate information in these patients, but its use requires considerable expertise.

Practical aspects

• CVP is normally estimated using a central venous catheter whose tip lies in the superior vena cava (check this on the CXR). It must not be measured using a catheter with a tip lying outside the thorax, as venous valves will distort the reading.
• Lie the patient flat when reading the CVP.
• The CVP line may be connected to an electronic transducer, which may give useful information from the display of its waveform.
• Bedside CVP can be measured with a saline manometer. The zero point should be marked on the patient in the mid-axillary line in the fourth interspace. (This is the surface marking of the right atrium.) Ensure when using a saline manometer that the fluid is able to rise and fall, and swings with respiration.
• Always measure CVP with the patient in the same position.

Indications for measuring the CVP

• Hypotensive patients who are not responding to adequate volume loading.
• When large volume transfusions/fluid administration are being given.
• Patients with pre-existing cardiovascular compromise who are being given fluid loading.
• When the state of the circulating volume is unclear, particularly if there are signs of compromise such as hypotension or oliguria.
• In order to deliver inotropic or vasodilator drugs.

In addition, central lines are often inserted to facilitate TPN or when peripheral veins are inadequate.

Interpretation of the CVP in a hypotensive patient

A single level is often unhelpful, unless it is well outside the normal range. The trend during resuscitation is more important; see Table 37.6.

Difficulties in interpreting CVP readings

Whenever the CVP does not correlate with the clinical examination check the whole central venous cannulation set up and calibration, with particular reference to the zero point being used. The CVP should always be used in conjunction with careful clinical examination, and the patient should never be transfused to a pre-set CVP.

- The patient appears hypovolaemic but has a CVP in the normal range: This is one of the limitations of CVP measurement. It is possible that the patient may normally run with a higher CVP (e.g. cor pulmonale) or that they have intense vasoconstriction as a physiological response to hypovolaemia. Manage these patients with a fluid challenge. Give 250 ml of colloid over 10 min and if the CVP rises and remains raised by more than 2 cmH$_2$O this suggests that the circulation is reasonably well-filled. If, as more commonly occurs, there is no change in CVP, repeat the fluid challenge regularly until a response in the circulatory signs and venous pressures are seen.

- The CVP never seems to rise despite a lot of fluid being given: There may be continuing hypovolaemia, the measuring system is faulty, or the patient is vasodilated (as in sepsis). Ask for expert assistance from the ICU team. The venous circulation is capable of significant vasodilatation as a reservoir of circulating volume.

- The patient is clinically hypovolaemic but has a high CVP: Ensure that the saline manometer is functioning correctly. If it is, it is likely that more than one clinical condition exists. Consider the diagnoses suggested in Table 37.6 and ask for expert assistance from your senior colleagues or the ICU team. Some of these patients will require a pulmonary artery catheter.

Colloids versus crystalloids – the debate

For decades controversy has existed as to whether crystalloids or colloids are more effective for volume expansion of shocked patients. Traditionally it is believed that if crystalloid (Hartmann's solution or 0.9% saline) is to be effective as a plasma expander, around three times the volume of intended plasma expansion needs to be given. This commonly results in widespread peripheral oedema some days later. Supposed advantages of colloids include the ability to give effective plasma expansion faster and a reduced overall fluid loading. Disadvantages include potential allergic reactions. Hypertonic saline is another plasma expanding treatment under review.

Hypovolaemic patients are far from homogenous: causes include major trauma, peritonitis, burns, and septic shock. Whether results obtained from research in one subset of patients can be used on another is unclear. An attempt to reach clinical consensus has been made by using the crude tool of meta-analysis, but the inclusion of widely differing clinical trials has muddied rather than clarified the central issue of whether colloid or crystalloid offers specific benefits or risks. Trials on hypovolaemia in surgical patients (excluding trauma, burns, and major sepsis) suggest benefits of colloid over crystalloid, and it is only in other categories of patients that major doubts have surfaced.

This book reflects UK practice at the time of writing; namely, that rapid volume expansion of surgically shocked patients is usually best achieved initially with a plasma expander, but with early blood transfusion and early surgery to control haemorrhage.

Practice will change according to the results of future randomized controlled trials, meta-analyses, and fashion. However, all experts agree that hypovolaemia requires i/v fluid therapy to maintain tissue O_2 delivery. In our opinion loss of crystalloid is best replaced with crystalloid, loss of blood or plasma with crystalloid and/or colloid and when necessary blood products. Albumin solutions should not be used as a colloid for the purpose of volume expansion. The indications for their use are changing and again their use in this book represents our hospital practice in 1999.

Recent meta-analyses are referenced below for further reading.

Further reading

Cochrane Injuries Group Albumin Reviewers (1998). Human albumin administration in critically ill patients: systematic review of randomized controlled trials. *British Medical Journal* 317:235–40 (see also correspondence *British Medical Journal* 1988;317:882–6).

Evans PW (1998). Anaphylaxis. *British Medical Journal* 316:1442–5.

Fisher M (1996). Treatment of acute anaphylaxis. *British Medical Journal* 311:731–3.

Gomez CMH, Palazzo MGA (1998). Pulmonary artery catheterization in anaesthesia and intensive care. *British Journal of Anaesthesia* 81:945–56.

Joint Task Force on Practice Parameters, American Academy of Allergy, Asthma and Immunology, American College of Allergy, Asthma and Immunology, and the Joint Council of Allergy, Asthma and Immunology (1998). The diagnosis and management of anaphylaxis. *Journal of Allergy and Clinical Immunology* 101:S465–528.

Mark JB (1991). Central venous pressure monitoring: clinical insights beyond the numbers. *Journal of Cardiothoracic and Vascular Anesthesia* 5:163–73.

Schierhout G, Roberts I (1998). Fluid resuscitation with colloid or crystalloid solutions in critically ill patients: a systematic review of randomized trials. *British Medical Journal* 316:961–4 (see also correspondence *British Medical Journal* 1988;317:277–9).

Chest pain

Anthony Nicholls

Differential diagnosis

Chest pain after surgery is relatively common. Apart from those patients who have had thoracic surgery, the important causes to consider are MI, angina, PE, pneumonia, pneumothorax, and (in those who have had oesophageal dilatation or repeated vomiting) oesophageal rupture. 50% of patients given suxamethonium develop chest, neck, and/or shoulder pain.

As in medical practice, benign oesophageal disease (acid reflux or spasm) is common, often provoked by abdominal surgery, and sometimes difficult to differentiate from cardiac pain on the history.

The rarer causes of chest pain – aortic dissection, pericarditis, and pain referred from the spine – are uncommon in surgical practice and only need brief consideration.

- *Acute myocardial infarction* (AMI): Consider this diagnosis in any patient with central chest pain/tightness/heaviness. It is more likely with a previous history of IHD or in a high risk group: diabetes, hypertension, peripheral vascular disease, heavy smoker. Typical triggers are hypotension, hypertension, major haemorrhage, hypoxia, and sepsis.

- *Angina*: This is usually clear from the history. The patient will describe pain identical to their normal angina. Triggers are as for

AMI, and distinction from it will hinge on ECG and cardiac enzymes.

- *PE*: A major PE causes central chest pain with dyspnoea and hypotension. Smaller PEs cause pulmonary infarction, characterized by pleuritic pain and haemoptysis but lesser dyspnoea and preserved BP.

- *Pneumonia*: Postoperative pneumonia does not normally cause the picture of classical lobar pneumonia (sudden pleuritic chest pain with dyspnoea and fever). It normally presents with dyspnoea with or without fever.

- *Pneumothorax*: Occurs most commonly following central venous cannulation or chest trauma. In other settings more likely in: tall, thin young men, asthmatics, and those with emphysema. Occasionally follows abdominal or thoracic endoscopic procedures.

- *Oesophageal rupture*: A life-threatening complication of patients who have either recently had oesophageal instrumentation, particularly dilatation of a stricture, or those who have had severe vomiting. The pain is typically worse on swallowing. Often accompanied by palpable air in the neck or in the mediastinum on CXR.

- *Oesophagitis and oesophageal spasm*: These problems are common postoperatively in those who have suffered from them previously. A new presentation is more difficult to diagnose, and may first require exclusion of IHD.

- *Aortic dissection* may occur by chance in a perioperative situation, possibly triggered by severe hypertension. Characteristics are severe unremitting chest pain, conducted through to the back, unrelieved by opioids, with lack of evidence of acute MI. Management is outside the scope of this book.

- *Pericarditis* is common after cardiotomy, but otherwise is uncommon in surgical patients.

Immediate priorities

- Assess and treat the ABC.
- Administer O_2 at high flow rates through a face mask if the patient is breathless or suffering major distress. Check O_2 saturation by pulse oximetry.
- Check the circulation.
- Gain i/v access. If the patient is hypotensive and does not have signs of acute pulmonary oedema, give a rapid infusion of fluid (0.9% saline, gelatine, etherified starch) as in the section on hypotension, p. 251. Check for signs of surgical haemorrhage.
- Check for bilateral air entry: if a tension pneumothorax is diagnosed, decompress it as described on pp. 257, 286.
- Connect the patient to an ECG monitor.

- Request a 12-lead ECG. Do not rely on a monitor trace for accurate diagnosis.
- Request a portable CXR.
- After immediate management, take time to obtain a proper history and examine the patient properly.

History

Relevant features of the history include the previous history and risk factors. If the patient is distressed, they may be unable to give a coherent history. Has the patient had a similar pain before, was it investigated and what happened? Check for information in the admission clerking.

Usually it is possible to differentiate cardiac, pleuritic, and oesophageal pain on clinical grounds. However, postoperatively many patients present in an atypical fashion and further investigation is often necessary. Ask specifically for associated symptoms (dyspnoea, haemoptysis, vomiting), exacerbating and relieving factors. The exact sequence of events that triggered the chest pain may be evident from the nurses or from scrutiny of the observation charts.

Shoulder tip pain is often a sign of diaphragmatic irritation, common after laparoscopic surgery, and may occur with traumatic diaphragmatic rupture. Shoulder and chest pain often follow suxamethonium.

Examination

Assess the circulation (pulse, BP, peripheral perfusion, JVP), check for a new cardiac murmur (typical of MI involving the mitral valve mechanism), and look for any physical signs in the chest. An early CXR will assist in making the diagnosis in many patients. However postoperative chest films are often abnormal, which may confuse the clinical picture.

Investigations

- *12-lead ECG*: Diagnostic of AMI in 50% of cases at onset. May be normal in angina if the pain has settled. A normal ECG during severe chest pain argues against angina. Marked ST depression during angina indicates possible impending AMI. Arrhythmias may precipitate angina.
- *Arterial blood gases*: The combination of central chest pain, a clear CXR, and acute hypoxia is virtually diagnostic of major PE in a postoperative patient.
- *CXR* will assist in the diagnosis of oesophageal rupture, pneumonia, pneumothorax. Pulmonary oedema that may not be evident clinically may be visible on CXR.
- *Hb*: Bleeding/haemodilution may be the trigger to angina or MI.
- *Full sepsis screen* if pyrexial. Fever, chest pain and breathlessness suggests pneumonia. Sepsis at any site may trigger angina or MI in patients with underlying IHD.

· *Serial cardiac enzymes*: A retrospective diagnosis of AMI can be based on elevation of cardiac enzymes with a history of chest pain and ST/T wave changes on ECG. CK may be elevated postoperatively from muscle damage; measure the MB fraction.

Myocardial infarction (MI)

Diagnosis

Rests solely on ECG and cardiac enzyme changes. The development of left bundle branch block on ECG in association with cardiac chest pain is of the same diagnostic importance as the appearance of Q-waves.

Management

· *Pain*: Treat the pain with i/v morphine or diamorphine in incremental doses of 2.5 mg.
· *Aspirin*: Give aspirin 300 mg po or n/g (or by suppository if oral route unavailable).
· *CCU*: Move the patient to the CCU or ICU for rhythm monitoring.
· *Triggers*: Treat any factors that might have precipitated the infarct: bleeding, hypotension, hypoxia, sepsis.
· *Thrombolysis* is contraindicated within 4–5 days of major surgery, longer after neurosurgery. Thrombolysis in the postsurgical patient should only be given with the agreement of a senior surgeon.
· *Heparin* is generally safe in the postoperative situation and can be given if thrombolysis is contraindicated.
· *Electrolytes*: Check the serum Mg^{2+}, Ca^{2+} and K^+. Disorders of these electrolytes are common after surgery, and predispose to arrhythmias.
· *Nitrates*: Treat continuing pain with i/v nitrates.
· *Medical referral*: The medical team should take over the care of the cardiac problem. If the patient is kept on a surgical ward, notify the cardiac team so that the patient can be referred for cardiac rehabilitation and further investigation as needed.
· *Immediate coronary arteriography* with stenting of the occluded vessel may be feasible in some specialized centres.

Angina

Diagnosis

This will depend on the history, exclusion of AMI, and possibly ECG changes during pain.

Further investigations such as treadmill testing and coronary arteriography are generally inappropriate in the immediate postoperative situation, but unstable angina with deep ST depression may herald a major MI, and these patients may need coronary arteriography during their surgical hospitalization.

Management

- *Nitrates*: Unless sublingual nitrates promptly relieve the pain, start a nitrate infusion: isosorbide dinitrate 0.1% (1 mg/ml) should be infused at an initial rate of 2 mg/h, increasing progressively if pain persists. The maximum dose is 10 mg/h. The BP should be monitored every 30 min on a nitrate infusion: reduce the dose if the systolic BP falls below 100 mmHg. This may have to be done on a normal surgical ward but transfer to CCU/HDU/ICU is safer.
- *Opioids*: Treat the pain with i/v morphine or diamorphine in incremental doses of 2.5 mg if it is unrelieved by nitrates.
- *Aspirin*: Give aspirin 300 mg po or n/g (or by suppository if oral route unavailable).
- *Trigger factors*: Treat any factors that might have precipitated angina: bleeding, hypotension, hypoxia, sepsis.
- Refer to the medical/cardiac team.

Pulmonary embolism (PE)

Diagnosis

- *Hypoxia*: PE is the most likely cause of acute hypoxia with a clear CXR in a postoperative patients. Airflow obstruction (asthma or emphysema) should be excluded clinically.
- *ECG*: T-wave inversion across the chest leads is more common than the 'S1-Q3-T3' pattern. Tachycardia is usual.
- *CXR*. Minor changes – a small pleural effusion, plate atelectasis – are common.
- *Lung scan*: Minor PE is more difficult to diagnose. An isotope lung scan may be helpful, but unless it is totally normal it cannot exclude the diagnosis of PE.
- *Spiral CT*: This new modality is the best diagnostic test for PE but is not yet widely available. It is a rapid thoracic CT which can image the pulmonary arteries more accurately and rapidly than a conventional pulmonary angiogram.
- *Pulmonary arteriography*: This has remained the 'gold standard' test for PE, but is time consuming and cumbersome. It is rarely needed in surgical patients.
- In many patients the diagnosis of PE will be made on a *probability basis*: the risk associated with surgery, the suggestive clinical scenario and a lung scan that is consistent with (rather than diagnostic of) the diagnosis.

Management

- *O₂*: Give high flow O_2 by mask. Monitor pulse oximetry.
- *Fluids*: Start i/v fluid resuscitation as for any hypotensive patient if BP low. A raised venous pressure is typical of a major PE and in this situation does not indicate fluid overload. **Diuretics are dangerous.**
- *Anticoagulation*: Start i/v heparin and subsequently warfarin as for DVT (see p. 350). The target INR is the same.
- *Thrombolysis* can be considered in unstable patients, but the risk of major bleeding after surgery may rule it out except in occasional circumstances.
- *Caval filter*: Occasionally anticoagulation is contra-indicated in a surgical patient. If such a patient has proven thromboembolism, a temporary or permanent filter may be inserted percutaneously into the inferior vena cava.
- *Emergency embolectomy* may rarely be undertaken for life-threatening PE.

Pneumonia

Diagnosis

Usually made by CXR. Fever and purulent sputum are usually present. Pleuritic pain may occur. Laboratory markers of infection (WCC, CRP) will be raised.

Management

Refer to section on p. 284.

Pneumothorax

Chest pain (± dyspnoea) in a surgical patient may be due to spontaneous pneumothorax. More commonly pnemothorax in surgical patients is traumatic or iatrogenic. CXR is usually diagnostic, but a small pneumothorax may be missed unless an expiration film is taken. The management is addressed in Chapter 41, p. 286.

Ruptured oesophagus

Diagnosis

This hinges upon the CXR with a typical history. The CXR will show pleural fluid together with gas. Air is often seen in the mediastinum and the neck tissues. A barium swallow is diagnostic.

Management

- Keep patient nil-by-mouth.
- i/v access and fluid resuscitation.

- *Antibiotics*: Gentamicin 3–5 mg/kg i/v (single dose) plus metronidazole 500 mg i/v 8 hourly plus cefotaxime 1 g i/v 8 hourly.
- *Surgery*: Discuss further management with surgeon or endoscopist
  who performed the dilatation. Avoid n/g tube insertion.

Oesophagitis and oesophageal spasm

Diagnosis

- History: Usually similar pain experienced before.
- Exclude cardiac cause if in doubt.
- Therapeutic trial of antacids is popular and safe.
- May be aggravated by NSAIDs.

Management

- *Acid suppression*: Usually best with a proton pump inhibitor (e.g.
  lansoprazole 30 mg, omeprazole 20 mg). If nil-by-mouth, pantoprazole 40 mg i/v (slowly) or ranitidine 50 mg tds i/v is appropriate.
- *Motility agents*: Metoclopramide or cisapride (avoid with erythromycin) are both useful.

Further reading

Goldhaber SZ (1998). Pulmonary embolism. *New England Journal of
Medicine* **339**:93–104.

Uncontrolled postoperative hypertension

Anthony Nicholls

Simple postoperative hypertension rarely needs acute emergency treatment in surgical patients unless BP >220/120, or complications of hypertension develop – LVF, cardiac ischaemia, bleeding. Lesser degrees of hypertension may indicate an underlying physiological problem that needs solving. Neuro-, cardiac and vascular surgery may require tighter blood pressure control.

Causes of postoperative hypertension

- rebound from withdrawal of previous medication
- pain, anxiety, confusion
- arousal from anaesthesia
- retention of urine
- hypoxia, hypercarbia
- hypothermia and shivering
- raised intracranial pressure
- volume overload secondary to excessive blood transfusion or fluid replacement
- exaggeration of previously untreated mild hypertension by any of the above factors
- drug error (check that a vasopressor has not been administered).

Risks

- AMI
- LVF with pulmonary oedema
- cerebral haemorrhage, encephalopathy
- postoperative bleeding.

Investigations

- ECG to exclude acute ischaemia
- electrolytes and creatinine to exclude renal failure. Ensure the patient is passing adequate volumes of urine (>30 ml/h).

Treatment

- Check blood pressure personally using the correct size of cuff.
- Look for and treat all precipitating factors.
- Treat pain and anxiety.
- Palpate bladder to exclude retention of urine.
- Sit the patient partially up if possible.
- Review intravenous fluid therapy, give frusemide if overloaded or evidence of pulmonary oedema.
- Check whether regular antihypertensive therapy has been administered. Resume normal regime orally or via n/g tube if possible. If patient unable to absorb from gut give hydralazine 5 mg i/v over 5 min and repeat every 10–15 min to a total of 20 mg until diastolic pressure <110 mmHg. Labetolol (see below) can be given if the patient is in the recovery room or other area capable of monitoring the patient.
- Brittle hypertensives, especially those with target organ involvement, should be considered for ICU/HDU care.

Emergency therapy of severe hypertension

- This is only applicable if the patient has a BP >220/120 mmHg and has evidence of a life-threatening complication such as hypertensive encephalopathy, retinal haemorrhages, heart failure, or MI.
- There is no proven benefit of rapid blood pressure reduction in the absence of complications. These patients can be treated by standard oral therapies, e.g. atenolol 50 mg, nifedipine LA 30 mg.

In HDU/ICU or recovery, if precipitating factors have been excluded and urgent therapy is needed, hypertension can be treated with a fast acting rapidly titratable intravenous drug such as:

- *β-blockers*: Labetolol (5–100 mg slowly i/v) may be used but beware long half-life (2–4 h). Esmolol has a short duration of action: give

0.5 mg/kg loading dose followed by maintenance infusion of 50–200 μg/kg per min. Avoid β-blockers in asthma, heart failure, or heart block.

- *Hydralazine* 5–10 mg i/v over 20 min.
- *Nitrates*: Glyceryl trinitrate can be given by infusion at 1–4 μg/kg per min. Isosorbide dinitrate is given at 2–10 mg/h by infusion. Both may have limited efficacy in patients with moderate to severe hypertension.
- Sodium nitroprusside is occasionally used, starting at 0.25 μg/kg per min. May cause coronary steal, increased intrapulmonary shunting, and reflex tachycardia. High doses and prolonged infusion increases the risk of cyanide and thiocyanate toxicity. Intra-arterial pressure monitoring in ICU is essential.

Note: Nifedipine 5–10 mg sublingually has been associated with a an increased risk of myocardial infarction when used in hypertensive crises. It should no longer be used. Oral long-acting nifedipine (Adalat LA) is safe.

Further reading

Editorial (1989). Severe symptomless hypertension. *Lancet* ii:1369.

Gifford RW (1991). Management of hypertensive crises. *Journal of the American Medical Association* 266:829–35.

Grossman E, Messerli FH, Grodzicki T, Kowey P (1996). Should a moratorium be placed on sublingual nifedipine capsules for hypertensive emergencies or pseudoemergencies? *Journal of the American Medical Association* 276:1328–30.

Cardiac arrhythmias

John Dean

Risks

The haemodynamic consequences of the arrhythmia determine the urgency of the treatment. The same rhythm disturbance may have little or no impact on one patient, but cause cardiovascular collapse in another. Patients with compromised LV function are at the greatest risk, and may develop arrhythmias without provocation even when all appropriate measures for prevention have been taken.

Major surgery such as aortic aneurysm repair imposes a higher risk of arrhythmia than a minor procedure such as cataract surgery. Any abrupt change in heart rate, particularly if there is a fall in BP, should raise the possibility of an arrhythmia. Whenever possible a 12-lead ECG of the arrhythmia should be recorded; failing this a rhythm strip may be obtained by using the ECG monitor of the ward defibrillator. Patients with life-threatening arrhythmias should be managed on CCU/ICU/HDU.

When assessing patients with arrhythmias look for any precipitating factors that need controlling. These include hypovolaemia, cardiac failure, respiratory failure, sepsis, electrolyte imbalance (especially K^+, Ca^{2+}, Mg^{2+}) and PE.

Tachycardias

Sinus tachycardia

This commonly occurs perioperatively and is invariably secondary to some other process such as pain, volume depletion, sepsis, β-blocker

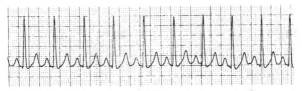

Fig. 40.1 Sinus tachycardia. Each QRS complex is preceded by a normal P-wave.

withdrawal, etc. Tachycardia may induce ischaemia in patients with coronary disease and may precipitate heart failure in those with compromised LV function.

Treat the underlying cause. β-blockers are useful if angina or ECG evidence of ischaemia occurs.

Atrial fibrillation (AF)

AF is commonly precipitated (often for the first time) by surgery. It is more likely to occur in elderly patients, following cardiac or thoracic surgery (due to pericardial irritation) and in those with known heart disease. Treatment is aimed at controlling the ventricular rate to <100/min, restoring and sustaining sinus rhythm, and preventing complications, particularly arterial thromboembolism.

- Check for precipitating factors such as hypovolaemia, hypoxia, hypokalaemia, hypomagnesaemia.
- Digoxin is still one of the most valuable drugs for treating AF. A loading dose of 0.5–1.0 mg will quickly slow the ventricular rate with an average daily maintenance dose of 0.25 mg according to age, size, renal function, serum K^+ and co-administration of other drugs especially β-blockers and Ca^{2+} antagonists. Digoxin can be given parenterally, preferably by intravenous infusion (loading at 0.5 mg/h), to patients who cannot tolerate oral therapy.
- Alternative drugs to control ventricular response are β-blockers or Ca^{2+} channel blockers. The short acting intravenous beta blocker esmolol (500 μg/kg bolus, then 50–300 μg/kg per min as a maintenance infusion), is useful in an emergency to control the ventricular

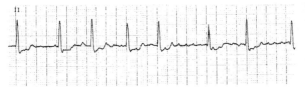

Fig. 40.2 Atrial fibrillation. Rapid irregular rhythm with erratic baseline due to F-waves.

rate in patients with IHD, and has been shown to facilitate cardioversion to sinus rhythm.

- Flecainide is an alternative where β-blockers are contraindicated (e.g. asthma or peripheral vascular disease), given as a slow bolus of 10 mg/min up to a maximum of 150 mg. The onset of action is more rapid than amiodarone. Do not use if LV function is compromised.

- Amiodarone is the best alternative in patients with severely compromised LV function. It should be given i/v through a central line (5 mg/kg over 1 h, followed by 500 mg every 12 h by maintenance infusion).

- Synchronized DC cardioversion ($\geq$200 J) to restore sinus rhythm may be necessary in patients who are severely compromised by AF. General anaesthesia or careful sedation with diamorphine and midazolam is necessary if the patient is conscious. Anticoagulation with intravenous heparin should be given to all patients with AF where practicable to reduce the risk of arterial thromboembolism.

Atrial flutter

Closely related to AF. The principles of treatment are similar. The coordinated atrial conduction pattern imposes a lower risk of thromboembolic complications.

- *DC cardioversion*: Atrial flutter is very electrically sensitive and successful conversion to sinus rhythm by DC shock is virtually 100%. Low-energy synchronized DC cardioversion (<200 J) is pointless for any arrhythmia; the widely held belief that high energy DC shocks (200–360 J) damage the myocardium is untrue. Although atrial flutter may be successfully treated by 50 J or less, energies below 200 J may convert it to atrial fibrillation so multiple shocks may become necessary.

- Carotid sinus massage or intravenous adenosine (0.2 mg/kg by rapid bolus injection) with ECG monitoring, rarely converts the rhythm to sinus, but slowing the ventricular rate will expose the flutter waves on the ECG if these were not obvious before.

- The same drugs as are used for AF may be used to slow the ventricular response in established atrial flutter.

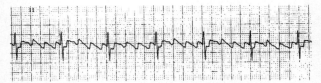

Fig. 40.3 Atrial flutter. Rapid regular/irregular rhythm with characteristic 'sawtooth' baseline.

Junctional tachycardia

Sometimes referred to as supraventricular tachycardia (SVT) and can occur in patients of any age, including children. The QRS complexes are usually, but not always, narrow. There may be features of Wolff–Parkinson–White syndrome on the ECG in sinus rhythm (short PR with δ-wave).

- Simple vagal stimulating manoeuvres such as carotid sinus massage may be effective in terminating the tachycardia.

- If these are not successful try i/v adenosine (0.2 mg/kg) by rapid intravenous bolus injection, while recording the ECG. This can be simply done by attaching the patient to the ECG monitor of the ward defibrillator and running the paper recorder. Adenosine is a potent, but very short-acting AV nodal blocking agent. The dose required to achieve AV block varies according to the site of injection (peripheral injections reach the heart in a more diluted form) whereas heart transplant recipients and patients taking dipyridamole are more sensitive. Patients should be warned of the unpleasant effects of adenosine which coincide with the AV nodal blocking effect. These include flushing, dyspnoea, and chest tightness. The patient should keep as still as possible to minimize motion artefact on the ECG. Adenosine should be used with extreme caution in asthma, as it can trigger bronchospasm.

- If the rhythm reverts to sinus after adenosine but then relapses, a longer-acting AV nodal blocking agent such as verapamil (5–10 mg over 1–2 min) may be given.

- If adenosine has no effect and the QRS complexes on the ECG during tachycardia are narrow, then a higher dose of adenosine is required. However, if the QRS complexes are broad consider whether ventricular tachycardia is present.

- DC cardioversion is rarely needed for junctional tachycardia as adenosine at high dose is so effective. If needed, a brief general anaesthetic is preferable to sedation: call the anaesthetist and medical specialist registrar.

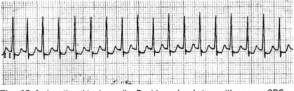

Fig. 40.4 Junctional tachycardia. Rapid regular rhythm with narrow QRS complexes.

Ventricular tachycardia (VT)

VT may present as anything from mild palpitations to cardiac arrest. The ECG shows a broad QRS complex tachycardia (Fig. 40.5). Complex algorithms have been produced to distinguish broad complex SVT from VT, but these are largely valueless. **Any patient presenting with a regular, broad complex tachycardia, particularly if there is a history of myocardial infarction or ventricular disease should be treated as VT until proved otherwise, particularly if there is a history of MI or ventricular disease.**

- If the patient is haemodynamically stable give a rapid intravenous bolus of 0.2 mg/kg adenosine while monitoring the ECG.
- If there is no change, proceed to DC cardioversion.
- **Do not give intravenous verapamil** if adenosine fails. In VT, verapamil is ineffective and the negative inotropic and vasodilatory effects may result in cardiovascular collapse.
- Lidocaine (lignocaine) may be given intravenously (100 mg bolus) and will restore sinus rhythm in about 60% of cases. If conversion does not occur, it may result in haemodynamic deterioration, owing to its negative inotropic effect.
- DC cardioversion is safe and effective at restoring sinus rhythm in virtually 100% of cases. Reserve prophylactic therapy for recurrent VT.
- If the patient relapses back into tachycardia, drugs such as lidocaine (lignocaine), flecainide, or amiodarone may be necessary to sustain sinus rhythm. Expert assistance should be sought from a cardiologist.

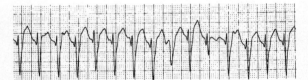

Fig. 40.5 Ventricular tachycardia. Rapid broad QRS complex rhythm.

Ventricular fibrillation (VF)

VF results in cardiac arrest and is usually due to acute myocardial ischaemia. It is managed with emergency DC cardioversion. Following successful resuscitation, transfer the patient to CCU/HCU/ICU. If VF is recurrent, give intravenous Mg^{2+} (10 mmol bolus, 1–3 mmol/h infusion). *Torsades de pointes* is a form of polymorphic VT which responds to i/v Mg^{2+}, but is aggravated by lidocaine (lignocaine). See Chapter 30 for further management of cardiac arrest.

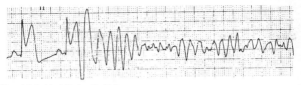

Fig. 40.6 Ventricular fibrillation.

Bradycardias

Vagal stimulation

This is common during abdominal, head, neck, eye, and thoracic surgery and may produce profound bradycardia in otherwise healthy individuals. The effect can be either on the sinus node causing sinus bradycardia, or sinus arrest (Fig. 40.7), or on the AV node causing AV block (Fig 40.8). This does not imply cardiac disease. Highly trained athletes will have a high resting vagal tone and are prone to periods of bradycardia that may need no treatment. The effects of excessive vagal stimulation are usually easy to counter by using anticholinergic agents such as atropine (0.5–1 mg i/v). Patients receiving β-blockers are more at risk of bradycardia and may be resistant to atropine. They may be managed with intravenous isoproterenol (isoprenaline) (i/v infusion 0.5–10 μg/min) on CCU/ICU.

Fig. 40.7 Sinus arrest.

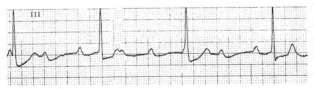

Fig. 40.8 Complete heart block.

Symptomatic bradycardia

Treat bradycardia resulting in syncope or hypotension by cardiac pacing. The causes are either sinus node disease with sinus arrest or heart block. Both are due to cardiac conducting tissue disease.

- Temporary pacing may be necessary as an emergency measure, particularly when atropine or isoproterenol is ineffective or cannot be tolerated. The strongly preferred approach is transvenous, using the internal jugular or subclavian vein. If it is likely that the patient will require permanent pacing, use the right sided veins for right-handed patients and vice versa, as this leaves the opposite (non-dominant) side free for the permanent system. Flotation electrodes are easy to use and do not require X-ray screening facilities.

- Using an aseptic technique pass the electrode through the central vein to the 20 cm mark. Attach a pulse generator and inflate the balloon. Use the demand mode and set the pacemaker rate 10–20 beats/min higher than the intrinsic ventricular rate with an output of 5 V. Advance the electrode slowly watching the ECG tracing. As the electrode makes contact with the right atrium, pacing spikes with atrial capture may be seen. Ventricular ectopic beats are usually seen as the electrode passes across the tricuspid valve into the right ventricle and then ventricular capture will be seen (broad QRS complexes preceded by a pacing spike). Deflate the balloon at this point and advance a further 5 cm. If the electrode reaches 50 cm without ventricular capture, it is likely to be coiled within the right atrium. Deflate the balloon, withdraw to 20 cm, and attempt a further 'pass'.

- Transcutaneous or oesophageal pacing may be used in an emergency if the transvenous approach is not immediately available. Transcutaneous pacing can be very painful if the threshold required to achieve capture is high and should only be given to patients who are unconscious or heavily sedated.

The breathless patient

Iain Wilson and Chris Sheldon

Dyspnoea in a surgical patient is normally caused by hypoxia. It always requires urgent investigation and treatment. The cause of the hypoxia can usually be diagnosed on the basis of history, examination, and CXR.

Anaesthesia affects respiratory function in a variety of ways, but these are largely over within 24 h. A thoracic or upper abdominal incision affects respiration for several days. Lung atelectasis, diaphragmatic and chest wall splinting, and sputum retention occur commonly. Uncontrolled pain worsens the situation.

- Dyspnoea that develops over a few minutes is suggestive of pulmonary oedema, PE, pneumothorax, anaphylaxis, aspiration, or a cardiac disaster such as a valve rupture.

- Breathlessness developing over a few hours suggests lung collapse/atelectasis/consolidation, pulmonary oedema from LVF or excessive fluid therapy, asthma, pulmonary contusion, or ARDS, which may follow a variety of problems such as sepsis, aspiration, fat embolism, and massive transfusion.

- Slowly worsening dyspnoea should suggest the possibility of a pleural effusion, lung collapse/consolidation, or pneumonia.
- Breathlessness may be due to a non-respiratory cause, sometimes without hypoxia. Assessment should consider septicaemia, bleeding, acidosis, pain, and anxiety as possible causes.

Immediate management

- Assess the airway to ensure that it is patent; remove any obstruction.
- Administer O_2 at high flow rates through a face mask – see section on O_2 therapy p. 293.
- Check that the breathing is adequate. Assess both tidal volume and the quality and equality of breath sounds on auscultation. Assist respiration with a self-inflating bag if necessary.
- Check the circulation. If the pulse disappears commence chest compressions and call for the cardiac arrest team.
- If a tension pneumothorax is diagnosed, decompress it (see p. 257).
- If the situation is life threatening or the conscious level is depressed immediately contact the anaesthetist on call for ICU.
- Connect a pulse oximeter; O_2 saturations < 95% in a previously fit patient are significant, < 90% indicate serious hypoxia.
- Gain i/v access.

When stabilized

- *Obtain a history.* Did the dyspnoea follow any specific event, such as drug administration (possible anaphylaxis)? Could the dyspnoea be related to the surgical condition or an underlying medical problem? Was there any cough, chest pain, haemoptysis, or wheeze?
- *Examine the whole patient* including the conscious level and look for signs of confusion. An altered conscious level due to respiratory failure is critical. Look for abnormal physical signs in the chest – there may be none, which is also important. Record the temperature and examine the abdomen for distension or tenderness.
- *Reassess the circulation.* Check the heart (rate, murmurs, gallop rhythm), and assess the peripheral circulation and blood pressure. In the postoperative patient sudden cardiovascular instability accompanied by dyspnoea is suggestive of PE. Obtain an ECG.
- *Request an urgent CXR*, on the ward if necessary. Do not confuse a tension pneumothorax with lung collapse on the opposite side.
- *Measure arterial blood gases* whilst waiting for the radiographer. These will reveal the severity of hypoxia, the $PaCO_2$ and the acid/base balance. A PaO_2 < 8 kPa needs urgent treatment. If this is obtained on

a high inspired concentration of O_2, the patient will usually need admission to HDU/ICU and perhaps mechanical ventilation. The gases will reveal whether the patient is acidotic due to hypercarbia or a metabolic problem. A chronically raised $PaCO_2$ may occur in some patients with underlying chest disease. This may deteriorate with the effect of anaesthesia and surgery in a compromised patient.

- *Decide on a plan of action.* If an expert opinion is required then ask for this as early as possible. The most useful people are likely to be the ICU medical staff, consultant surgeon, or a respiratory physician. Continuing management will depend on the specific diagnosis.

Acute asthma

Asthma presenting postoperatively for the first time (i.e. no history of asthma) is extremely unlikely. If you suspect that the patient has an attack of asthma, try to assess severity:

- Able to talk in full sentences?
- Respiratory rate.
- Signs of respiratory distress, use of accessory muscles, hyperinflation, or agitation. Remember the chest may be silent in severe asthma.
- Able to use a peak flow meter? (Compare with preoperative value).
- Check arterial blood gases (a rising $PaCO_2$ or a low PaO_2 are ominous).
- CXR – to exclude causes other than asthma, especially pneumothorax complicating asthma.

Treatment

- 60% O_2 via face mask, humidified if possible.
- Monitor SpO_2 (should be >95%).
- Nebulized salbutamol 2.5–5 mg repeated after 30 min if still very short of breath.
- Nebulized ipratropium bromide (Atrovent) 500 μg 6 hourly.
- If severe, consider giving hydrocortisone 200 mg i/v bolus and increase or start systemic steroids.
- **Patients with asthma may suddenly deteriorate. Call for advice from either a physician or the ICU if there is no improvement after 45 min. Ask for help immediately if patient is becoming tired or more breathless despite treatment.**
- Physiotherapy is not normally helpful in acute asthma.

Lung collapse, consolidation, and pneumonia

These complications arise most commonly after abdominal or chest surgery. They are more frequent in smokers, those with underlying chest disease, or the elderly and frail.

Atelectasis

- Usually occurs at the bases of the lungs due to the inability to expand the lung efficiently. Occurs immediately after surgery and typically lasts for several days. May be detected on auscultation and confirmed on a CXR.

- Treatment involves humidified O_2, pain control, posture, physiotherapy to promote lung expansion and clearance of secretions, and early mobilization. Sputum retention is a frequent problem and if it does not resolve with simple measures, a mini-tracheostomy (placed through the cricothyroid membrane) may help clear secretions. These are usually performed by the ICU team and used by the physiotherapists and nursing staff. Any coincidental bronchospasm, cardiac failure, or fluid overload should be managed vigorously.

- If infection is thought to be present (fever, raised WCC and CRP) manage as pneumonia. Aggressive early treatment of these patients appears to prevent many late problems.

Pneumonia

Postoperative pneumonia is more common in those patients with any serious underlying illness but particularly obesity, prolonged surgery and ventilation, pre-existing respiratory disease, immobility, and prior antibiotic treatment.

Presentation

Pneumonia generally develops 36–72 h postoperatively. Patients frequently feel non-specifically unwell with increased breathlessness, sweating, and cough. There may be pleuritic pain. Haemoptysis is relatively infrequent and is usually mixed with purulent sputum.

The first signs are generally pyrexia followed by an increase in respiratory rate, tachycardia, and hypotension. Confusion may occur but is more common in those with underlying cerebral pathology such as early dementia. Cough with sputum production is a relatively late phenomenon.

Investigations

- Pulse, BP, pulse oximetry (blood gases if pre-existing lung disease or SpO_2 <95%).
- CXR: Consolidation is necessary to make the diagnosis of pneumonia.
- FBC, electrolytes, CRP, liver function tests.
- Blood cultures.
- Sputum microscopy, culture and sensitivity (sometimes only obtainable after physiotherapy).
- Tracheal suction specimen, where appropriate.
- Consider sending MSU if source of fever is unknown and diagnosis of pneumonia is in doubt.

Likely pathogens

- Much more commonly gram −ve organisms than in community-acquired pneumonia.
- Commonest gram −ve organisms are *Pseudomonas aeruginosa*, *Klebsiella* species and *Escherichia coli*. Anaerobes may become pathogenic after aspiration.
- *Staphylococcus aureus* should also be considered as this may account for up to 15% of postoperative pneumonia.
- Patients with COPD may develop pneumonia due to *Streptococcus pneumoniae* or *Haemophilus influenzae* 1–3 days after operation.
- Immunocompromised patients (those on immunosuppressive therapy, with neutropenia, with AIDS) may develop infection with opportunist organisms such as *Pneumocystis pneumoniae*, CMV, fungi, *Pseudomonas*. Always refer such patients to a respiratory physician for further management, which will probably include diagnostic broncho-alveolar lavage.

Treatment

- O_2 to maintain saturation >92% (see O_2 therapy below, p. 293).
- Antibiotics as described on p. 343.
- Give first dose of antibiotics i/v. After this, many patients may be able to take them orally. If severely unwell with hypotension or unable to take orally, continue i/v until pyrexia has resolved for at least 24 h.
- Once sputum cultures and sensitivities are available antibiotic therapy can be more appropriately targeted. Wherever possible use an effective drug with the narrowest spectrum of activity to prevent complications of treatment such as *Clostridium difficile* enterocolitis and the emergence of resistant organisms.
- Physiotherapy is helpful in mobilizing secretions and preventing further atelectasis.
- i/v fluids may be required to maintain blood pressure and urine output.

Complications

Many patients recover with no complications. However the commonest complications are:

- respiratory failure (detected clinically or by falling SpO_2 in the face of increasing inspired O_2 concentrations); check blood gases
- cardiac arrhythmias, most commonly atrial fibrillation
- renal failure associated with septicaemia or hypotension
- pleural effusion/ empyema may be detected on CXR; differentiate between lung consolidation, effusion and empyema by chest ultrasound
- sepsis syndrome requiring ICU support.

Pneumothorax

Pneumothorax may follow insertion of a central line or a surgical procedure, complicate an attack of asthma, or be caused by IPPV. Alternatively, the presentation in a postoperative patient may simply be with pleuritic pain and dyspnoea. Either way, the symptoms will always trigger the need for a CXR, so the diagnosis should not be missed. However, iatrogenic pneumothorax after central venous cannulation typically presents some hours after cannulation and is not ruled out by a normal CXR immediately after insertion.

Management

- *Tension pneumothorax* is usually characterized by both dyspnoea and hypotension. The management is described under hypotension on p. 257.

- *Intercostal drain or aspiration?* Spontaneous pneumothorax is normally treated intially by aspiration (Box 41.1). Pneumothorax in a surgical patient is typically secondary to central line insertion, trauma or positive pressure ventilation. These patients usually need an intercostal drain.

- *Aspiration or observation?* Some patients can be managed by inpatient observation alone. Observation is all that is required for the management of a patient without significant dyspnoea who has incomplete lung collapse. Patients with underlying COPD are usually breathless even after a small pneumothorax. They can still be treated initially by aspiration, although many will subsequently need a chest drain.

- *Chest drain insertion:* An intercostal chest drain must be inserted into three categories of patients: those on ventilators, tension pneumothorax, and failed aspiration. The technique for drain insertion

Box 41.1 Technique for pneumothorax aspiration

1. Lie the patient flat or propped up on several pillows according to comfort.
2. Ask the patient to put their hands behind their head.
3. Identify the third or fourth intercostal space in the mid-axillary line.
4. Infiltrate lidocaine (lignocaine) 1% down to the pleura. You will recognize the pleural space by aspirating air into the syringe. Replace the needle with an 18 gauge cannula. Insert the needle and cannula into the space and then withdraw the needle leaving the cannula in the space.
5. Attach a three-way tap and 60 ml syringe.
6. Aspirate air into the syringe and expel it via the three-way tap. A medium pneumothorax may contain a litre or more of air, so many syringe-fulls are required to drain it.
7. Get a CXR to confirm resolution or improvement of the pneumothorax.

should not be learnt from a book – get someone who has been trained to teach you.

- *Ventilated patients*: Beyond the scope of this book. Always require a chest drain.

Left ventricular failure (LVF) and pulmonary oedema

Pulmonary oedema impairs gas exchange causing hypoxia and acute dyspnoea, typically with orthopnoea. In addition, the lungs are 'stiff' and difficult for the patient to expand.

Pulmonary oedema is usually due to LVF, but the two terms are not synonymous: pulmonary oedema may develop due to changes in both LV function and volume status. Causes include:

- an acute deterioration of LV function (e.g. AMI, arrhythmia)
- deterioration in LV function due to extracardiac causes (hypoxia and anaemia are typical postoperative triggers)
- a combination of fluid overload and chronic LV dysfunction
- less commonly a pulmonary capillary leak – ARDS (see below).

The aetiology and therapy of pulmonary oedema should be considered in terms of LV function, triggering factors, and volume status.

Presentation

- Dyspnoeic, cold, clammy, sweating, anxious, cyanosed patient with pink frothy sputum.
- Bilateral lung crackles, sometimes audible wheeze, and tachycardia. Raised JVP. Angina may develop.
- Often a history of previous MI or episodes of pulmonary oedema.

Investigations

- The initial diagnosis is clinical.
- CXR should confirm pulmonary oedema, and possibly show upper lobe blood diversion (if radiograph taken sitting), enlarged heart on PA film, pleural effusion. Rethink the diagnosis if CXR is clear.
- ECG may be normal or reveal arrhythmia, ischaemia or MI.
- Arterial blood gases.
- Haemoglobin.
- Ensure patient is not in renal failure. Check the urine output, and check creatinine if patient oliguric.

Management

The treatment aims to reduce pulmonary oedema and LV filling pressures.

- 60% O_2: measure SpO_2 continuously.
- Sit the patient up.
- Stop i/v fluids.
- Frusemide (furosemide) 20–50 mg i/v slowly.
- Diamorphine 5 mg or morphine 10 mg i/v slowly (reduces preload and anxiety).
- GTN spray 1–2 puffs under tongue (unless systolic BP < 90 mmHg or known aortic stenosis).
- Consider the underlying cause – IHD or valvular heart disease, arrhythmia, MI, fluid overload, anaemia. Correct any reversible factors.
- If the patient is hypoxic (SpO_2 < 93%) and does not improve with these basic measures ask for immediate help either from the on-call medical team who may admit the patient to CCU (vasodilator therapy), or the ICU team (vasodilator, CPAP, or ventilation). If the patient continues to deteriorate, cardiac arrest is likely; delays in therapy will prove fatal.
- Patients in renal failure will need haemofiltration or haemodialysis and possibly ventilation. Urgent referral to the renal or ICU team is appropriate.
- If a new murmur is heard, arrange for an echocardiogram to detect valve failure and ventricular function.

Pulmonary embolism (PE)

Major PE classically present as circulatory collapse and/or acute dyspnoea 7–10 days after surgery or immobilization. Minor PE produce the syndrome of pulmonary infarction, with pleuritic pain, but less prominent dyspnoea and normal BP.

Untreated, PE will be followed by a recurrent PE in 50% of cases, and 50% of these recurrences will be fatal. It is safer to initially over-diagnose PE in a postoperative situation than allow the patient to run the risk of dying. **The diagnosis of PE cannot always be 100% accurate, so unless there is a clear-cut alternative to PE for a postoperative patient's symptoms of breathlessness, start a heparin infusion. Check with the surgeon who performed the operation that there are no contraindications for heparinization.**

Diagnosis

- There may be pleuritic chest pain, hypoxia, dyspnoea, haemoptysis, tachycardia, raised JVP, and evidence of a DVT.
- An ECG may show an S wave in lead SI, Q wave in lead III, T wave inversion in lead III, (S1-Q3-T3 pattern); right ventricular strain pattern; T-wave inversion in the chest leads; or right bundle branch

block. The ECG is normal in 50% of patients. Sinus tachycardia is the commonest finding; a proportion of patients develop AF.

- A V/Q scan is the best investigation, but takes time to organize and can be difficult to interpret, particularly if there is pre-existing pulmonary disease. Spiral CT scans may be diagnostic.
- Pulmonary angiography is occasionally performed.
- A CXR is often unhelpful, although with a large PE an oligaemic area may be seen.
- The diagnosis is frequently made on a high index of clinical suspicion.

Management

- Check airway, breathing and circulation (ABC), administer high flow O_2.
- If the patient is *in extremis* consider immediate embolectomy if facilities allow, otherwise contact ICU.
- Anticoagulate using heparin according to the schedule on p. 350. A loading dose of 5000 U by i/v bolus is followed by an infusion at an initial rate of 17 500 units 12 hourly.
- Consider streptokinase with consultant.
- Analgesia – i/v morphine 5–15 mg slowly.
- With repeated PE, or if anticoagulation totally contraindicated, consider an inferior vena caval filter.

Fat embolism syndrome

- Fat embolism presents with confusion, coma, dyspnoea, and skin petechiae 24–48 h after any major trauma with fractures. Massive fat embolism may resemble thrombotic embolism, but smaller amounts of fat released into the circulation cause little pulmonary distress.
- Fat that passes through the lungs and occludes small systemic capillaries may cause confusion or other cerebral signs and skin petechiae.
- The diagnosis is made clinically and may be difficult to confirm. Occasionally fat globules may be detected in the urine.
- Treatment is supportive. Assessment by the ICU staff will be required as severe hypoxia due to ARDS may occur. DIC and multi-organ failure may follow immune system activation.
- The incidence of fat embolism syndrome has been reduced by the increasing practice of early long bone fixation.

Acute respiratory distress syndrome (ARDS)

Results from abnormal pulmonary capillary permeability developing in response to a variety of non-specific problems such as massive transfusion, sepsis, major trauma, fat embolism, aspiration, or pancreatitis.

Non-hydrostatic, proteinaceous pulmonary oedema develops which may resolve with treatment of the underlying problem, but in a few patients progresses rapidly to alveolar fibrosis. It is often associated with a general capillary leak within the systemic circulation and multiple organ dysfunction or failure.

Presentation

Patients present with dyspnoea and hypoxia. The CXR may be unimpressive in the early stages but always goes on to develop a ground glass/pulmonary oedema appearance. Blood gases demonstrate hypoxia, often with hypocarbia due to hyperventilation. The diagnosis should be suspected when a surgical patient fails to respond to treatment for pulmonary oedema.

Management

An underlying cause should always be looked for and treated, as the resolution of ARDS depends on this. Patients suspected of developing ARDS should always be referred to the ICU team as the management is complex and often requires considerable physiological support. It includes:

- treatment of the underlying problem (e.g. antibiotics)
- respiratory support (CPAP/ventilation)
- optimization of the circulation with inotropes and detailed attention to fluid balance to ensure adequate O_2 delivery
- haemofiltration if renal failure develops

Steroids are not useful in the early stages.

Upper airway obstruction (stridor)

Obstruction of the upper airway is an occasional cause of respiratory problems in the postoperative period. It may be simple upper airway obstruction caused by a depressed conscious level, which usually presents, and is dealt with, in the recovery unit. However, it may also arise as a complication of surgery or anaesthesia presenting as acute respiratory distress. Airway obstruction is an emergency and should always be responded to immediately.

Immediate postoperative airway obstruction due to sedation/anaesthesia/depressed conscious level

These patients present with noisy/obstructed breathing caused by obstruction at the level of the pharynx due to a depressed conscious level.

Management

- Immediate airway manoeuvres – chin lift + oropharyngeal airway (normally size 3 for men, size 2 for women) and/or jaw thrust.
- Give O_2 and support breathing if clinically indicated.

- Call for help – anaesthetist on call or ICU staff.
- Assess reason for depressed conscious level and treat.
- If conscious level depressed by opioids give i/v naloxone 200 μg and repeat until effective.
- If conscious level depressed by benzodiazepines give i/v fluma-zenil 200 μg.
- For other causes of coma see p. 326.

Upper airway obstruction not related to anaesthesia/sedation

These patients present with stridor and are normally conscious, dis-tressed, and hypoxic. The cause is related to obstruction in the upper airway. The history and nature of the surgery performed may assist in the diagnosis.

Management

- Added O_2 – high flow. Assess airway – foreign body?
- Sit up, if not already doing so.
- Call for help – anaesthetist on call or ICU staff and surgical consultant. Alert theatres in case operation needed.

Possible diagnoses

- Trauma to the upper airway following intubation – rare, usually settles spontaneously, anaesthetist will advise.
- Injury to the upper airway following trauma: Anaesthetist and ENT/thoracic surgeon will advise. Normally presents on arrival at hospital.
- Following thyroid/parathyroid surgery there may be haemorrhage into the neck. Immediately remove skin staples/sutures, and sutures holding strap muscles to decompress trachea.
- Following thyroid/parathyroid surgery there may be damage to the recurrent laryngeal nerve. Usually presents as stridor whenever patients exerts themselves and characterized by a hoarse (bovine) cough. Consider also tracheomalacia.
- Tumour of upper airway: Swelling may follow biopsy or manipula-tion. History will help. Treatment may include tracheostomy.
- Infection – including epiglottitis.

Other measures

- Heliox is a mixture of 20% O_2 in 80% helium. It has a lower density than air and is sometimes used as it causes less respiratory resist-ance than air O_2. Although it may reduce airway resistance, **it is never a solution to an obstructed airway.**
- The peak flow, if obtainable, is a good measure of the severity of large airway obstruction causing stridor; a peak flow < 200 l/min is

worrying, < 100 l/min may indicate critical airway narrowing and approaching asphyxiation.

Arterial blood gas analysis

Taking the sample

- Use a pre-heparinized blood gas syringe. Expel excess heparin before use. If possible use a specifically designed blood gas syringe (e.g. Pulsator).
- When sampling from the radial artery a small amount of 1% lidocaine (lignocaine) injected subcutaneously will make the procedure more comfortable. After sampling, expel air bubbles and note the time of sampling and the FiO_2.
- Apply pressure over the artery for 5 min, longer in anticoagulated patients. If immediate analysis is not possible, store the sample in ice for transport.

Interpreting the blood gas result

Table 41.1 gives normal blood gas values. Interpretation of blood gases must take account of the clinical picture and any previous blood gas results.

- *pH*: If abnormal, decide whether acidosis or alkalosis.
- *PaO_2*: < 8 kPa indicates significant hypoxia (particularly if the patient is receiving O_2 therapy), and is classed as respiratory failure. If this does not fit the clinical picture consider whether a venous sample has been obtained or if there could be a cardiac shunt present. Levels > 15 kPa indicate high inspired O_2.
- *$PaCO_2$*: A low $PaCO_2$ indicates hyperventilation, a raised $PaCO_2$ hypoventilation.
- *HCO_3^-* and base excess are derived values giving information about the metabolic condition of the blood. Low HCO_3^- or negative base excess levels suggest a metabolic acidosis; a raised bicarbonate or positive base excess indicates a metabolic alkalosis.
- *O_2 saturation* is usually a calculated value unless the blood gas analyser is fitted with a co-oximeter. A calculated Hb saturation is less accurate than values obtained by pulse oximetry.

Table 41.1 Normal arterial blood gas values

pH	7.36–7.44
PaO_2	11–13 kPa (83–98 mmHg)
$PaCO_2$	4.8–6.0 kPa (36–45 mmHg)
HCO_3^-	22–32 mmol/l
Base excess	−3 to +3
Haemoglobin O_2 saturation	>94%

Interpretation of acid–base changes

An acidosis may be respiratory (raised $PaCO_2$) or metabolic (base deficit). With an acute respiratory acidosis there will no be time for metabolic compensation. A metabolic acidosis is usually accompanied by an immediate respiratory compensation that is often incomplete.

A respiratory alkalosis commonly results from hypoxic hyperventilation but may also have metabolic causes. Sometimes a metabolic alkalosis is accompanied by CO_2 accumulation to allow pH compensation. The history will differentiate this from chronic CO_2 retention with metabolic compensation.

Causes

- *Respiratory acidosis*: respiratory failure or depression (consider excessive sedation from opioids or other drugs).
- *Metabolic acidosis*: renal failure, lactic acidosis (circulatory failure, liver failure, biguanides), chronic loss of HCO_3^- (bowel), diabetic ketoacidosis.
- *Respiratory alkalosis*: hyperventilation secondary to hypoxia, central (neurological) causes of hyperventilation, e.g. anxiety, head injury, subarachnoid haemorrhage.
- *Metabolic alkalosis*: loss of acid (e.g. pyloric stenosis), diuretics, hypokalaemia.

Special circumstances

In metabolic acidosis the anion gap may be calculated as $[Na^+] + [K^+] - [Cl^-] - [HCO_3^-]$. The normal is 16–18 mmol/l. An elevated anion gap suggests accumulation of anions (phosphates, lactate, or ketones) within the circulation (e.g. lactic acid).

- Carbon monoxide poisoning: measure blood gases using an analyser with a co-oximeter to estimate the carboxyhaemoglobin percentage.
- Hypothermia and pyrexia: temperature correction is not normally required.
- Capillary gases are sometimes used in small children: The PaO_2 is lower than arterial, but other parameters are the same if sampling is done correctly.

O_2 administration

O_2 is routinely administered to patients recovering from surgery and anaesthesia. Most require 30–40% O_2 until awake and in control of their airway. Those who have had major surgery; who are receiving morphine; who have respiratory or ischaemic heart disease; or who are elderly will need O_2 for longer – possibly up to 24–48 h after major abdominal or thoracic surgery. This may be administered by facemask (28–35%) or nasal cannulae 2–4 l/m. O_2 is required due to respiratory depressant drugs, V/Q mismatch produced by areas of lung atelectasis, and other respiratory changes that occur perioperatively. As with any drug it should be prescribed in the patient's drug chart. Administration is best guided by measuring the SpO_2.

Oxygen for dyspnoeic patients

There is sometimes confusion regarding appropriate O_2 therapy to breathless patients. The principles are:

- Hypoxia will kill a patient by causing cardiac arrest. An alert patient may be critically hypoxic.
- Hypercapnia will make a patient drowsy but only kills if cerebral depression causes the patient to stop breathing and become critically hypoxic. An alert patient cannot possibly have critical hypercapnia.
- **If in doubt give 60% O_2** via a face mask and check O_2 saturation, or if patient is seriously unwell, blood gases.
- Pulse oximetry is very useful as a saturation of >92% will usually correspond to a PaO_2 >8.0 kPa. However, pulse oximetry gives no information about the $PaCO_2$ level. Arterial blood gases are essential if you need to know the $PaCO_2$.
- The PaO_2 can be considered to measure perfusion (V/Q) mismatch within the lungs whereas the $PaCO_2$ is a measure of alveolar ventilation.
- Figure 41.1 provides a guide when to use pulse oximetry and when to check blood gases. High concentrations of inspired O_2 are rarely a problem except when the patient is in respiratory failure with a rising $PaCO_2$ – this is uncommon postoperatively.

Further reading

Bateman NT, Leach RM (1998). ABC of oxygen. Acute oxygen therapy. *British Medical Journal* 317:798–801.

Miller AC, Harvey JE (1993). Guidelines for the management of spontaneous pneumothorax. *British Medical Journal* 307:114–16.

Rees PJ, Dudley F (1998). Oxygen therapy in chronic lung disease. *British Medical Journal* 317:871–4.

Tai NRM, Atwal AS, Hamilton G (1999). Modern management of pulmonary embolism. *British Medical Journal* 86:853–68.

Williams AJ (1998). ABC of oxygen: assessing and interpreting arterial blood gases and acid-base balance. *British Medical Journal* 317:1213–6.

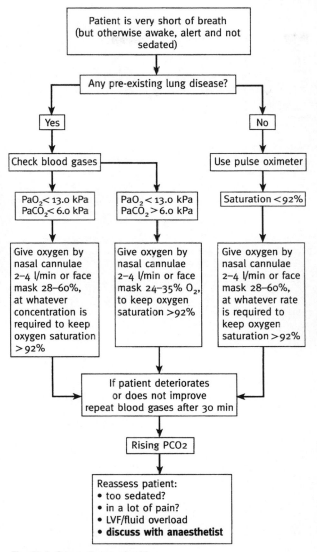

Fig. 41.1 Oxygen therapy algorithm.

Haemoptysis

Anthony Nicholls and Iain Wilson

- Postoperative haemoptysis is rare, but alarming and important. It may be the only clue to PE when this presents as minor pulmonary infarction. This is the major diagnosis to exclude.
- True haemoptysis is bleeding from below the larynx. After endotracheal intubation apparent haemoptysis may arise from oral, nasal, or pharyngeal bleeding.
- Exclude haematemesis. Stomach contents are acid.

Causes and investigation

- *PE*: Pulmonary infarction may present with expectoration of frank blood clots or blood-stained sputum. Dyspnoea may be relatively mild unless a major PE supervenes. Is the patient at high risk of PE? Get CXR, ECG, and blood gases. Haemoptysis with hypoxia and a clear CXR is highly suggestive of a PE and should be treated as such (p. 288).
- *Pulmonary oedema*: Haemoptysis here is typically pink frothy sputum, but may be frank blood from a ruptured pulmonary vein. CXR should show oedema. Exclude AMI with ECG and cardiac enzymes.
- *Acute bronchitis*: Haemoptysis is accompanied by symptoms of upper respiratory infection: cough, purulent sputum, fever. If CXR is clear then antibiotics are not needed.
- *Pneumonia*: Sputum in pneumonia may be rusty with blood or blood mixed with pus. CXR is diagnostic. Staphylococcal pneumonia may result in tissue destruction and haemoptysis.
- *Lung abscess*: Rare as a postoperative problem unless previous aspiration and/or pneumonia.
- *TB, cancer*: May be seen by chance on CXR, but routine preoperative films are no longer taken.

Oliguria and renal failure

Anthony Nicholls

Diagnosis

Renal failure is diagnosed when the serum creatinine rises rapidly by 20% or more above the preoperative value. Oliguria is typical but not invariable. Postoperative acute renal failure can also occur in the presence of a urine flow of 50 ml/h or greater (non-oliguric renal failure).

Renal failure should be suspected when postoperative urine output is low: the diagnosis is confirmed biochemically. The preoperative biochemistry allows certainty in the diagnosis of acute or acute-on-chronic renal failure.

Causes of renal failure

The differential diagnosis of postoperative acute renal failure is commonly limited to the following:

- *Pre-renal factors*: Renal hypoperfusion. Common in shock, aortic surgery, sepsis, and hepatorenal syndrome.
- *Renal causes*:
  - acute tubular necrosis: typical triggers are prolonged pre-renal hypoperfusion, sepsis, rhabdomyolysis (crush injury, ischaemia)
  - interstitial nephritis due to drugs such as NSAIDs, antibiotics, radiological contrast (very rarely).

- *Postrenal problems*: Ureteric damage following pelvic surgery or trauma.

Other causes, such as glomerulonephritis, or obstruction in the absence of pelvic surgery or trauma, are very rare. Renal infarction after aortic surgery may occur occasionally due to embolism of renal tissue during mobilization of vessels.

Postoperative renal failure is important for two quite different reasons:

- the direct effect of renal failure, with biochemical and fluid balance problems, potentially culminating in the need for dialysis
- rather like a fever or raised ESR, oliguria is a non-specific sign of underlying problems: attention to renal failure and its consequences alone is insufficient. Close identification and correction of the underlying causes are vital if the patient is to survive. Patients do not die of renal failure, but those who develop renal failure have a mortality approaching 50%.

Risk factors for the development of postoperative renal failure

Although renal failure is unusual, the risk is associated with several clearly identifiable factors, some preoperative, some postoperative, some medical, and some surgical (Table 43.1).

Patients identified as being at risk of renal failure should have particular attention paid to monitoring urine output and renal function perioperatively. They should not be dehydrated preoperatively, and potentially nephrotoxic drugs (particularly NSAIDs) should be avoided.

One third of patients with postoperative renal failure have hypovolaemia as the dominant cause, one third have sepsis, and one third have multiple factors including surgery itself. The more complex the surgery, the more likely that it is the sole cause of renal failure.

Table 43.1 Classification of risk factors for renal failure

Preoperative risk factors		Postoperative risk factors	
Medical	**Surgical**	**Medical**	**Surgical**
Renal impairment	Emergency or urgent surgery	Hypovolaemia	Haemorrhage
Increasing age	Perforated viscus	Sepsis	Anastamotic dehiscence
Obstructive jaundice	Sepsis	Cardiac failure	Biliary leak
Liver failure	Shock on presentation	NSAIDs	
Diabetes	Cardiac surgery		
Cardiac disease	Abdominal surgery		
Hypertension	Vascular surgery		
NSAIDs			

Approach to postoperative oliguria

The normal physiological response to surgery is reduced urine volume, mediated by the secretion of antidiuretic hormone. A urine output of < 400 ml/day or < 30 ml/h for 3 consecutive hours is abnormal. It may herald the development of renal failure. The following steps should be taken:

- Think immediately about haemorrhage or inadequately treated hypovolaemia following surgery.
- Pass a urethral catheter and monitor urine output hourly.
- Send blood for urgent (result within 3 h) electrolytes, creatinine, urea, and Hb.
- Assess the circulation: what is the blood pressure, both lying and sitting? – a postural fall in BP usually indicates hypovolaemia; what is the cardiac rhythm and cardiac output clinically? – oliguria and renal failure may be secondary to cardiac failure.
- Look for sepsis: chest, wound, septicaemia (blood cultures), urine.
- Consider a major complication of surgery itself: intestinal anastomotic leak, biliary leak, gangrenous tissue – gut, limb, muscle.

Immediate management

Give a rapid fluid challenge with 500 ml fluid – crystalloid or colloid – over 15–30 min (except in patients with signs of heart failure).

Subsequent management of acute renal failure

If simple volume replacement fails to restore urine output, and no underlying cause can be found, further assessment is needed. Either there is persisting prerenal failure or the patient has developed acute tubular necrosis (ATN), ie established acute renal failure. Simple biochemical tests on blood and urine (Table 43.2) can sometimes distinguish these diagnoses, but their value is often overstated as diuretic therapy or pre-existing renal impairment may make the results difficult to interpret.

Further measures in prerenal uraemia

(See also the chapter on hypotension, p. 249)

- Consider admission to HDU/ICU.
- Insert a central venous catheter and infuse fluids to normalize the circulating volume. Depending on the Hb and whether there is any evidence of bleeding, either blood or clear fluids may be appropriate.
- If the BP is low with a normalized or high CVP, then cardiac failure or major PE are possible. Get an ECG, CXR, and check arterial blood gases.

Table 43.2 Biochemistry in oliguric states

Test	Pre-renal failure	ATN
Serum urea	Disproportionately raised compared with creatinine	Raised proportionately to creatinine
Serum creatinine	Normal or slightly raised	Raised proportionately to urea
Urinary sodium (mmol/l)	<20	>40
Urine osmolality (mosmol/kg)	>500	<350
Urine: serum urea ratio	>8	<2
Urine: serum creatinine ratio[a]	>40	<20

[a] NB: Urine creatinine in mmol/l, serum creatinine in μmol/l.

- If there is fever with hypotension and oliguria, then septic shock is likely. See p. 255.
- Ask for help from the medical or renal team at this stage. Further therapy may include inotropic support and high dose diuretics.
- Do not give diuretics until you are sure that hypovolaemia is excluded. When the circulation has been optimized it is reasonable to give a large single i/v dose of frusemide (80–160 mg). Although this never prevents renal failure developing it occasionally results in non-oliguric renal failure developing instead of anuria/oliguria.
- Scan the drug chart and stop any drugs that may be nephrotoxic or may impair renal blood flow: NSAIDs, ACE inhibitors. Suspect any new therapy started in the previous week as a possible cause of allergic interstitial nephritis, and either stop it or switch to an alternative agent.

Management of established renal failure

At this stage, there should be collaboration from the medical, intensive care or nephrology team. Transfer for extracorporeal therapy (dialysis or haemofiltration) is not always necessary. Many patients with postoperative renal failure will improve in as little as 3–5 days before dialysis is needed. When the diagnosis of established renal failure has been made:

- avoid over-infusion of fluids with resultant pulmonary oedema
- avoid giving excess K^+ in infusions or diet
- check biochemistry daily, and ensure K^+ remains < 6 mmol/l
- modify the dose of drugs that are renally excreted (BNF Appendix 3)
- avoid drugs that may prolong renal failure – NSAIDs, aminoglycosides, ACE inhibitors

- beware of the accumulation of morphine metabolites that cause respiratory depression and prolonged sedation.

Specialist referral

Referral for dialysis (renal unit) or haemofiltration (ICU) will be necessary if the following are present:

- hyperkalaemia >6.5 mmol/l (see electrolyte disorders, p. 309 for more details)
- pulmonary oedema
- oliguria such that there is no room for adequate enteral or parenteral nutrition
- acidosis with pH <7.1
- rapidly rising urea >30 mmol/l and creatinine >500 μmol/l.

Clinical uraemic features – vomiting, drowsiness, confusion, pericarditis – are late features of renal failure. Refer to ICU or renal unit before the development of these features. The management of established renal failure is outside the scope of this book.

Further reading

Thadhani R, Pascual M, Bonventre JV (1996). Medical progress: acute renal failure. *New England Journal of Medicine* 334:1448–52.

44

Electrolyte imbalance

Anthony Nicholls

Hyponatraemia

Hyponatraemia is both common and potentially fatal. The resultant fall in plasma osmolality causes water to move into cells. This can cause cerebral oedema, and is responsible for the neurologic symptoms seen. If the serum Na^+ is < 120 mmol/l the patient is likely to have a reduced level of consciousness and/or confusion, and be at risk of seizures. Modest hyponatraemia (> 125 mmol/l) may indicate an underlying disorder needing attention, but in itself is unlikely to be clinically important as it is well tolerated.

Preoperative hyponatraemia may be either acute or chronic, and this affects both the urgency for and type of therapy. Ideally significant hyponatraemia detected preoperatively should be diagnosed and corrected before surgery and anaesthesia.

Acute postoperative hyponatraemia is much more likely to cause cerebral symptoms and may prove fatal. The rate of change of serum Na^+ is of more importance than the actual level.

Causes

The laboratory result may be spurious if the blood was sampled proximal to an infusion of dextrose or dextrose/saline. Whenever possible try to access previous blood results.

Preoperative hyponatraemia

- Hyponatraemia commonly accompanies dehydration. In a surgical setting, this will usually be from gastrointestinal losses.
- Chronic hyponatraemia may occur in patients on regular diuretics.
- Rarely, chronic hyponatraemia may result from inappropriate secretion of ADH from a tumour.
- Adrenal insufficiency is an uncommon cause of hyponatraemia (though ideally should be prevented by a steroid boost in susceptible patients). History and examination, and if necessary a short synacthen test will exclude this.
- Oedematous states (heart failure, liver failure, nephrotic syndrome) often result in hyponatraemia.

Postoperative hyponatraemia

- True postoperative hyponatraemia is usually due to excessive intravenous administration of 5% dextrose or dextrose 4%/saline 0.18%. Postoperative pain, hypotension, nausea, and some drugs can increase the secretion of antidiuretic hormone (ADH), thereby impairing free water excretion by the kidney.
- If the patient has had TURP or TCRE, there may be a dilutional state due to absorption of 1.5% glycine irrigating solution through open venous sinuses.
- The syndrome of inappropriate secretion of ADH is unusual as an acute finding in a postoperative situation but may occasionally complicate pneumonia. (NB: ADH is secreted as a normal physiological response to major surgery. It is appropriate, and does not cause hyponatraemia.)

Risks

- Hyponatraemia with severe neurological symptoms (confusional state, reduced conscious level, seizures) is a medical emergency.
- A Na^+ level < 120 mmol/l needs urgent therapy as there is a risk of neurological catastrophe.
- A Na^+ level of 120–130 mmol/l rarely causes any adverse complication. It usually needs no urgent intervention. If the patient exhibits disordered mental functioning an alternative cause should be sought, but occasionally the only explanation may be a Na^+ concentration in the low 120s.

Diagnostic approach

The various causes of hyponatraemia are best considered according to the clinical volume status of the patient: normovolaemic, volume depleted or fluid overloaded. The time-scale (acute or chronic) affects the rate at which hyponatraemia should be corrected.

- Normovolaemic hyponatraemia: This is a dilutional state with normal circulating volume. There is no oedema and BP is normal.

This is the commonest clinical setting for postoperative hyponatraemia and is usually due to inappropriate i/v therapy with 5% dextrose or dextrose/saline.

- Hyponatraemia with volume depletion: There will be evidence of gastrointestinal losses. Skin turgor is reduced, the tongue dry. BP may be low; if normal it may show a postural fall (if the patient cannot stand, even sitting the patient up in bed may reveal postural hypotension).

- Hyponatraemia with fluid overload: The patient will have peripheral or pulmonary oedema. Cardiac failure is the likeliest cause. Renal or hepatic failure can be excluded by simple laboratory tests. Appropriate therapy is normally to slow or stop i/v fluids and/or restrict oral intake. Diuretics will be needed.

Treatment

Much confusion surrounds the therapy of hyponatraemia. The options are either to give salt (usually as a saline solution), or to restrict water intake. The key message is that aggressive therapy of asymptomatic hyponatraemia may do more harm than good, but tardy therapy of hyponatraemia with neurological complications can be fatal. If you know hyponatraemia is of acute onset (24–36 h), or if the patient is exhibiting major cerebral complications, then rapid correction is necessary. Otherwise, act more slowly, as the syndrome of central pontine myelinolysis (osmotic demyelination) can be caused by rapid correction of chronic (> 2–3 days) hyponatraemia.

Urgent therapy for those with coma or seizures

Apply standard resuscitation measures for coma – check airway, give O_2, monitor O_2 saturation; check BP; check blood glucose with BM-stick test. Call senior help and consider admission to ICU. Subsequent therapy will depend on volume status of patient.

- Volume depletion: The therapy here is to give i/v normal saline as fast as is necessary to restore circulating volume to normal. This is best judged by inserting a central line and monitoring CVP.

- Normovolaemia: Give hypertonic saline (see Box 44.1).

- Volume overload (or cardiac failure): Give hypertonic saline (see Box 44.1) together with i/v loop diuretics. Place a bladder catheter, and give repeated doses of 20–40 mg frusemide i/v aiming to establish a diuresis fast enough to remove the volume of saline being infused, plus the estimated volume overload.

Therapy for asymptomatic or chronic hyponatraemia

Hypertonic saline is not indicated: Give 0.9% saline if volume depleted. Otherwise simply restrict water intake and allow homeostasis to be restored slowly.

Box 44.1 Hypertonic (3%) saline therapy for acute hyponatraemia with severe neurological symptoms

---

Not applicable if volume depleted

The aim is to increase the serum Na+ by 20 mmol/l or to 130 mmol/l and to restore conscious level.

The patient should be in HDU or ICU.

1. Estimate total body water (TBW):
   TBW ranges from 35% of body weight in elderly fat women to over 60% in muscular young men. 50% of body weight in women and 60% in men is a rough guess.

2. The volume (in ml) of 3% saline which will raise the serum Na+ by 1 mmol/l is twice TBW (in litres). (This is because 3% saline contains 1 mmol Na+/2 ml.)

3. The maximum rate of correction is 1.5 to 2 mmol/l per hour for the first 3–4 h. Thereafter the rate of rise of the serum Na+ should not exceed 1 mmol/l per hour, nor > 12 mmol in the first 24 h.

5. A volumetric infusion pump should be used. *Write your calculations down. Use a pocket calculator. Get someone to check your maths. Doctors have ended up in court for getting simple sums wrong in the middle of the night!*

Example

Sodium concentration: 115 mmol/l
Patient weight: 70 kg
Sex: male

TBW = $70 \times 0.6 = 42$ l

Thus 84 ml 3% saline will raise serum Na+ by 1 mmol/l

Total volume of 3% saline to be given in first 24 h is 12×84 ml = 1008 ml

Give 126 ml/h (1.5 mmol/l per hour) for the first 3 h

Give the remaining 730 ml over the next 21 h (35 ml/h)

This should correct the serum sodium to 127 mmol/l in 24 h, and more 3% saline can be given subsequently according to lab results.

Hypernatraemia

Hypernatraemia is due to increased body Na+, water deficiency, or both. In a surgical setting water loss in excess of Na+ loss is typical, but in order to produce hypernatraemia water intake has to be deficient as well. This may be due to lost of normal thirst from postoperative sedation, or the patient being nil-by-mouth. Evidence of water deficiency (reduced skin turgor, hypotension, vasoconstriction) is usually obvious.

Causes

Preoperatively

- Dehydration with water losses exceeding Na^+ losses, e.g. GI losses without fluid intake.
- Uncontrolled diabetes causing osmotic diuresis.
- Other causes rare in most surgical settings (primary hyperaldosteronism, cranial diabetes insipidus). May follow neurosurgery or brain trauma.

Postoperatively

- Incorrect i/v fluid replacement with 0.9% saline in excess of Na^+ losses. Many fluid losses – diarrhoea, intestinal contents, burns – are hypo-osmolar, and in the absence of normal thirst or oral intake fluid replacement with normal saline alone is inappropriate.
- Patients who have received large volumes of i/v fluid containing saline (Hartmann's solution, colloids, or 0.9% saline) and who have been given diuretics for oedema may develop hypernatraemia.
- Nephrogenic diabetes insipidus after relief of chronic urinary obstruction. Renal tubular function is damaged by chronic obstruction and urinary concentrating ability may be permanently lost. Loss of water in excess of Na^+ in this situation leads to hypernatraemia if the patient does not receive sufficient water.

Risks

- Excess Na^+ can cause confusion or coma due to cellular dehydration resulting from osmolar shrinkage of brain cells. Secondary venous rupture and subarachnoid haemorrhage can occur. This is unlikely unless the Na^+ is >158 mmol/l.
- A lesser degree of hypernatraemia is not itself usually a hazard, but the underlying water deficiency and hypovolaemia may cause vascular complications due to a sluggish circulation of hyperviscous blood. Cerebral and coronary insufficiency are most likely, with renal failure possible if circulating volume is not rapidly restored.

Diagnostic approach

- Exclude diabetes: BM-stick.
- Has the patient had urinary obstruction relieved: prostate, tumour, stones?
- Has the i/v fluid regime been predominantly saline? Check fluid balance charts.
- Is the patient unable to drink normally?
- Are there excessive water losses from the GI tract?

Treatment

Calculation of water deficit

Hypernatraemia is treated by calculating the estimated body water deficit and then replacing it. The water deficit can be calculated according to the steps in Box 44.2.

Rate of correction

- If hypernatraemia is chronic, correction should be slow. As with hyponatraemia, rapid correction can do more harm than the physiological derangement itself. Hypernatraemia initially causes brain shrinkage, but after 1–3 days brain volume is restored by uptake of solutes. If water is then given fast, cerebral oedema can occur, with seizures, permanent neurological damage, and death.

- In a surgical setting hypernatraemia is likely to be acute, and there will be laboratory proof of the rapidity of onset. It can then safely be corrected rapidly. Aim to lower the serum Na^+ no faster than 0.5 mmol/l per h; and there is no need to carry on with therapy once the Na^+ has fallen to 145 mmol/l.

- In the example in Box 44.2, the 28 mmol/l Na^+ excess should be corrected by providing the necessary 4.8 l of water over 56 h (86 ml/h). In addition, insensible losses are ~40 ml/h and urinary water loss will be at least another 40 ml/h, so water can be given in this example at 160 ml/h.

Box 44.2 Calculation of water deficit in hypernatraemia

Assumptions

Normal serum Na^+ is 140 mmol/l.

Total body water is 50% of body weight in women, 60% in men.

In a dehydrated state, body water is 10% less.

Normal body water (NBW) = current body water (CBW) $\times \left(\dfrac{\text{serum } Na^+}{140} \right)$

Water deficit = NBW − CBW

Therefore

$$\text{water deficit} = \left[CBW \times \left(\frac{\text{serum } Na^+}{140} \right) - CBW \right] = CBW \times \left[\left(\frac{Na^+}{140} \right) - 1 \right]$$

Example

Female patient, body weight 60 kg, serum Na^+ 168 mmol/l.

CBW = 40% × 60 = 30 l

$$\text{Water deficit} = 40\% \times 60 \times \left[\left(\frac{168}{140} \right) - 1 \right] = 4.8\,l$$

Route of water administration and monitoring
- If the patient can drink, encourage water orally.
- If not, give 5% dextrose i/v.
- Monitor hourly urine output via a bladder catheter and aim for at least 30 ml/h.
- Check serum Na^+ 6 hourly to ensure the rate of fall does not exceed 0.5 mmol/l per h.
- Resume normal fluid replacement when serum Na^+ is < 145 mmol/l.

Hypokalaemia

Hypokalemia is common in surgical patients. K^+ < 2.5 mmol/l is dangerous, and will need urgent treatment before anaesthesia and surgery.

A deficit of 200–400 mmol is necessary to lower the K^+ from 4.0 to 3.0 mmol/l, and a similar deficit lowers the K^+ from 3.0 to 2.0 mmol/l.

Causes

- *Decreased intake*: Normal K^+ intake is 40–120 mmol/day. This is commonly reduced in surgical patients who have been anorexic and unwell.
- *Increased entry into cells*: Alkalosis, excess insulin, β-agonists, stress, and hypothermia all cause a shift of K^+ into cells. There is no true state of K^+ deficiency if this is the sole cause.
- *Increased GI loss*: Vomiting, diarrhoea, and tube drainage are typical of a patient before or after abdominal surgery. Laxative abuse in the elderly is common, and may cause preoperative hypokalaemia.
- *Increased urinary loss*: Loss of gastric secretions, diuretics, metabolic acidosis, low Mg^{2+}, and mineralocorticoid excess cause urinary K^+ wasting. The mechanism of hypokalaemia in gastric fluid loss is complex. When excess gastric fluid is lost (by vomiting or via n/g tube), increased $NaHCO_3$ is delivered to the renal collecting tubules. Na^+ is exchanged for K^+ with a consequential increase in K^+ loss. The renal loss of K^+ in response to severe vomiting is the major factor causing hypokalaemia, as little K^+ is present in gastric secretions. Metabolic acidosis results in increased tubular delivery of H^+. This is exchanged along with K^+ for Na^+, and urinary K^+ increases.
- *Increased sweating* may exacerbate hypokalaemia.

Risks

- cardiac arrhythmias, particularly in patients taking digoxin
- prolonged paralytic ileus
- muscle weakness
- cramp.

Diagnostic approach

· History usually enables the causal factor(s) to be identified.

· pH of blood is needed to interpret a low K^+. Alkalosis commonly accompanies hypokalemia and results in K^+ shifting into cells. Acidosis causes direct urinary K^+ loss.

Treatment

· KCl is normally used to replace K^+ deficiency, as there is normally Cl^- deficiency in addition.

· If chronic diarrhoea is the cause, $KHCO_3$ or potassium citrate may be more appropriate.

· Oral therapy with K^+ salts is appropriate if there is time for correction and clinical manifestations are absent.

· Replacement of 40–60 mmol K^+ leads to a rise of 1–1.5 mmol/l in the serum K^+, but this is transient as K^+ is shifted back into cells. Regular monitoring of serum K^+ is necessary to ensure full correction of the deficit.

i/v potassium

· KCl should be given i/v if patients are unable to eat and have severe hypokalemia.

· In general, **do not add KCl to a bag of fluid. Use a manufactured prepack.**

· Saline rather than dextrose should be used. Administration of dextrose with K^+ can lead to a transient fall in serum K^+ of 0.2–1.4 mmol/l due to stimulation of insulin release by glucose.

· 'KCl 0.3% and NaCl 0.9% i/v infusion' provides 40 mmol K^+/l. This should be the standard i/v K^+ replacement fluid.

· Large volumes of saline may cause fluid overload. If severe cardiac arrhythmia is present, then a more concentrated K^+ solution can be given through a central venous line with ECG monitoring. Regular monitoring of serum K^+ is vital. Seek advice before giving >20 mmol K^+/h.

· A concentration >60 mmol/l through a peripheral vein should avoided as pain and sclerosis of the vein are likely.

· If you do add KCl to an i/v infusion, check the dose with another doctor as well as the nurse who will administer the infusion. Patients have died from the wrong concentration of K^+ replacement.

Hyperkalaemia

A serum K^+ above the normal range but <6.5 mmol/l is not in itself a medical emergency but the underlying cause may be (e.g. adrenal insufficiency). Remember that by the time you receive a laboratory report of hyperkalaemia the situation will have changed by a few hours. **Always repeat the estimation at the same time as starting therapy.**

K^+ above 6.5 needs rapid correction. Tradition dictates that ECG changes should be looked for, but by the time the T-wave is peaked or QRS widened cardiac arrest is imminent. Do not wait for an ECG before starting treatment, but start monitoring the ECG during treatment.

Causes

- *The result may be an artefact*: was the sample old when it reached the lab or was the venepuncture difficult (haemolysis)?
- *Acidosis causes a shift of K^+ from cells to plasma*. Typical causes include diabetic ketoacidosis, renal impairment, or any other cause of metabolic acidosis.
- *Renal failure*, particularly when accompanied by acidosis.
- *Drugs that inhibit K^+ excretion in mild renal impairment*: ACE inhibitors, non-steroidals, K^+-sparing diuretics (amiloride, spironolactone, etc).
- *Insulin deficiency* in a diabetic patient with hyperglycaemia.
- *Adrenal insufficiency*.
- *Massive blood transfusion*: K^+ leaches from cells when blood is stored. Occasionally a massive blood transfusion may result in a K^+ load beyond the rate of renal excretion – this is more common in an acidotic, shocked patient.
- *Severe tissue necrosis* (burns, gangrene, crush injury) leads to release of intracellular K^+.

Risks

- The risk of cardiac arrest relates not just to the degree of hyper-kalaemia but is compounded by the following factors which commonly coexist: acidosis, hypoxia, hypocalcaemia and sympathetic overactivity (due to pain or shock). Cardiac arrest is rare with K^+ <7 mmol/l unless other factors are present. Above that level K^+ alone is sufficient to cause arrest.
- Since resuscitation of a patient who has suffered cardiac arrest due to hyperkalaemia is usually unsuccessful, severe hyperkalaemia should be treated **immediately**.

Diagnostic approach

- Was there pre-existing renal impairment preoperatively? If so, has hyperkalaemia been precipitated by acidosis, an abnormal K^+ load, or use of a drug inhibiting K^+ excretion (see above)?
- Has the patient developed postoperative renal failure? Is the patient still passing urine?
- Has the patient developed diabetic ketoacidosis? Check a BM-stick.

- Is adrenal insufficiency possible? Look for low Na^+ and low BP. Is the patient at risk of adrenal suppression from previous steroid therapy?

Treatment

See Box 44.3 for summary.

Block the direct cardiac effects of K^+

- Ca^{2+} blocks the effect of K^+ on the heart.
- Give 10 ml calcium gluconate 10% i/v over 1–2 min. This is entirely safe and can be repeated every 5 min for 4 doses if the ECG continues to show features of hyperkalaemia – tall peaked T-waves, widened QRS complexes.
- Ca^{2+} can be life-saving when given immediately.

Lower K^+

Three drugs lower K^+ by different mechanisms: insulin, β-agonists such as salbutamol, and $NaHCO_3$.

- Insulin moves K^+ into cells.
  - 15 U soluble insulin should be given by bolus along with 50 ml of 50% dextrose to prevent hypoglycaemia unless the patient has uncontrolled diabetes. This will usually lower K^+ for 30–60 min.
  - Follow this by an infusion of insulin at a rate of 4 U/h with sufficient dextrose to maintain normal blood sugar. 50% dextrose given at a rate of 50 ml/h is usually satisfactory but blood glucose must be monitored.
  - NB: 50% dextrose is strongly irritating to tissues (vesicant). A large-bore peripheral cannula or preferably a central line should be used for 50% dextrose infusions.
- β-adrenoceptor agonists such as salbutamol are under-used as a therapy for hyperkalaemia.
  - Salbutamol reliably lowers K^+ by about 1 mmol/l and is effective when given by nebulizer.
  - 5 mg salbutamol nebulized by facemask is as effective at lowering K^+ as insulin and is additive to it. It also avoids the risks of i/v 50% dextrose extravasation.

Box 44.3 Emergency treatment of hyperkalaemia (see text for details)

1. Give 10 ml *calcium gluconate* 10% intravenously over 1–2 min.
2. Give 15 u soluble *insulin* by bolus with 50 ml of 50% dextrose.
3. Give 5 mg nebulized *salbutamol* by mask.
4. Correct acidosis with *$NaHCO_3$*.
5. *Stop offending drugs*
6. Give *resonium* 15 g 6 hourly by mouth or 30 g bd rectally by enema.
7. Consider need for *dialysis*.

- NaHCO$_3$:
  - it is vital to correct acidosis as increases the risk of cardiac arrest
  - correction of acidosis lowers K$^+$ by causing movement of K$^+$ into cells
  - correction of acidosis lowers the ionized Ca^{2+} concentration, and tetany can be provoked if Ca^{2+} is not given before NaHCO$_3$.
- Box 44.4 shows how to calculate total base deficit and how to correct it.

Box 44.4 Correction of acidosis <pH 7.2 in patients with coexisting hyperkalemia

---

1. Give Ca^{2+} intravenously before correcting acidosis (see text above).

2. Check arterial blood gases and calculate the total HCO$_3^-$ deficit:

$$\text{total HCO}_3^- \text{ deficit (mmol)} = \text{base deficit} \times \left(\frac{\text{body weight in kg}}{3} \right)$$

(The volume of distribution of bicarbonate is one third of body weight.)

3. Correct half the base deficit over 15–30 min.

4. Use isotonic (1.26%) NaHCO$_3$, if the patient is volume depleted (the usual scenario). 1.26% NaHCO$_3$ contains 150 mmol HCO$_3^-$/l. Hypertonic solutions (4.2% and 8.4%) are not usually appropriate.

Example

Patient weight 60 kg
Base deficit 10 mmol/l

$$\text{Total HCO}_3^- \text{ deficit} = \frac{(10 \times 60)}{3} = 200 \text{ mmol}$$

Thus, 100 mmol HCO$_3^-$ can be replaced fast to correct half the deficit.

$$\text{Volume of 1.26% NaHCO}_3^- \text{ to be infused} = \frac{100}{150}\text{l} = 667 \text{ ml}$$

Other risk factors
- Give O$_2$.
- Treat pain or anxiety.

Treat underlying causes
The underlying causes (listed in a previous section) need correction:

- Stop offending drugs: NSAIDs, ACE inhibitors, K$^+$-sparing diuretics.
- Treat diabetes.
- Consider and treat adrenal insufficiency.
- Remove necrotic tissue, e.g. amputate dead limb.

Prevent rebound
- Hyperkalaemia may rebound if the patient is in renal failure and not diuresing.

- If the patient is passing urine, the above measures will be adequate therapy until the underlying cause has been corrected.
- A patient in renal failure can be kept alive until transfer to a dialysis unit by the above measures, but they are not definitive solutions.
- Resonium (a resin to absorb K^+) can be given by mouth (15 g 6 hourly or 30 g rectally by enema twice daily) can be given if the patient is not passing urine and is awaiting transport to a renal unit. It does not need to be given routinely.

Hypercalcaemia

Clinical features

Hypercalcaemia may be detected for the first time on admission to a surgical ward. It may be the cause of the presenting symptoms: abdominal pain, nausea, vomiting, constipation, anorexia, weight loss, or kidney stones. It may be a consequence of the primary surgical problem, particularly if this is malignant disease: bony metastases from breast, prostate, colon, kidney, thyroid, lung, or ovarian cancer. Often it may be an unrelated finding, typically primary hyperparathyroidism in a middle-aged or elderly woman.

- Modest hypercalcaemia (<3 mmol/l) rarely causes clinical problems beyond thirst, polyuria and modest dehydration, but may be aggravated by dehydration and immobilization. Primary hyperparathyroidism is the commonest cause of a slightly elevated Ca in an otherwise fit patient. There are no particular risks provided dehydration is prevented or corrected.
- Severe hypercalcaemia (>3 mmol/l) should normally be corrected before surgery to minimize the risks of cardiac arrhythmias, depression of consciousness, and severe dehydration. Malignancy is the usual cause.
- Spurious hypercalcaemia can arise if blood is taken from a dehydrated patient, or with prolonged application of a tourniquet. These circumstances lead to elevation of the Ca along with the serum albumin. Most laboratories correct for the albumin concentration so that the result can be interpreted sensibly. It is wise, however, to repeat the estimation if the Ca is raised and there was difficulty taking the blood sample.

Laboratory interpretation

- Biologically active Ca is the ionized fraction (Ca^{2+}), that which is unbound to protein. The normal range for Ca^{2+} is 1.07–1.27 mmol/l. Although few laboratories offer this test routinely on serum, most arterial blood gas analysers report the ionized Ca^{2+}. Hypercalcaemia is serious if Ca^{2+} is >1.5 mmol/l.
- Interpretation of the total serum Ca needs to taken into account the serum albumin concentration, as Ca is bound to albumin. If

the total Ca is low, together with a low albumin, the Ca may be biologically normal. There are several formulae to correct for the serum albumin, and the one in Box 44.5 is simple and fairly accurate. It should be applied only if the laboratory result is uncorrected for the albumin. Most laboratories already correct the Ca, so don't manually 'correct' it a second time!

Box 44.5 Corrrection of serum Ca

'Corrected' Ca $\cong$ uncorrected Ca – 0.025 × (serum albumin 40)

(The formula also applies in the interpretation of apparently low Ca levels when the albumin is low.)

For example, suppose the uncorrected Ca is 2.8 mmol/l with an albumin of 48 g/l:

corrected Ca = 2.8 – 0.025(48 – 40) = 2.8 – 0.2 = 2.6 mmol/l

Never write down in the notes a total Ca level as being 'Ca^{2+} = 1.8 mmol/l'; the symbol 'Ca^{2+}' means ionized Ca, and the result would indicate severe hypercalcaemia, whereas a total Ca of 1.8 mmol/l is low.

Causes (in order of frequency)

- primary hyperparathyroidism
- bony metastases
- myeloma
- iatrogenic – usually vitamin D or a derivative (alfacalcidol, dihydroxycholecalciferol); the milk–alkali syndrome is excessively rare
- sarcoid (rare)
- thyrotoxicosis (very rare).

Risks

- polyuria, dehydration, hypotension
- drowsiness, confusion.

The long-term risks of hypercalcaemia (kidney stones, renal failure, corneal calcification) are not relevant to the acute management of surgical patients.

Investigations

- Na^+, K^+, urea, creatinine (hypercalcaemia can cause polyuria and renal failure)
- phosphate (low in primary hyperparathyroidism)
- albumin (usually low in metastases)
- alkaline phosphatase (raised in bony metastases, sarcoid, thyrotoxicosis)

- prostate specific antigen (raised in metastatic prostate cancer)
- ESR (very high in myeloma, may be raised in metastases)
- serum protein electrophoresis, bone marrow for myeloma
- PTH (raised in hyperparathyroidism, suppressed in other causes).

Management

- Ideally hypercalcaemia should be diagnosed and corrected before surgery. The risks of surgery in mild hypercalcaemia are modest. Simply ensure adequate hydration with i/v 0.9% saline administered during preoperative fasting and continued postoperative.
- Elective surgery should be deferred in the presence of Ca levels >3 mmol/l.
- Emergency or urgent surgery in the face of severe hypercalcaemia should be postponed until the following measures have been undertaken:
  - bladder catheter for hourly urine output
  - rehydration with 1000 ml 0.9% saline over 1 h and then 4–6 l over the next 24 h
  - CVP to guide i/v fluid replacement
  - pamidronate 60 mg i/v in 500 ml saline over 4 h (the Ca will fall over 2 days except when primary hyperparathyroidism is the cause).
- Hypercalcaemia may appear or increase postoperatively due to dehydration and immobilization, typically in the elderly. Treatment is rehydration, monitoring renal function, and pamidronate as above.

Hypocalcaemia

- Rare postoperatively unless the patient has had thyroid or parathyroid surgery. It may arise as a complication of acute renal failure, pancreatitis, or crush injury syndrome.
- The risks are neuromuscular excitability predisposing to fits and a prolonged Q-T interval on ECG predisposing to ventricular arrhythmias. The development of tetany during repeated BP measurement is an important clinical clue.
- Spurious hypocalcaemia may cause concern if an apparently low Ca is not corrected for the albumin concentration (see hypercalcaemia section above).
- The ionized Ca^{2+} is again a more direct way of assessing the true impact of a low Ca (see above). Blood gas analysers often measure the ionized Ca^{2+}, the normal range being 1.07–1.27 mmol/l. Hypocalcaemia is dangerous if the total Ca is <2.0 mmol/l or the ionized Ca^{2+} <0.9 mmol/l.

Management

- If corrected Ca >2 mmol/l (or $Ca^{2+} > 0.9$ mmol/), give oral Ca supplements and monitor Ca daily.
- If corrected Ca <2 mmol/l (or $Ca^{2+} < 0.9$ mmol/), give the following:
  - 10 ml 10% calcium gluconate i/v over 1–3 min
  - alfacalcidol or dihydroxycholecalciferol 1–5 μg orally (seek medical advice).
- Check Ca 4 h later: if not rising, start a Ca infusion of 2– 5 ml/h 10% calcium gluconate by continuous infusion using a syringe driver.
- Recheck Ca daily.
- Temporary overcorrection of hypocalcaemia is not harmful.

Hypomagnesaemia

Prevalence

- Estimated to affect 7% of inpatients, but many of these are asymptomatic, and do not need aggressive therapy.
- Frequently associated with both hypocalcaemia and hypokalaemia. Always check Mg^{2+} levels if Ca or K^+ levels are low.
- Common in surgical patients: reduced food intake, increased GI losses from diarrhoea, vomiting, or intestinal fistulae.
- Other high-risk patients include chronic alcoholics and patients on chronic diuretic therapy.

Clinical features

Risks similar to hypocalcaemia and hypokalaemia: fits, tetany, ventricular arrhythmias. These are only likely if $Mg^{2+} < 0.5$ mmol/l.

Management

- Monitor Mg^{2+} 3 times a week in high-risk patients.
- Replace or prevent deficiency with Mg^{2+} salts added to enteral or parenteral nutrition.
- Give a Mg^{2+} infusion in symptomatic patients (Box 44.6).

Box 44.6 Intravenous magnesium for correction of severe symptomatic hypomagnesaemia

---

Magnesium sulphate injection 50% contains 2 mmol Mg^{2+}/ml.
Give 8 mmol Mg^{2+} (4 ml 50% solution) over 10–15 min.
Repeat the injection once if the clinical problem (arrhythmia, fit) persists.
Replace the Mg^{2+} deficiency by infusing 50–72 mmol Mg^{2+} (25–36 ml 50% solution) over 24 h.

Hypophosphataemia

Epidemiology and pathophysiology

10–15% of hospital inpatients have a low serum phosphate (<0.8 mmol/l). A smaller proportion has profound hypophosphataemia (<0.3 mmol/l).

The chronic effects of a low serum phosphate on bone metabolism are irrelevant in the acute situation. It is the biochemical impact of phosphate depletion on cellular metabolism that is potentially dangerous in surgical patients:

- red cell 2,3-DPG (diphosphoglycerate) levels fall with reduced tissue O_2 delivery
- intracellular ATP levels fall and cellular functions involving energy-rich phosphate compounds may be affected.

Symptoms and signs

- *Nervous system:* A metabolic encephalopathy can occur leading to irritability and confusion or even delirium and coma.
- *Heart:* Cardiac output may be reduced secondary to impaired myocardial contractility.
- *Respiration* may be impaired due to weakness of the diaphragm.
- *Muscle function:* Proximal myopathy, dysphagia, and ileus can occur. Rhabdomyolysis is a risk in alcoholic patients with hypophosphataemia.
- *Red cells:* The risk of haemolysis is increased but rarely occurs with hypophosphataemia alone.
- *White cells:* Severe hypophosphataemia can impair granulocyte phagocytosis and chemotaxis.
- *Platelet numbers* and function may be diminished.

Causes

In surgical patients several factors typically contribute to hypophosphataemia. The first three are the most important.

- *Increased insulin secretion during re-feeding:* Glycolysis promotes the phosphorylation of carbohydrates in the liver and skeletal muscle with a consequent rapid fall in the serum phosphate. This is particularly likely in malnourished or alcoholic patients, or in patients receiving TPN.
- *Respiratory alkalosis* (for example in ventilated patients) causes a rise in intracellular pH that leads to enhanced glycolysis. Alkalosis is the most common cause of hypophosphataemia in hospitalised patients.
- *Diarrhoea* can cause mild phosphate depletion.
- *Reduced intake of phosphate* does not cause hypophosphataemia as cell catabolism releases phosphate from cells and renal retention of phosphate can compensate for reduced intake.

- *Drugs*: antacids containing Al^{3+}, Ca^{2+}, or Mg^{2+} can bind intestinal phosphate and lead to modest phosphate depletion.
- **Primary hyperparathyroidism** causes increased urinary phosphate excretion.
- *Vitamin D deficiency* causes secondary hyperparathyroidism, which also increases urinary phosphate loss.
- *Acute volume expansion* diminishes proximal tubular Na^+ resorption and increases urinary phosphate loss.

Treatment

The treatment of hypophosphataemia is predominantly the treatment of the underlying cause. Oral supplementation is inappropriate except for those with chronic untreatable urinary losses.

i/v phosphate supplementation is usual in all patients receiving TPN, and a phosphate infusion is occasionally needed in alcoholic patients who are at risk of rhabdomyolysis from hypophosphataemia. The i/v dose of phosphate should not exceed 0.08 mmol/kg body weight 6 hourly. I/v phosphate is potentially dangerous and can cause cardiac arrhythmias.

Further reading

Bushinsky DA, Monk RD (1998). Calcium. *Lancet* 352:306–11.

Gennari FJ (1998). Hypokalemia. *New England Journal of Medicine* 339:451–8.

Gluck SL (1998). Acid-base. *Lancet* 352:474–9.

Halperin ML, Kame KS (1998). Potassium. *Lancet* 352:135–40.

Kumar S, Berl T (1998). Sodium. *Lancet* 352:220–8.

Rose BD (1986). New approach to disturbances in the plasma sodium concentration. *American Journal of Medicine* 81:1033–7.

Weisinger JR, Bellorín-Font E (1998). Magnesium and phosphorus. *Lancet* 352:391–6.

45

Postoperative jaundice and abnormal liver function tests (LFTs)

Anthony Nicholls and Iain Wilson

Postoperative jaundice results from an accumulation of bilirubin. It may occur in any patient, but is commonest in patients who have had biliary, hepatic, or pancreatic surgery. This is often related to the nature of the surgery performed and resulting hepatobiliary problems: obstruction or leakage.

Jaundice may also develop after procedures unrelated to the biliary system, e.g. orthopaedic, gynaecological, or bowel surgery. In such patients jaundice is usually multifactorial in origin, and medical rather than surgical in nature.

Although jaundice itself may be relatively benign, it should always be investigated carefully as it may be manifestation of a serious problem outside the liver. Patients with postoperative hepatocellular dysfunction have a poor prognosis and need urgent investigation and management.

Causes

- *Biliary obstruction* or leakage must be considered after hepatobiliary surgery.
- *Medical causes* include haematoma resorption, hepatotoxic drugs, sepsis, parenteral nutrition, postoperative hypoxia, or hypotension,

and possibly newly acquired viral hepatitis. If renal failure develops, jaundice will worsen.

- Patients with *chronic liver disease* may suffer hepatic decompensation after surgery, particularly if complicated by sepsis, shock, or an acute GI bleed. Jaundice in these patients appears as part of the picture of liver failure.
- *Gilbert's syndrome* (or other congenital bilirubin metabolism disorders) may become apparent postoperatively.
- *Cardiac failure* is one of the commonest causes of mild jaundice and deranged LFTs postoperatively.
- *Haemolysis* should be excluded.

Resorption of haematomas

Extravasated blood is phagocytosed by macrophages, which degrade haem to biliverdin and then bilirubin. Serum unconjugated bilirubin may rise to ~60 mmol/l, unaccompanied by a rise in liver enzymes. Urinary urobilinogen is elevated. Tests for haemolysis are negative, but reticulocytosis is a response to blood loss as well as haemolysis.

Drugs

- *Antibiotics*: Penicillin derivatives are a common cause of jaundice. Erythromycin, clindamycin, and fusidic acid are more rarely the culprit.
- *Halothane hepatitis* is rare, but extremely serious and potentially fatal. It typically occurs after repeated exposure to the agent, usually within a few months, but sometimes over years. Jaundice with raised liver enzymes appears 1–3 weeks after halothane exposure. Hepatitis following other volatile inhalational anaesthetic agents is exceptionally rare.
- *Phenothiazines* can cause cholestatic jaundice even after brief exposure. Antihistamines that are structurally related can cause a similar problem.
- *Other drugs*: In an unexpectedly jaundiced patient, it is worth checking all prescribed drugs in the BNF to see if jaundice is a reported side-effect.

Sepsis

Bacterial sepsis at any site may be accompanied by cholestatic jaundice and often elevated liver enzymes. Associated factors include hypotension, drugs, and bacterial endotoxins.

Total parenteral nutrition (TPN)

- Fatty change and cholestasis are common in patients receiving TPN. Changes in LFTs (e.g. alkaline phosphatase) may occur after 2–3 weeks TPN, and jaundice occasionally accompanies this.

- TPN promotes intestinal bacterial overgrowth, which has three potential mechanisms of promoting cholestasis: increased portal endotoxaemia, bacterial sepsis, and increased production of secondary bile acids.
- TPN also contributes to cholestasis by the increase in biliary sludge that occurs after 6 weeks of TPN, and possibly by hepatotoxicity from tryptophan degradation products.

Hypotension and hypoxia

Cholestasis is a common reaction to a low perfusion state of the liver, such as occurs in heart failure or hypotension. Hypoxia causes a similar hepatic reaction. This complication of shock falls short of overt hepatic necrosis. The clinical picture is of raised liver enzymes and, less commonly, jaundice and elevated prothrombin time.

Chronic liver disease

Jaundice may develop (or worsen) after any surgery in patients with chronic liver disease. This is discussed further on p. 197.

Gilbert's syndrome

Gilbert's syndrome (unconjugated hyperbilirubinaemia) is an inherited disorders of bilirubin metabolism leading to fluctuating low-grade jaundice which may be made worse by starvation or infection. Jaundice in these patients will worsen after surgery. Liver enzymes are always normal. The diagnosis is made from the history of previous episodes of mild jaundice after typical triggers, and after exclusion of other causes (including haemolysis). The condition is benign.

Infective

Viral hepatitis should be excluded by serology; until this is done take precautions as described on p. 97.

Haemolysis

Characterized by unconjugated hyperbilirubinaemia, increased urinary urobilinogen, reticulocytosis, reduced haptoglobin, elevated LDH, usually abnormal blood film (polychromasia, spherocytes, fragmented cells).

Approach to the patient with postoperative jaundice

History

- *Biliary surgery*: If the patient has had hepatobiliary surgery, then postoperative jaundice is likely to be surgical in origin.
- *Shock*: Has the patient been shocked or hypoxic?

- *Haematomas*: Has the patient a large collection of extravasated blood, e.g. after pelvic fracture or ruptured aortic aneurysm?
- *Drugs*: Has the patient been exposed to halothane, phenothiazines, erythromycin?
- *TPN*: How long has this been given?
- *Sepsis* is the most important causal factor to consider. Regard jaundice as a marker of potential infection, and initiate a sepsis screen.
- *Chronic liver disease*: Was this present preoperatively? Perhaps the patient was alcoholic, but not recognized to have liver disease.
- *Heart failure* may be the sole cause.

Investigations

- Liver function tests, coagulation screen (INR is the most sensitive test of liver synthetic function), glucose (patients may become hypoglycaemic due to impairment of glycogenolysis in the liver), creatinine and electrolytes, FBC. The serum urea is typically low in liver failure.
- Investigate the biliary tree if the primary surgical problem was hepatic/pancreatic/biliary/duodenal. Ultrasound is usually needed to exclude obstruction unless blood tests clearly point to another cause. A further operation may be needed.
- Sepsis screen if relevant
- Advice of gastroenterologist may be needed if the problem is not immediately surgical in nature

Treatment

- Manage underlying cause if identified.
- Monitor glucose 6 hourly.
- Daily coagulation screen, FBC and U&E.
- Catheterize and measure urine output.
- If hypotension or encephalopathy develops, consult ICU immediately.

Postoperative diarrhoea

Anthony Nicholls and Iain Wilson

Diarrhoea is common on all hospital wards and often arises as a post-operative problem. It consumes many hours of nursing time, puts patients at risk of fluid and electrolyte loss, and predisposes to pressure sores.

Diarrhoea is technically the passage of >300 ml stool daily. Patients may refer to diarrhoea when they simply have frequent stools. It is the volume and consistency of a diarrhoeal stool that matters.

Differential diagnosis of diarrhoea

Spurious diarrhoea

- Common in the elderly.
- Usually caused by a combination of opioids, dietary change, and immobility.
- May present with copious incontinence of mucoid stools.
- Diagnosed by rectal examination (occasionally aided by a plain abdominal radiograph).

Drug-induced diarrhoea

- May simply be due to overenthusiastic prescription of laxatives to pre-empt opioid-induced constipation.
- May be a side-effect of some antacids.
- Enteral tube feeding may cause osmotic diarrhoea. This is minimized by increasing the volume and strength of feed progressively. May need and anti-motility agent for control.

Table 46.1 Causes of postoperative diarrhoea

Spurious	Faecal impaction with overflow
Drug-induced	Laxatives
	Antacids
	Enteral tube feeding
	Many other agents – always check side effects of drugs in the BNF
Antibiotics	Simple bacterial overgrowth
	Clostridium difficile associated diarrhoea
After GI surgery	Lactose intolerance
	Bile acid malabsorption
	Dumping
Endocrine	Diabetes
	Hypoadrenalism
	Thyrotoxicosis
	Hypocalcaemia
Vascular	Mesenteric ischaemia

- Common side-effect of many drugs. Look in the BNF at the side-effects of any drug on the prescription sheet.

Antibiotic-induced diarrhoea

- May be due to simple bacterial overgrowth.
- *Clostridium difficile* needs to be excludes in all cases by stool culture and assay of stool for *C. difficile* toxin.
- See Chapter 17 for further details of management.

Diarrhoea after GI surgery

- May arise after vagotomy, pyloroplasty, cholecystectomy, small- and large-bowel resection.
- Due to lactose intolerance, bile acid malabsorption, or dumping.

Endocrine causes

The endocrine causes of diarrhoea can be diagnosed by the appropriate blood tests: glucose, cortisol, thyroxine, Ca.

Mesenteric ischaemia

May present in critically ill patients, particularly in ICU, with diarrhoea. There is evidence of widespread arterial disease at other sites.

Management of postoperative diarrhoea

- Exclude faecal impaction.
- Consider prophylactic brewer's yeast in high risk patients (diabetes, immunosuppression) given antibiotics.

- Exclude *C. difficile* if patient treated with antibiotics.
- Start brewer's yeast before *C. difficile* results available.
- Consider drug side-effects.
- Exclude endocrine causes.
- Avoid anti-motility agents unless a functional disturbance is the cause (e.g. associated with enteral feeding or after GI surgery). Anti-motility agents worsen infective diarrhoea.
- The simplest anti-motility agents are codeine phosphate 15–30 mg 4–6 hourly or loperamide 4–8 mg initially followed by 2–4 mg bd.
- Increase pressure sore care.
- Encourage continuing nutrition.

Drowsiness, coma, and delirium

Julia Munn and Richard Hardie

Definitions

Coma is defined as a state of impaired consciousness, progressing from mild drowsiness to unrousable coma. The Glasgow coma scale (GCS, see Table 47.1) affords an objective way of assessing the depth of coma and thereby monitoring its progress.

Delirium typically presents with irrational behaviour and agitation. Technically, it is defined as global cognitive impairment with impaired levels of attention and consciousness. Speech and movement may be increased or diminished, with disorientation, and disturbance of the normal sleep/wake cycle, and of perceptions leading to misinterpretations, illusions and hallucinations.

- The onset in a postsurgical patient is usually acute, and often at night.

- Being called to assess a drowsy, comatose, or delirious patient postoperatively is one of the most taxing tasks for a junior doctor. The patient will typically have been mentally normal on admission to hospital, only to deteriorate rapidly postoperatively.

- Such patients have an increased risk of cardiac arrest and death, the relatives may panic and other patients on the ward may be disturbed. Rapid assessment and correction of underlying causes is essential in this critical situation. **Call for the anaesthetist or medical registrar to help you at an early stage.**

Table 47.1 Glasgow coma scale

Eye opening	Score
Spontaneous	4
To voice	3
To pain	2
None	1
	Eye opening score _____
Verbal response	
Normal	5
Confused/disorientated	4
Inappropriate words	3
Incomprehensible sounds	2
None	1
	Verbal score _____
Motor response	
Obeys commands	6
Localizing	5
Withdrawal	4
Abnormal flexion	3
Extension	2
None	1
	Motor score _____
	Total score /15

- Studies of elective surgery in geriatric patients show that as many as 40% have a degree of postoperative delirium. A single treatable reason is not always found, but a diligent search for a serious underlying cause is mandatory.

Causes and investigation

Anaesthesia and analgesia

- Most patients start to regain consciousness within minutes of the end of surgery. If a patient has woken up to the point of communicating, but subsequently becomes unrousable, the anaesthetic itself is unlikely to be the sole cause.

- Opioid analgesics given intra- or postoperatively can cause drowsiness and respiratory depression. This is most likely when administered by infusion – i/v, s/c, or epidural – and particularly in patients with hepatic or renal impairment. Narcotized patients characteristically have slow, deep respiration, and small pupils. Start resuscitation along the usual lines, discontinue the opioid, and give naloxone (100 μg increments to 400 μg i/v) if necessary.

- The signs of cerebral oedema and raised intracranial pressure can be delayed for 24 h following head injury. If a patient with a head injury undergoes emergency surgery for other injuries, cerebral oedema may increase during anaesthesia, resulting in neurological deterioration postoperatively. The ICU team should be informed and CT scan may be indicated.

Direct complications of surgery

- A deteriorating conscious level after craniotomy may be due to intracranial bleeding or cerebral oedema. Either will require prompt surgical or medical intervention after initial resuscitation. The neurosurgeon should be informed as CT scan and further surgery may be indicated.

- Stroke is a recognized complication of carotid endarterectomy but permanent neurological damage may be averted by immediate further surgery if the carotid is occluded in the neck by haematoma or an intraluminal blockage. Frequent neurological observations should always be recorded after carotid surgery and the surgeon informed immediately of any deterioration.

Other perioperative problems

Blood gas disturbances

- Hypoxia initially produces agitation and confusion before drowsiness.

- Hypoventilation will cause hypercapnia which can result in unconsciousness when the CO_2 reaches very high levels (>10 kPa). This can occur solely from an accumulation of opioid but may also be seen in patients with pre-existing hypercapnic respiratory failure when precipitated by a number of factors including opioids, pain, chest infection, and loss of hypoxic drive from oxygen therapy. Hypoventilation is difficult to detect clinically.

- **Arterial blood gases must be checked in any unconscious patient.**

Metabolic disturbances

Metabolic conditions that can cause confusion, drowsiness, or coma include:

- hyponatraemia
- hypernatraemia
- hypoglycaemia
- hyperglycaemia (rarely)
- uraemia (unlikely if renal function normal preoperative and patient still passing urine)
- hypercalcaemia
- hepatic failure.

Clinical features may narrow the differential diagnosis but serum creatinine, electrolytes, and glucose should be tested on all patients with an altered mental state postoperatively. Hyponatraemia with cerebral oedema and pulmonary oedema is a specific complication of TURP and TCRE (see p. 302).

Cerebrovascular disease

- Patients with arterial disease at any site are prone to cerebrovascular accidents in the intra- and postoperative period.
- Examine the patient for lateralizing signs to help distinguish from other causes of coma. Correct systemic factors such as hypoxia and hypotension that worsen cerebral ischaemia. If anticoagulation is considered, arrange a CT to exclude haemorrhagic stroke. Cerebral infarction is often not apparent on CT for a few days.

Epilepsy

Epileptic control may worsen if patients are unable to take anti-convulsants for some days postoperatively. If a fit is not witnessed, only the post-ictal drowsiness may be evident.

Sepsis

Septic shock can cause any mental disturbance from mild confusion to deep coma. Look for other signs of sepsis and its source. Sepsis as a cause of postoperative delirium is unlikely without fever, but may occur in the elderly. The combination of any degree of fever with acute confusion may herald overt septic shock with circulatory collapse. Manage these patients as if septic shock had already developed (see Chapter 37, p. 255).

Alcohol withdrawal

Alcohol withdrawal is a common precipitant of delirium after surgery. Few heavy drinkers are totally honest about previous consumption. Mild confusion may pass in a day or two, but progression to delirium tremens (DTs) is a medical emergency, which carries a significant mortality.

Previously unrecognized mild dementia

Many elderly patients will have mild dementia that has not been documented or been severe enough to affect normal activities. Middle class, well-spoken elderly patients may retain their normal social interactions while in a state of fairly advanced dementia. It may merely take the disruption of a hospital admission to unmask severe confusion and disorientation, particularly after anaesthesia and surgery.

Undiagnosed space occupying lesions (SOL)

Rarely, an intracranial SOL may present in the postoperative period due to increased peri-tumour oedema. Presentation is with signs of raised intracranial pressure, which may have been exacerbated perioperatively

Management

Coma

Coma is a medical emergency. Unexplained drowsiness is just one step away from coma. Resuscitate the patient along the usual lines of ABC.

- Establish and maintain airway patency by positioning, jaw lift, oral airway or consider intubation by an anaesthetist.
- Assess breathing, give O_2 and monitor SpO_2.
- Impaired respiratory drive may cause profound respiratory failure, which is easy to miss, as the patient will not appear dyspnoeic. Pulse oximetry will not detect respiratory depression until the minute ventilation is extremely low and then the O_2 saturation will fall precipitously. Blood gas analysis must be performed to look for a rising $PaCO_2$. Hypercapnia and acidosis will worsen any cerebral oedema and rapid intubation and ventilation may be indicated.
- Circulation – monitor heart rate and BP and initiate treatment if hypotensive.
- Hypoxia and/or hypotension will worsen any cerebral ischaemia or oedema. The prevention or rapid correction of these secondary insults is mandatory if further permanent neurological damage is to be avoided.
- Exclude hypoglycaemia.
- After initial resuscitation examine the patient neurologically, document the findings and record the GCS. Start a neurological observation chart.
- If there is any doubt about the patient's ability to protect his/her airway (i.e. GCS <8) or breathe adequately, and if the coma is not readily reversible (e.g. hypoglycaemia) the HDU/ICU team should be informed.
- After basic assessment of gas exchange and the circulation, send a metabolic and sepsis screen.
- If coma persists or deepens without clear explanation, ask for assessment by the on-call medical/ICU team.

Delirium

Postoperative delirium affects over 25% of elderly patients, and a single causal factor is often not identified. Once metabolic, respiratory, septic, and cerebral causes of delirium have been excluded, the patient may still have a behavioural problem that disturbs the ward, and places the patient at risk (of falling over or out of bed, for example). The patient may pull out intravenous lines or n/g tube, and safe care may become impossible.

- Before forcefully sedating a patient, try simple calm talking in a quiet single room first. Talk the problem over with the nursing staff and see if they can manage the patient with increased care rather than drugs.
- Explain the problem to relatives who are likely to be anxious themselves, and see if they can calm their relative.
- If these measures fail, the administration of a tranquillizing drug such as haloperidol (2.5–10 mg i/m) is perfectly justifiable, even if

the patient resists. You are not assaulting the patient in such circumstances, as you are acting in his/her best interests.

- Document your actions in the notes, and ensure that the patient is adequately monitored. A sedative drug may calm the patient, but places him/her at risk of respiratory depression. Inform the on-call anaesthetic team if you are concerned.

- If alcohol withdrawal is the likeliest cause, chlordiazepoxide 10 mg 4–6 times per day can be used both to calm the patient and to prevent alcohol withdrawal seizures (see p. 231). Some clinicians treat mild alcohol withdrawal by allowing patients some alcohol. This may be acceptable as a short-term measure in patients who are otherwise well and who are able to drink. Sedation with intravenous chlormethiazole is potentially hazardous. It should only be given in a well-monitored setting, as patients can become deeply comatose for a prolonged period.

Postoperative seizures

Richard Hardie

The management of postoperative seizures differs between patients with and without a pre-existing seizure disorder (see p. 186). In someone with a poorly controlled chronic seizure disorder, one or two seizures should not normally be regarded as an emergency, although it may be prudent to seek expert advice before discharging the patient back home. Do not over-react to this situation.

Avoid drugs which lower the seizure threshold in patients with epilepsy. The management of a single seizure should be according to that of convulsive epileptic status, described below.

Although uncommon, non-convulsive status does occur, and may present as postoperative confusion in patients with established epilepsy. It can only be diagnosed by electroencephalography.

Repeated seizures

Convulsive epileptic status (status epilepticus) is defined as prolonged or recurrent seizures lasting more than 30 min. Although rare, this medical emergency carries a significant morbidity and a mortality of 5–10%, mainly determined by the underlying condition.

Complications

The potential complications of epileptic status should be considered if it is to be managed optimally.

- The primary problem is widespread and excessive neuronal metabolic activity, which may lead to cerebral anoxia and oedema, exhaustion of neurotransmitters, and potentially permanent brain damage.
- The secondary complications are mainly respiratory and autonomic. Massive release of adrenaline and noradrenaline leads to

increases in body temperature and sweating, increased cardiac rate and output with the risk of arrhythmia or arrest, and early hypertension. In addition, excess salivary and bronchial secretion may add to inefficient ventilation, and central respiratory depression makes cerebral anoxia more likely. Pulmonary hypertension and oedema may develop along with a progressive decline in blood pressure. Increased metabolic demands result in variable changes in K^+ levels, hypoglycaemia, hyponatraemia, and lactic acidosis. Tonic–clonic movements themselves may result in fractures and rhabdomyolysis, even leading to renal failure.

Management principles for convulsive status

- *ABC of basic life support*: O_2, safe positioning of patient.
- *Time*: When did it start? Keep a record of the time as you would for a cardiac arrest.
- *Is emergency therapy needed?* Satisfy yourself that intervention is necessary, and that as far as you can the diagnosis is correct. One of the commonest causes of apparently uncontrollable epilepsy is pseudo-seizures, but always seek expert help in diagnosis.
- *Treat the epilepsy* (Table 48.1).
- *Precipitating factors*: Suspect inadequate drug treatment or compliance in a known epileptic recently admitted, and/or drug withdrawal including alcohol. Send blood for urgent FBC, clotting studies; biochemistry including renal and liver function tests, glucose, Ca and Mg; and arterial blood gases. Take extra blood for routine toxicological screen and baseline anticonvulsant drug levels.
- *Treat the underlying cause* (if any): Give 50% glucose if hypoglycaemia is suspected, with iv thiamine if alcohol abuse or malnutrition may be relevant.
- *Look for complications*: aspiration pneumonia, soft tissue injuries.

Emergency management of prolonged or recurrent seizures

- *Initial first aid*: note time, secure airway, administer O_2.
- *Basic observations*: confirm diagnosis, check TPR & BP, look for lateralizing neurological signs.
- *Emergency steps*: establish i/v access and 0.9% saline infusion.
- *First line anti-convulsant drug treatment*, e.g. diazepam or lorazepam.
- *Investigations*: glucose, Na^+, Ca, Mg^{2+}.
- *i/v glucose and/or thiamine* if appropriate.
- *Summon expert medical assistance*: consider requesting HDU/ICU admission.

Table 48.1 Emergency anti-epileptic drug treatment

Drug	i/v dose (mg/kg)	Typical adult dose	Remarks
Diazepam	0.2–0.3	10 mg over 3–4 min	*Standard therapy*
			Slow i/v injection; repeat once after 15 min
Lorazepam	0.07	4 mg bolus injection	*Safer than diazepam if hypotensive*
			Repeat once after 15 min
Phenytoin	15–18	1000 mg over 20 min	*For those not previously on the drug*
			Slow i/v infusion; then 5–6 mg/kg per day po or i/v
Chlormethiazole	5–10	90 ml of 0.8% solution over 6 min	*Can cause profound respiratory depression: move patient to HDU/ICU*
			Slow i/v infusion followed by 0.5–4 ml/min
Phenobarbital	10	700 mg over 7 min	*Consider if other measures fail*
			Slow i/v injection then 1–4 mg/kg per day

Intravenous doses should be calculated by body weight.

With the exception of lorazepam, all i/v drugs can cause hypotension and/or respiratory depression if administered too quickly, and phenytoin may precipitate arrhythmias so ECG monitoring is advisable.

If i/v access is difficult, the following options may be considered:

- Diazepam is available as a special rectal formulation (Stesolid), and the i/v solution can be given rectally in an emergency.
- Paraldehyde is less commonly used nowadays in UK hospitals, but can also be given rectally or by i/m injection.
- Midazolam is well absorbed after i/m injection, typically 5–10 mg in adults.

- **If seizures continue:**
  - repeat first line anti-convulsant after 10–15 min.
- **Establish likely aetiology:**
  - complete examination
  - review blood results
  - initiate specific treatment where appropriate
  - organize further investigations, e.g. brain scan, EEG, CSF examination, ECG and monitor.
- **If seizures still continue:**
  - second-line anti-convulsant drug, e.g. i/v phenytoin loading dose.

- **Seizures continue:**
  - transfer to ICU
  - general anaesthesia
  - long-term prophylactic anti-epileptic therapy will be needed.

Further reading

O'Brien MD (1990). Management of major status epilepticus in adults. *British Medical Journal* 301:918.

Shorvon S (1993). Tonic-clonic status epilepticus. *Journal of Neurology Neurosurgery and Psychiatry* 56:125–34.

Headache in surgical patients

Paul Thomas

**Physiology and management of headache
sub-types** *337*
Investigations *338*

Headache is common on surgical wards (Table 49.1). Mostly benign
and self-limiting, it may occasionally be a serious symptom. The
history will normally exclude serious underlying pathology, and
the patient can then be reassured and treated with appropriate
analgesia.

Headaches that are associated with altered neurology require urgent
investigation.

Table 49.1 Clinical features of types of postoperative headache in order
of frequency of occurrence

Cause	Features
Tension headache	A feeling of pressure over the head or ache around the neck and shoulders. Often gets worse over the course of the day. Anxious patient. Previous similar headaches.
Migraine	Those regularly afflicted can often detect when an episode is about to occur. May be associated with a prodromal phase during which flashing lights, blind spots and hemianopia may be experienced. Common migraine may not be preceded by these auras: it most commonly presents as unilateral facial pain with associated nausea and vomiting.
Hypoxia and/or hypercapnia	Hypoxia ± hypercapnia can cause arterial dilatation and hence headache in the immediate post operative period. Hypoventilation should be considered as the cause of headache in patients receiving regular opioids.

Table 49.1 Continued

Cause	Features
Caffeine withdrawal	May develop if the patient normally drinks a lot of tea and coffee every day. Similar characteristics to tension headache.
Vasodilating drugs	Nitrates, Ca^{2+} channel blockers and other antihypertensive agents may give rise to headache. Check if the patient has suffered ill effects before.
Hypertension	Severe hypertension (>180/>100) may cause headaches if left unchecked.
Sepsis	Systemic infection is often associated with headache. Mild neck stiffness may accompany the headache and give rise to concern over meningitis. Further investigation to elucidate the source of infection is indicated.
Dehydration	Only if the patient is clinically dry. Causes headaches due to shrinkage of brain tissue with subsequent traction on the venous sinuses.
Post dural puncture	Presents as a severe throbbing pain over the occiput. Exacerbated by movement and an upright posture.
Referred pain	Headache may be the only outward clinical sign of underlying facial and skull fractures in patients who have fallen or suffered trauma. Similar headache may arise after maxillofacial surgery. Acute otitis media and sinusitis also cause headache by referred pain.
Raised intracranial pressure	Pain worse on lying flat, coughing or straining. Papilloedema is sometimes present, but this is not invariable. Intracranial haemorrhage can present with a headache prior to neurological deterioration. Patients on anticoagulants are at particular risk. Intracranial tumours may rarely present for the first time perioperatively as a headache or a change in conscious level.
Subarachnoid haemorrhage	Sudden onset severe ('thunderclap') occipital headache ± altered neurology. Diagnosed by CT scan.
Meningitis	Patients at risk are those who have recently had ENT, maxillofacial, or neurosurgical procedures. Likely to be systemically unwell with prominent drowsiness. Extremely rarely, spinal anaesthesia may be followed by meningitis.

Physiology and management of headache sub-types

Tension headache: muscle spasm

- The perioperative period is stressful. Tension headaches account for most headaches in surgical patients. They are benign but may cause a disproportionate amount of stress. The pain is often continuous, with no obvious exacerbating or relieving factors.

• If simple analgesics and NSAIDs are ineffective, reassurance and education in the use of relaxation techniques may help. Occasionally, organic causes of muscle spasm (such as temporomandibular joint occlusion and arthritis of the cervical spine) give rise to tension headaches.

Migraine

• Try simple analgesics (e.g. paracetamol, aspirin) and an anti-emetic (e.g. metoclopramide, prochlorperazine) first.

• The specific $5HT_1$ agonists sumatriptan, naratriptan, and zolmatriptan are more potent than simple analgesics for acute migraine. Sumatriptan 6 mg subcutaneously or 20 mg by intranasal spray can be given to those unable to take oral medication.

• Sumatriptan may cause minor drowsiness and hypotension.

Post dural puncture headache

Loss of CSF after a spinal anaesthetic or inadvertent puncture of the dura after an epidural anaesthetic may result in a post dural puncture headache. The CSF is less able to cushion the brain within the skull and traction develops on the venous sinuses.

• Post dural puncture headaches are usually self-limiting, resolving spontaneously within a few days.

• If suspected, the anaesthetist involved in the patient's care should be informed.

• Treatment is conservative initially, with bed rest and the administration of regular simple analgesics, and active hydration with oral or intravenous fluids. Caffeine tablets (which increase CSF production) or coffee may be a useful adjunct in pain management if the patient is able to take oral fluids.

• Sumatriptan has been reported to be effective in some patients.

• If symptoms become intolerable or are persistent, further treatment may be appropriate in the form of a 'blood patch.' This procedure involves taking ~30 ml of the patient's blood by venepuncture and injecting it slowly into the epidural space adjacent to where the dural puncture is suspected. The fibrin plug that forms will stop the leak of CSF with rapid resolution of symptoms in ~90% cases.

Investigations

The cause of a headache in surgical patients can usually be decided by the history. Most settle spontaneously with reassurance and simple analgesia. If they do not, further investigation should be considered.

- If the headache is thought to be associated with an inflammatory process or sepsis then routine blood tests including FBC, ESR, CRP, U&E are appropriate.
- In cases where there is an associated neurological element, a CT scan should be considered.
- Further specific tests should be used as indicated by the clinical presentation. Lumbar puncture may be needed in suspected meningitis, but only when there is no suspicion of accompanying raised intracranial pressure.

Further reading

Carp H, Singh PJ, Vadhera R, Jayaram A (1994). Effects of the serotonin-receptor agonist sumatriptan on postdural puncture headache: report of six cases. *Anesthesia and Analgesia* 79:180–2.

Razis PA, Robinson DL, Alberry R (1995). Clinical presentation of 'silent' meningiomas after general anaesthesia. *British Journal of Anaesthesia* 74:335–7.

Sprigge JS (1999). The use of sumatriptan in the treatment of postdural puncture headache after accidental lumbar puncture complicated a blood patch procedure. *Anaesthesia* 54:95–6.

Fever

Julia Munn and Marina Morgan

The timing of postoperative fever suggests the diagnosis in most patients. Typical timings for the common causes of fever are given in Table 50.1, together with comments on frequency.

Table 50.1 Causes of fever

Cause of fever	Typical timing	Typical temperature	Incidence
Surgery itself	0– 2 days	<38°C	Up to 30% after major surgery
Sepsis	> 2 days (unless present preoperatively or after certain procedures, e.g. urinary catheterization)	Usually >38°C	Common: see below
Febrile blood transfusion reaction	During transfusion and < 6 h afterwards	<39°C	2% of all transfusions
Venous thromboembolism	> 2 days	Usually <38°C	Up to 30% in orthopaedic surgery, 1–5% after abdominal and gynaecological surgery
Malignant hyperpyrexia	During anaesthesia and < 6 h after	>39°C	Rare

Surgery as a cause of fever

A mild self-limiting fever is common during the first 2 postoperative days. Immediately after major surgery most patients have a low body temperature due to heat losses in theatre and impaired temperature regulation caused by anaesthesia. This is followed by a systemic response in which the metabolic rate is increased and energy stores are mobilized. This frequently causes mild pyrexia (<38°C). If temperature exceeds this, is prolonged, or is associated with systemic upset, other causes must be sought.

Sepsis

All bacterial infections can result in bacteraemia. The main risks of sepsis are the development of septic shock (the sepsis syndrome) and contamination of prostheses – joints, vascular grafts, heart valves, etc.

Sepsis must always be considered as a cause of pyrexia, and is the likeliest cause after the second postoperative day. It may occur earlier if infection was present preoperatively or if there is breakdown of a bowel anastomosis.

Typical sites of infection

- *Wound*: Increased risk in malnutrition, obesity, diabetes, steroid therapy. Very common.
- *Urine*: Predominantly if catheter is present. Unlikely if no catheter nor urinary tract instrumentation.
- *Chest*: Especially after abdominal or thoracic surgery, or in smokers or those with chronic bronchitis. Unlikely if no cough, sputum production, dyspnoea, tachypnoea, or signs of consolidation. Reduced air entry at lung bases is common after abdominal surgery but it does not necessarily imply the presence of pneumonia.
- *Intravenous cannulae*: Usually obvious with a peripheral line (clinical signs of inflammation); more hazardous with central lines. Very common.
- *Intra-abdominal*: Only after laparotomy. Highest risk after perforated viscus. Spiking fever is classical but not universal, particularly in the elderly. Consider subphrenic collection, pelvic collection, biliary leakage, anastamotic leakage, further perforation.

Examination

- Abdomen if laparotomy performed. A leaking intestinal anastomosis is likely to cause peritonism and severe sepsis, but abdominal signs may be hard to interpret after surgery or in patients on steroids.
- Wound.
- Chest.

- Line sites: Peripheral and central.
- Vital signs: Temperature, pulse, BP, respiratory rate, conscious level.

Investigations

- *Blood cultures* always.
- *Wound swab*: Send pus rather than swab if possible.
- *MSU/CSU* but visual inspection of urine useful as crystal clear urine has virtually no likelihood of being the cause of postoperative fever.
- *CXR* if signs/symptoms of chest infection or pre-existing lung disease. Compare with preoperative film in these cases. Radiographic changes appear later than physical signs so a normal CXR does not exclude infection.
- *CRP* will be raised after major surgery or trauma but a later increase may indicate sepsis.
- *Cannula culture*: If peripheral or central lines are removed, cut off the tips with sterile scissors for culture.
- *FBC*: A white cell count has little differential diagnostic value in isolation (low specificity and sensitivity) but the trend may be more useful.
- *Sputum culture* has a low diagnostic yield (low sensitivity) and is often contaminated by oral flora but a heavy growth of one organism is usually significant.

Management

- Remove central lines if *in situ* for more than a few days or if site inflamed and if only being used as venous access. If a CVP line is still required (e.g. for CVP measurement or TPN) it should be re-sited if line sepsis is likely. Inserting a new line over a guide-wire ('railroading') can remove source of sepsis (unless skin site infected) but it is better to insert a new line in a fresh site.
- Remove/re-site peripheral lines unless clinically clean and <48 h old.
- Drain wound infections by removing some sutures or by surgical exploration.
- Start antibiotic therapy if high risk patient (vascular surgery, prosthesis, steroids/immunocompromised) or clinically ill (delirium, hypotension, tachycardia, tachypnoea, oliguria). Otherwise, monitor vital signs 2 hourly for 24 h while awaiting clinical developments and/or the result of cultures. Guidelines on appropriate prescribing are given on p. 256, and the management of septic shock is discussed on p. 255.
- If a patient develops a new pyrexia while on antibiotics seek guidance from a microbiologist who may advise either to change to a

different class of antibiotic or to stop antibiotics and repeat all cultures. Also, think of alternative explanations for fever (e.g. DVT).

- Metastatic infection of a prosthesis can be lethal or prejudice the survival of the implant. Treat infection in these patients with the utmost vigour. In these circumstances even organisms normally of low pathogenicity such as enterococci or coagulase −ve staphylococci can cause severe infection.

Table 50.2 Rational prescribing and management of common postoperative infections

Likely site of infection	Likely organisms	Specimens	Suggested antibiotics for initial therapy	Comments
Urinary tract/post urological surgery	Gram –ves	MSU/CSU Blood cultures if clinically septicaemic	If seriously ill: gentamicin 3– 5 mg/kg i/v stat, then cefotaxime 2 g tds i/v Otherwise: ciprofloxacin 250 mg bd po or ampicillin 500 mg qds i/v	Do not rely on previous catheter urine results because of organism and resistance changes
Chest infections (esp. if post intubation or in ITU)	Gram –ves (including *Pseudomonas, E.coli, H. influenzae*) *Strep. pneumoniae* unlikely postoperative	Sputum for microscopy and culture (physiotherapy assisted) Blood cultures Tracheostomy site swab if relevant – often colonized	If gram –ves predominate in the Gram film: cefotaxime 2 g tds i/v + gentamicin 3–5 mg/kg i/v stat If Gram +ves predominate: cefuroxime 1.5 g tds i/v + gentamicin 3–5 mg/kg i/v stat	If MRSA likely add vancomycin 1 g bd (monitor levels)
Wound infection (inflammation/pus/ tender)	*Staphylococcus*, gram –ves, anaerobes	Wound swab for culture and sensitivity? Pus from (fresh) drainage bag Blood cultures	cefotaxime 2 g tds i/v + metronidazole 500 mg tds i/v (or 1 g bd pr)	If MRSA add vancomycin 1 g bd i/v, infuse over 2 h (monitor levels)
CVP line/venflon site/TPN feeding line (Pus at exit site, or line blocked or temperature coincides with infusion)	*Staphylococcus*, especially coagulase –ve Occasional gram –ves Fungi, especially *Candida* if on TPN	Wound swab if exit site purulent Blood cultures from central and peripheral lines If very septic remove line and send tip for culture	vancomycin 1 g bd i/v + cefotaxime 1 g tds i/v	If evidence of candidiasis – (oral or other sites) add fluconazole 400 mg i/v and culture fully for *Candida* spp. Check fundi for evidence of infarcts. Do not 'railroad' a new line into an infected site

Condition	Organisms	Specimen	Treatment	Notes
Post ERCP sepsis/biliary sepsis/post cholecystectomy	*Pseudomonas, enterococcus,* anaerobes	Bile from drainage bag, Blood cultures, Wound swab	piperacillin 2 g tds i/v + gentamicin 3–5 mg/kg i/v stat + ciprofloxacin 400 mg bd i/v (or 750 mg bd po) + metronidazole 500 mg tds i/v (or 1 g bd pr)	34% of associated septicaemias have >1 organism liberated
Faecal peritonitis	Enterobacteria, anaerobes	Blood cultures, Wound swab or pus from drainage bag or operation	gentamicin 3–5 mg/kg i/v stat + cefotaxime 2 g tds i/v + metronidazole 500 mg tds i/v	
Neurosurgical shunt	Ventriculo-peritoneal: gram –ves more likely. Ventriculo-atrial: gram +ves more likely	CSF from 'button' tap if possible (not routine LP), Blood culture, Wound swab	vancomycin 1 g bd i/v + cefotaxime 2 g tds i/v + metronidazole 500 mg tds i/v	Consult with microbiologist
Post prosthesis insertion (vascular or orthopaedic)	Staphylococci both Staph aureus (usually flucloxacillin sensitive) + coagulase –ve staphylococci (often flucloxacillin resistant)	Blood cultures, Wound swab	vancomycin 1 g bd i/v + cefuroxime 1.5 g tds i/v	
Offensive diarrhoea after recent antibiotic treatment	*C. difficile*	Stool for *C. difficile* toxin testing	metronidazole 400 mg tds po or vancomycin 125 mg qds po	Oral more effective. No need to measure vancomycin levels

Febrile transfusion reactions

Fever occurs in 2% of patients receiving blood transfusion. Commonly due to immune reaction to white cells or allergens in plasma.

Management

- Stop transfusing the individual unit of blood if any of the following features are present: fever (<39°C), rigors, hypotension, urticaria, bronchospasm. Return the residual blood or plasma to the blood bank.
- Cool the patient with a fan.
- Give paracetamol 1 g orally or pr.
- Give an antihistamine intravenously (e.g. chlorpheniramine 4 mg).
- Fever <39°C without any other clinical manifestation can be treated by fan cooling, paracetamol, and cautious continuation of the transfusion.
- Reconsider the urgency for transfusion and restart another unit of blood when the patient has improved clinically.
- If a serious reaction occurs (hypotension, tachpnoea) give hydrocortisone 100 mg i/v (see also p. 209).

Venous thrombo-embolism

DVT/PE may cause a fever <38°C without any other signs. Fever without an obvious septic source should prompt exclusion of this diagnosis. Clinical signs are unreliable, and imaging may be needed. See p. 347.

Malignant hyperpyrexia

- An uncommon, potentially fatal, inherited disorder of striated muscle manifesting as acute hypercatabolism in response to certain anaesthetic agents. Most cases occur during anaesthesia, but a few arise afterwards.
- Clinical features: high and rapidly rising fever (may be >40°C), tachycardia, tachypnoea, hypoxia, acidosis, and hyperkalaemia.
- Dantrolene is the specific treatment. ICU is needed for cooling and supportive care. Investigation of the patient and family is needed after the acute event.

Further reading

Carli F, Aber VR (1987). Thermogenesis after major elective procedures. *British Journal of Surgery* 74:1041–5.

The swollen leg

Anthony Nicholls

- The development of a swollen leg in a surgical, orthopaedic, or gynaecology ward is common. The main concern is whether a deep venous thrombosis (DVT) is the underlying cause.

- PE only happens when thrombus extends into the femoral and iliac veins.

- Pelvic venous thrombosis can cause PE, particularly after gynaecological procedures.

- Venous thrombosis limited to calf veins does not cause PE. Unfortunately, clinical signs do not allow differentiation between calf vein thrombosis and proximal DVT. Calf vein thrombosis can extend above the knee if untreated.

- Not all swollen legs represent DVT, and many DVT are subtle, but the diagnosis is usually simpler than on a medical ward, because the change in the leg is usually observed.

- The greatest risk of DVT is after orthopaedic surgery and leg trauma. These patients are also most likely to develop leg swelling simply because of surgery or trauma itself.

- PE can occur without any clinical evidence of DVT.

- Any new leg swelling in a surgical patient must be taken seriously.

Differential diagnosis and clinical features of leg swelling after surgery

Table 51.1 is based on the assumption that a leg has suddenly become swollen in the perioperative period. All patients undergoing surgery

Table 51.1 Causes of postoperative leg swelling

Diagnosis	Clinical features
Common or important causes	
DVT: limited to calf veins	Unilateral calf oedema, calf pain/tenderness, warmth, and redness. Often low grade (<38°C) fever. Increased pain on foot dorsiflexion (Homan's sign) has no differential diagnostic power
DVT: above knee	Oedema of the entire leg, cyanosis, superficial venous engorgement, tenderness of the iliofemoral vein itself (in Hunter's canal and the groin). Often low grade (<38°C) fever. The signs of proximal DVT may be the same as calf vein thrombosis
Surgical or post-traumatic oedema	Leg swelling is universal after hip and knee surgery, and common after ankle and even foot procedures. The oedema develops painlessly, without fever, in the first day or two after orthopaedic surgery, and then slowly regresses. A degree of gravitational oedema may persist for a year or more after orthopaedic surgery. A DVT should be suspected when the oedema rapidly increases despite recumbency, or when there is pain, redness, warmth, or a fever
Cellulitis	Rapidly spreading intense redness and warmth of the skin, fever (less common in elderly), pain, blisters. May be no history of skin trauma
Compartment syndrome	Occurs after trauma/ischaemia to limb. Features are increasing pain, tense swelling, paraesthesiae. Needs urgent assessment. Compartment pressures should be measured using a transducer and fasciotomies performed if these are raised
Heart failure or fluid overload with unilateral venous insufficiency	Relatively common. Fluid resuscitation of shocked patients often leads to peripheral oedema in the recovery phase. In other patients, excess fluid therapy may precipitate heart failure. If these patients have underlying venous insufficiency (look for telltale signs of varicose eczema, healed ulcers, lipodermatosclerosis), the oedema may appear to be unilateral, but will be seen to be bilateral if the apparently normal leg is examined carefully
Acute gout	Exquisite joint tenderness with redness spreading around the joint. Often triggered by dehydration, sepsis and catabolism after surgery in a patient with a history of gout
Conditions more rarely seen in surgical practice	
Haematoma	Usually history of direct trauma. May be spontaneous in overanticoagulated patients. Relatively more common postoperatively after total knee or hip replacement
Thrombophlebitis	Tenderness directly over the course of palpable, lumpy superficial veins. Not often seen perioperatively

Table 51.1 *Continued*

Diagnosis	Clinical features
Conditions more rarely seen in surgical practice	
Ruptured popliteal cyst	Tenderness in popliteal fossa extending into posterior calf. Uncommon but may occur after trauma
Muscle tear	Only after obvious trauma
Post-phlebitic leg	Gravitational oedema in a patient with previous venous thrombosis and/or varicose veins. Venous insufficiency is improved by bed-rest, so this is an unlikely cause of a newly swollen leg in surgical practice

should have their legs assessed preoperatively so that postoperative changes can be elucidated.

Assessment of the swollen leg

New unilateral leg swelling in the postoperative period should always raise the possibility of DVT. Apart from orthopaedic patients having lower limb procedures, DVT is far more likely to be the cause of oedema than any other condition.

The main goal of investigation is to determine the extent of thrombosis; the diagnosis of thrombosis itself is often made on clinical grounds.

Investigations

Treatment of DVT depends on the extent of thrombosis. The extent of thrombosis cannot be determined clinically. **All patients suspected of having DVT require some form of imaging of the venous system.**

Compressive Döppler ultrasound of the femoral vein

This is the standard investigation of proximal DVT. Both sensitivity and specificity are high, and the test is non-invasive. It can be repeated to exclude possible above knee propagation of clot in selected patients.

Contrast venography

The 'gold standard' test for calf vein thrombosis. Time-consuming, inconvenient, and sometimes unpleasant for patients. Widely used in medical practice where the differential diagnosis of leg swelling is wider, but less relevant to surgical practice, where the clinical diagnosis of DVT is more secure. May be used to exclude calf vein thrombosis and so avoid short-term anticoagulation in patients judged at high risk of bleeding.

Impedance plethysmography

Not widely available, but gradually being introduced. The technique measures impedance changes in the thigh in response to leg compression. Allows accurate diagnosis and exclusion of proximal thrombosis.

New computer-assisted devices (e.g. the Belfast Scanner) are less oper-
ator-dependent than ultrasound. May replace ultrasound as the investigation of choice.

Other tests

- d-dimer shows that the clotting system has been activated. A raised
  d-dimer is of no value in diagnosing DVT in a surgical patient, but
  a normal d-dimer makes the diagnosis unlikely.
- C-reactive protein (CRP) is raised in DVT, but also after surgery
  and in sepsis. A normal value is useful in excluding DVT.
- If the clinical features are unimpressive, and d-dimer and CRP are
  both normal, then there is no need to image veins.

Treatment of venous thrombosis

- Unless a patient is at high risk of haemorrhage, it is better to treat a
  patient with suspected DVT than wait for definitive investigations.
- Treat proximal DVT with 6 months warfarin.
- Calf thrombosis needs only 6 weeks therapy unless risk factors for
  thrombosis still exist (e.g. advanced malignancy, immobility, etc.).
- Where possible, send blood for prothrombin time, activated partial
  thromboplastin (APT) time, platelet count, and LFTs before starting treatment.
- Commence therapy with heparin (unfractionated or LMWH
  according to hospital policy) and introduce warfarin when the risk of
  haemorrhage is low. If the patient is >4 days after surgery, and
  further surgery is unlikely, then start warfarin along with the heparin.

Heparin

- Give a bolus of 5000 U heparin i/v.
- Start a heparin infusion at a rate of 17 500 U over 12 h.
- Measure the APT ratio daily each morning and adjust the rate of
  heparin infusion according to Table 51.2.

Table 51.2 Adjustment of heparin infusion rate according to APTR ratio

APTR	Change in 12 hourly heparin dose
>5.0	Reduce by 6000 U
4.1–5.0	Reduce by 3500 U
3.1–4.0	Reduce by 1000 U
2.6–3.0	Reduce by 500 U
1.5–2.5	No change
1.2–1.4	Increase by 2500 U
<1.2	Increase by 5000 U

- Target range for APTR is 1.5–2.5.
- Give heparin for at least 4 days, and continue until the INR is in the target range.

Low-molecular-weight heparins (LMWH)

Several forms of LMWH have a product licence for treatment of DVT. They are given by subcutaneous injection. The dose is based on the weight of the patient. They are all more expensive than standard unfractionated heparin, but offer several advantages:

- convenience
- no monitoring needed
- at least as effective in preventing PE
- probably a lower rate of haemorrhage.

The dosage schedules of LMWHs licensed for DVT are given in Table 51.3.

Table 51.3 LMWH schedules for DVT

Agent	Dose
Dalteparin (Fragmin)	200 U/kg sc every 24 h (100 U/kg 12 hourly if high risk of haemorrhage)
Enoxaparin (Clexane)	1 mg/kg (100 u/kg) s/c every 12 h
Tinzaparin (Innohep)[a]	175 U/kg s/c every 24 h

[a] Tinzaparin doses are usually rounded up or down to standard ampoule sizes: 10 000, 14 000, 18 000 U.

Warfarin

- The standard loading dose of warfarin is 10 mg.
- Consider using a lower dose of warfarin to load patients if they are likely to be sensitive to warfarin: elderly (>75 years), congestive heart failure, liver disease, drugs that interact with warfarin (e.g. phenytoin, amiodarone. Check in BNF).
- Measure INR each morning and adjust the evening dose according to schedule in Table 51.4.

Further reading

Davidson BL, Deppert EJ (1998). Ultrasound for the diagnosis of deep vein thrombosis: where to now? *British Medical Journal* 316:2–3.

Grubb NR, Bloomfield P, Ludlam CA (1998). The end of the heparin pump? *British Medical Journal* 317:1540–2.

Heijboer H, Buller JR, Lensing AWA, Turpie AGG, Colly LP, ten Cate JW (1993). A comparison of real-time ultrasonography with impedance plethysmography for the diagnosis of deep-vein

Table 51.4 Warfarin loading schedule (only applicable to loading dose of 10 mg)

Day	INR	Warfarin dose (mg)
1	<1.4	10
2	<1.8	10
	1.8	1
	>1.8	0.5
3	<2.0	10
	2.0–2.1	5
	2.2–2.3	4.5
	2.4–2.5	4
	2.6–2.7	3.5
	2.8–2.9	3
	3.0–3.1	2.5
	3.2–3.3	2
	3.4	1.5
	3.5	1
	3.6–4.0	0.5
	>4.0	nil
4		(Predicted maintenance dose)
	<1.4	>8
	1.4	8
		7.5
	1.5	7
	1.6–1.7	6.5
	1.8	6
	1.9	5.5
	2.0–2.1	
	2.2–2.3	5
	2.4–2.6	4.5
	2.7–3.0	4
	3.1–3.5	3.5
	3.6–4.0	3
	4.1–4.5	Omit one dose, then give 2 mg
	>4.5	Omit 2 doses, then give 1 mg

thrombosis in symptomatic outpatients. *New England Journal of Medicine* 329:1365–9.

Lensing AWA, Prins MH, Davidson BL, Hirsh J (1995). Treatment of deep venous thrombosis with low-molecular-weight heparins: a meta-analysis. *Archives of Internal Medicine* 155:601–7.

Perioperative prescribing information

Anthony Nicholls and Iain Wilson

How to use the table 353

Section 15 of the BNF gives broad advice about the issue of long-term medication and general anaesthesia: the risk of stopping medication is often greater than the risk of continuing it during surgery, but surgery itself may alter the need for continued therapy for certain conditions.

Drugs that should not normally be stopped before surgery include analgesics, anti-epileptics, bronchodilators, cardiovascular drugs, glaucoma drugs, thyroid or anti-thyroid drugs, and peptic ulcer drugs.

Drugs that should be stopped include combined oral contraceptives (preferably 4 weeks before elective surgery, with appropriate alternative contraception), and lithium (2 days before major surgery, safe to continue with minor procedures). Controversy exists over monoamine oxidase inhibitors, which the BNF suggests stopping 2 weeks beforehand, and also ACE inhibitors. Hypoglycaemics are stopped perioperatively (see p. 165).

How to use the table

Table 52.1 gives specific advice on the perioperative prescribing of all commonly used classes of drugs together with rarer agents that have particular hazards. Where a drug is not listed, omission of therapy perioperatively is usually appropriate, but double-checking with the anaesthetist or a pharmacist is prudent.

- Check all drugs that a patient is taking, and look them up in the BNF.
- Look for specific interactions under the drug and in Appendix 1 of the BNF (Interactions).

- Check which section of the BNF contains the drug.
- Look up this section of Table 52.1.

Drug interactions are common. Those given here are not the only ones. Appendix 1 (Interactions) of the BNF should always be consulted. If in doubt, ask a pharmacist to check for more details.

Further reading

Dawson J, Karalliedde L (1998). Drug interactions and the clinical anaesthetist. *European Journal of Anaesthesiology* 15:172–89.

Table 52.1 Perioperative prescribing

BNF Section	Drug class	Examples	Typical indication	Perioperative prescribing (see footnote)	Specific hazards in surgical patients	Significant perioperative drug interactions
1 Gastrointestinal system						
1.2	Antispasmodics and other drugs altering gut motility	Mebeverine Alverine Propantheline Cisapride	Irritable bowel syndrome Non-ulcer dyspepsia Diverticular disease	3	Increased risk of ileus Risk of ventricular arrhythmias with cisapride if K^+ or Mg^{2+} low	Opioids may antagonize effect of cisapride on GI motility Clarithromycin and erythromycin associated with ventricular arrhythmias with cisapride
1.3.1	H_2-receptor antagonists	Cimetidine Ranitidine	Peptic ulceration	1 Consider 150 mg ranitidine the evening before anaesthesia and 150 mg 2 h preoperatively to reduce risk of acid aspiration		
1.3.5	Proton pump inhibitors	Omeprazole Lansoprazole	Oesophagitis Peptic ulceration	2 Consider 40 mg omeprazole the evening before anaesthesia and 40 mg 2–6 h preoperatively to reduce risk of acid aspiration		

Prescribing guidelines:
1 Continue therapy i/v until able to absorb from gut. 2 Give normal dose preoperatively and resume when stable postoperatively. 3 Omit preoperative dose and resume when stable postoperatively.

Table 52.1 Continued

BNF Section	Drug class	Examples	Typical indication	Perioperative prescribing (see footnote)	Specifc hazards insurgical patients	Significant perioperative drug interactions
1.4.2	Antimotility drugs	Codeine Loperamide	Diarrhoea	3		Possible tolerance to opioids with chronic codeine therapy
1.5	Aminosalicylates	Sulphasalazine Mesalazine	Ulcerative colitis Crohn's disease	3 Suppositories available		
1.6	Laxatives		Constipation, particularly in elderly	3 Suppositories may be needed postoperatively	Postoperative constipation	Constipation with opioid analgesia more likely if patient is previously prone to constipation
2 Cardiovascular system						
2.1	Cardiac glycosides	Digoxin	Atrial fibrillation Heart failure	1	Toxicity enhanced by hypokalaemia	
2.2	Diuretics	Frusemide (furosemide) Bumetanide Thiazides	Hypertension Heart failure Oedema	1 (heart failure) 2 (other indications)	Increased risk of electrolyte disturbance particularly hypokalaemia and hypomagnesaemia Hypovolaemia in elderly	Impaired glucose tolerance with thiazides Diuretic action antagonized by NSAIDs
2.3	Anti-arrhythmic drugs		Prophylaxis of chronic arrhythmias	1		Increased risk of both tachycardia and bradycardia under GA Enhanced effect of non-depolarizing muscle

2.4	β-blockers	Angina MI prophylaxis Hypertension Cardiac arrhythmia	2 (i/v preparation available if required)	relaxants in patients on quinidine, procainamide, flecainide Enhanced hypotension and bradycardia with GA Dangerous interaction with ketamine Bradycardia may mask physiological response to hypovolaemia Hypotension exaggerated Rebound of severe hypertension or angina if abruptly withdrawn
2.5.1	Vasodilators	Hydralazine Minoxidil	Hypertension	2	Reflex tachycardia under GA Enhanced hypotension with GA
2.5.2	Centrally acting antihypertensive agents	Clonidine Monoxidine Methyldopa	Hypertension	2	Abrupt withdrawal of clonidine or monoxidine may precipitate a hypertensive crisis Positive Coombs' test in 20% on methyldopa may affect blood cross-matching Enhanced hypotension with GA
2.5.3	Adrenergic neurone blockers	Bethanidine Debrisoquine	Hypertension (largely obsolete)	3	Exaggerated response to hypovolaemia Enhanced hypotension with GA

Prescribing guidelines:

1 Continue therapy i/v until able to absorb from gut.   2 Give normal dose preoperatively and resume when stable postoperatively.   3 Omit preoperative dose and resume when stable postoperatively.

Table 52.1 Continued

BNF Section	Drug class	Examples	Typical indication	Perioperative prescribing (see footnote)	Specific hazards insurgical patients	Significant perioperative drug interactions
2.5.4	α-adrenoceptor blocking drugs	Doxazosin Prazosin Terazosin	Hypertension Bladder outlet obstruction	2 (hypertension) 3 (urine flow)		Enhanced hypotension with GA
2.5.5.1	ACE inhibitors	Captopril Enalapril Perindopril	Hypertension Heart failure Proteinuric states	Controversial – discuss with anaesthetist	Increased risk of renal failure in shocked patients	Enhanced hypotension with GA NSAIDs enhance renal side-effects
2.5.5.2	Angiotensin-II receptor blockers	Losartan Valsartan Irbesartan	Hypertension Heart failure Proteinuric states	Controversial – discuss with anaesthetist	Increased risk of renal failure in shocked patients	Enhanced hypotension with GA NSAIDs enhance renal side-effects
2.6.1	Nitrates	Isosorbide mononitrate or dinitrate	Angina	2 Patches, sprays, i/v infusions available for postoperative angina	Need to take nitrates indicates increased cardiac morbidity and mortality Remove patch before defibrillation	
2.6.2	Ca²⁺ channel blockers	Nifedipine Verapamil Diltiazem	Hypertension Angina	2		Verapamil increases hypotensive effect of GA and risk of AV delay Isoflurane enhances hypotensive effects of

2.6.3	K+ channel activators	Nicorandil	Angina	2	The need to take nicorandil indicates increased cardiac morbidity and mortality
2.6.4.1	Peripheral vasodilators	Naftidrofuryl Nicotinic acid	Peripheral vascular disease	Little evidence for any benefit: stop therapy?	
2.8.2	Oral anticoagulants	Warfarin Nicoumalone	DVT/PE prophylaxis Artificial heart valve AF	See detailed guidance in Chapter 24 (p. 144)	Bleeding
2.9	Anti-platelet agents	Aspirin Dipyridamole	Prophylaxis of cerebrovascular and IHD (aspirin) Adjunct to anticoagulants (dipyridamole)	2 (the effect of aspirin on platelets is long-lasting)	Bleeding. Some surgery requires aspirin to be withdrawn 2 weeks prior to operation
2.12	Lipid-regulating drugs	Statins Fibrates	Raised cholesterol	3	

dihydropyridines (e.g. nifedipine)
β-blockers contra-indicated with verapamil, risky with diltiazem

Enhanced hypotension with GA

Many drug interactions including NSAIDs

Prescribing guidelines:

1 Continue therapy i/v until able to absorb from gut. 2 Give normal dose preoperatively and resume when stable postoperatively. 3 Omit preoperative dose and resume when stable postoperatively.

Table 52.1 Continued

BNF Section	Drug class	Examples	Typical indication	Perioperative prescribing (see footnote)	Specific hazards in surgical patients	Significant perioperative drug interactions
3 Respiratory system						
3.1.1.1	Selective β_2-adrenoceptor stimulants	Salbutamol	Asthma	Give regular inhalational therapy Convert tablets to inhalers/nebulizers		May result in hypokalaemia when used in high doses
3.1.2	Antimuscarinic bronchodilators	Ipratropium	Asthma	Give regular inhalational therapy		
3.1.3	Theophylline	Theophylline Aminophylline	Asthma	2 – discuss with anaesthetist	Toxicity enhanced by hypokalaemia	Increased risk of arrhythmias with halothane Blood levels raised by ciprofloxacin, clarithromycin, erythromycin, cimetidine
3.2	Corticosteroid inhalers		Asthma	Give regular inhalational therapy	Consider steroid supplementation when on very high dose	
3.4.1	Antihistamines	Chlorpheniramine Astemizole	Hay fever, urticaria	3	Astemizole and terfenadine associated with cardiac arrhythmias enhanced by hypokalaemia	Do not prescribe cisapride with terfenadine: cardiac arrhythmia risk

4 Central nervous system

4.1	Hypnotics and anxiolytics	Diazepam Temazepam Zopiclone	Insomnia Anxiety	2 Abrupt withdrawal of benzodiazepines may produce confusion, toxic psychosis or even convulsions up to 3 weeks after stopping therapy	Avoid attempting to rationalise or withdraw benzodiazepines immediately after major surgery	May potentiate opioids
4.2.1	Anti-psychotic drugs	Chlorpromazine Haloperidol Thioridazine	Schizophrenia Mania Agitated depression	2 or 1 (according to severity of behaviour disturbance)		Enhanced hypotensive effect of anaesthesia Enhanced sedation with opioids Effect of vasodepressor drugs enhanced
4.2.1	Anti-psychotic depot preparations	Flupenthixol Fluphenazine	Schizophrenia	Depot preparations are long acting and so will be pharmacologically active for up to 4 weeks	Hypothermia in elderly	Enhanced hypotensive effect of anaesthesia Enhanced sedation with opioids Effect of vasodepressor drugs enhanced

Prescribing guidelines:

1 Continue therapy i/v until able to absorb from gut. 2 Give normal dose preoperatively and resume when stable postoperatively. 3 Omit preoperative dose and resume when stable postoperatively.

Table 52.1 Continued

BNF Section	Drug class	Examples	Typical indication	Perioperative prescribing (see footnote)	Specific hazards in surgical patients	Significant perioperative drug interactions
4.2.3	Anti-manic drugs	Lithium	Mania	Stop 2 days before elective surgery Discontinue on admission with emergency cases	Toxicity enhanced by dehydration, hypovolaemia, sodium loss, renal failure Safe plasma level is 0.4–1.0 mmol/l; severe toxicity over 2 mmol/l	Excretion of lithium reduced by many NSAIDs Muscle relaxants enhanced Metoclopramide increases risk of extrapyramidal effects
4.3.1	Tricyclic and related antidepressants	Amitriptyline Dothiepin Trazodone	Depression Migraine prophylaxis Chronic pain	3		Increased risk of arrhythmias and hypotension with anaesthesia Use felypressin rather than epinephrine with local anaesthetics Effect of vasodepressor drugs enhanced
4.3.2	Monoamine-oxidase inhibitors (MAOIs)	Phenelzine Tranylcypromine	Depression	Controversial – discuss with anaesthetist	Associated with severe drug interactions but withdrawal may result in severe depression	CNS excitation or depression with pethidine Avoid nefopam and anticholinergics Hypertensive crisis with sympathomimetics such as dopamine, dopexamine, ephedrine

4.3.3	Selective serotonin re-uptake inhibitors (SSRIs)	Fluoxetine Paroxetine Sertraline	Depression	3	
4.3.4	Other antidepressants	Reboxetine Tryptophan	Depression	3	
4.4	Central nervous system stimulants	Dexamphetamine Methylphenidate	Narcolepsy Attention-deficit hyperactivity disorder	3	Possible cardiovascular instability
4.5.2	Centrally acting appetite suppressants	Phentermine	Obesity	3	Possible cardiovascular instability
4.6	Anti-emetics	Metoclopramide Domperidone Prochlorperazine	Nausea and vomiting	1	Young adults more likely to get extrapyramidal effects. Treat with procyclidine
4.7.2	Opioid analgesics	Morphine Pethidine Codeine	Pain	1	Tolerance may be present in patients taking opioids long term Drug addicts see p. 236
4.7.4	Anti-migraine drugs	Pizotifen	Migraine	3	
4.8	Anti-epileptics Phenytoin Sodium valproate	Carbamazepine	Epilepsy	1 See section on nervous system, section 4 (BNF)	Phenytoin levels increased by some NSAIDs

Prescribing guidelines:

1 Continue therapy i/v until able to absorb from gut. 2 Give normal dose preoperatively and resume when stable postoperatively. 3 Omit preoperative dose and resume when stable postoperatively.

Table 52.1 Continued

BNF Section	Drug class	Examples	Typical indication	Perioperative prescribing (see footnote)	Specific hazards in surgical patients	Significant perioperative drug interactions
4.9.1	Dopaminergic drugs used in Parkinsonism	Levodopa Apomorphine Pergolide	Parkinson's disease	2 No i/v preparation of levodopa available, but n/g therapy may be possible		Avoid metoclopramide and prochlorperazine which may worsen PD
4.9.2	Antimuscarinic drugs used in Parkinsonism	Benzhexol Orphenadrine Procyclidine	Parkinson's disease	2 N/g therapy may be possible; i/v preparations available		Avoid phenothiazines and butyrophenones
4.9.3	Drugs used in essential tremor, chorea, tics, and related disorders	Piracetam Riluzole Tetrabenazine	Miscellaneous disorders	3		
5 Infections						
5.1.1	Penicillins			Usually 1 (where i/v preparation available)		None serious
5.1.2	Cephalosporins and other β-lactams			Usually 1 (where i/v preparation available)		None serious
5.1.3	Tetracyclines			Usually 1 (where i/v preparation available)		None serious
5.1.4	Aminoglycosides	Gentamicin Netilmicin		Usually 1 (where i/v preparation available)		Enhanced effect of non-depolarizing muscle relaxants

				with NSAIDs
5.1.5	Macrolides	Erythromycin Clarithromycin	Usually 1 (where i/v preparation available)	Avoid concomitant use of cisapride: risk of ventricular arrhythmias
5.1.6	Clindamycin		Usually 1 (where i/v preparation available)	Enhanced effect of non-depolarizing muscle relaxants
5.1.7	Other antibiotics	Chloramphenicol Fusidic acid Vancomycin Teicoplanin Colistin	Usually 1 (where i/v preparation available)	Colistin causes enhanced effect of non-depolarizing muscle relaxants
5.1.8	Sulphonamides and trimethoprim		Usually 1 (where i/v preparation available)	None serious
5.1.9	Antituberculous drugs		2	None serious
5.1.10	Antileprotic drugs		2	None serious
5.1.11	Metronidazole		Usually 1 (where i/v preparation available)	None serious
5.1.12	Aminoquinolones	Ciprofloxacin Norfloxacin	Usually 1 (where i/v preparation available)	Ciprofloxacin and norfloxacin increase theophylline levels: risk of convulsions

Prescribing guidelines:
1 Continue therapy i/v until able to absorb from gut. 2 Give normal dose preoperatively and resume when stable postoperatively. 3 Omit preoperative dose and resume when stable postoperatively.

Table 52.1 Continued

BNF Section	Drug class	Examples	Typical indication	Perioperative prescribing (see footnote)	Specific hazards in surgical patients	Significant perioperative drug interactions
5.2	Antifungal drugs			Usually 1 (where i/v preparation available)		None serious
5.3	Antiviral drugs	Aciclovir Zidovudine Ritonavir		Usually 1 (where i/v preparation available)		Ritonavir potentiates sedative effect of benzodiazepines and phenothiazines
5.4	Antiprotozoal drugs			2		None serious
6 Endocrine system						
6.1.1	Insulins		Diabetes	See chapter 26 (p. 161)		
6.1.2	Oral antidiabetic drugs	Gliclazide Metformin	Diabetes	3 Discontinue long-acting agents (chlorpropamide, glibenclamide) 48 h before surgery See chapter on endocrine disorders (p. 165)	Hypoglycaemia with emergency surgery in the presence of long-acting agents	
6.2.1	Thyroid hormones	Thyroxine	Hypothyroidism	2		
6.2.2	Anti-thyroid drugs	Carbimazole Propylthiouracil	Hyperthyroidism	2		
6.3.1	Corticosteroid replacement therapy	Cortisone acetate	Adrenal insufficiency	Increase dose to hydrocortisone 100 mg 8		Increased risk of bleeding with NSAIDs

	Hydrocortisone				hourly perioperatively, starting with pre-med. Halve dose every day until maintenance dose is reached by day 5
6.3.2	Glucocorticoid therapy	Prednisolone	Asthma Rheumatoid arthritis Temporal arteritis	Steroid boost perioperatively as above. Reduce until back at or just above previous dose. See chapter 26 (p. 166)	Poor wound healing Increased infections	Increased risk of bleeding with NSAIDs May mask postoperative sepsis and abdominal signs
6.4.1.1	Oestrogens and HRT	Prempak-C® Cyclo-Progynova®	Vasomotor symptoms of menopause Osteoporosis prophylaxis	3	Increased risk of DVT and PE: cover with appropriate prophylaxis (see Chapter 13)	
6.4.1.2	Progestogens	Norethisterone	Endometriosis Menorrhagia	3		
6.4.2	Male sex hormones and antagonists	Testosterone Cyproterone acetate	Hypogonadism Prostatic cancer	3		Testosterone enhances effect of warfarin
6.4.3	Anabolic steroids	Nandrolone	Osteoporosis Body-building	3		Enhanced effect of warfarin

Prescribing guidelines:
1 Continue therapy i/v until able to absorb from gut. 2 Give normal dose preoperatively and resume when stable postoperatively. 3 Omit preoperative dose and resume when stable postoperatively.

Table 52.1 Continued

BNF Section	Drug class	Examples	Typical indication	Perioperative prescribing (see footnote)	Specific hazards in surgical patients	Significant perioperative drug interactions
7 Gynaecology						
7.3.1	Combined oral contraceptives	Logynon Loestrin Ovran 30	Oral contraception	Discontinue 4 weeks before major elective surgery and surgery to legs Discontinue on admission with emergency cases, and give DVT prophylaxis	Increased risk of DVT and PE: cover with appropriate prophylaxis unless stopped well in advance of surgery (see Chapter 13)	
7.3.2	Progestogen-only contraceptives	Levonorgestrel Norethisterone		3		
8 Cytotoxics						
8.1.2	Cytotoxic antibiotics	Bleomycin	Chemotherapy	N/A – discuss with anaesthetist	Previous exposure results in risk of pulmonary fibrosis with high inspired concentrations of O_2 during and after anaesthesia	
10 Musculoskeletal and joint diseases						
10.1.1	Non-steroidal anti-inflammatory drugs (NSAIDs)	Ibuprofen Naproxen Diclofenac	Arthritis	1 or 2 (suppositories may allow continued therapy)	GI haemorrhage – ranitidine may protect Oliguria or renal failure	

					especially with hypovolaemia
10.1.4	Drugs for gout	Allopurinol	Gout	2	

11 Drugs acting on the eye

Topical steroids Pilocarpine eye drops Timolol eye drops	Inflammatory eye disease Glaucoma	Continue all regular eye drops	Systemic absorption may follow topical application of β-blockers (for glaucoma)	Enhanced risk of bradycardia under anaesthesia.

Prescribing guidelines:

1 Continue therapy i/v until able to absorb from gut. 2 Give normal dose preoperatively and resume when stable postoperatively. 3 Omit preoperative dose and resume when stable postoperatively.

Table of normal values

Common haematology values

Haemoglobin	men:	13–18g/dl
	women:	11.5–16g/dl
Mean cell volume, MCV	76–96fl	
Platelets	150–400 × 10⁹/l	
White cells (total)	4–11 × 10⁹/l	
neutrophils	40–75%	
lymphocytes	20–45%	
eosinophils	1–6%	

Platelets $150–400 \times 10^9/l$

White cells (total) $4–11 \times 10^9/l$

Blood gases

	kPa	mmHg
pH	7.35–7.45	
PaO₂	>10.6	75–100
PaCO₂	4.7–6	35–54
Base excess	±2mmol/l	

U & E etc (urea and electrolytes)

sodium	135–145mmol/l
potassium	3.5–5mmol/l
creatinine	70–150μmol/l
urea	2.5–6.7mmol/l
calcium	2.12–2.65mmol/l
albumin	35–50g/l
proteins	60–80g/l

LFTs (liver function tests)

bilirubin	3–17μmol/l
alanine aminotransferase, ALT	3–35iu/l
aspartate transaminase, AST	3–35iu/l
alkaline phosphatase	30–300iu/l (adults)

'Cardiac enzymes'

creatine kinase	25–195iu/l
lactate dehydrogenase, LDH	70–250iu/l

Lipids and other biochemical values

cholestrol	4–<6mmol/l desired
triglycerides	0.5–1.9mmol/l desired
amylase	0–180somorgyi u/dl
C-reactive protein, CRP	<10mg/l
glucose, fasting	3.5–5.5mmol/l
prostate specific antigen, PSA	0–4ng/ml
T4 (total thyroxine)	70–140mmol/l
TSH	0.5–~5mu/l

Reproduced with permission of the authors of the Oxford Handbook of Clinical Medicine, fourth edition (1999), Oxford University Press.

INDEX